ADVANCES IN PHARMACEUTICAL SCIENCES

VOLUME 1

Advances in PHARMACEUTICAL SCIENCES

Edited by

H. S. BEAN, A. H. BECKETT and J. E. CARLESS

Chelsea College of Science and Technology, London

VOLUME 1

AN ACADEMIC PRESS REPLICA REPRINT

1964

ACADEMIC PRESS

A Subsidiary of Harcourt Brace Jovanovich, Publishers

New York London Toronto Sydney San Francisco

ACADEMIC PRESS, INC. (LONDON) LTD.
24/28 Oval Road, London NW1

U.S. Edition published by
ACADEMIC PRESS, INC.
111 Fifth Avenue, New York, New York 10003

Library of Congress Catalog Card Number: 64-21676
SBN: 12-032301-X

REPRODUCED AND PRINTED BY PHOTOLITHOGRAPHY AND BOUND IN GREAT BRITAIN AT THE PITMAN PRESS, BATH

80 81 82   9 8 7 6 5 4 3

CONTRIBUTORS TO VOLUME I

L. C. BAKER, *Allen & Hanburys Ltd., London, England*

GILBERT S. BANKER, *School of Pharmacy and Pharmacal Sciences, Purdue University, Lafayette, Indiana, U.S.A.*

A. H. C. CHUN, *Research Division, Abbott Laboratories, North Chicago, Illinois, U.S.A.*

ALFRED N. MARTIN, *School of Pharmacy and Pharmacal Sciences, Purdue University, Lafayette, Indiana, U.S.A.*

B. A. MULLEY, *School of Pharmacy, Chelsea College of Science and Technology, London, England*

DOREEN L. WEDDERBURN, *Unilever Research Laboratory, Isleworth, Middlesex, England*

G. R. WILKINSON, *Allen & Hanburys Ltd., London, England*

CONTRIBUTORS TO VOLUME [illegible]

[illegible]

[illegible] University, Lafayette, Indiana [illegible]

[illegible]

PREFACE

Considerable progress has been made during the last one or two decades in the field of pharmaceutics, and yet there is still very little literature dealing specifically with this area of knowledge. Undoubtedly this is because pharmaceutics embraces a wide range of disciplines, and much information of value to the pharmacist appears in journals having no obvious connection with pharmacy. The aim of this new series is to concentrate on areas of specific interest to the pharmaceutist; for example, it will consider the physical aspects of pharmaceutics, pharmaceutical microbiology and the influence of formulation on product stability and efficacy. Medicinal chemistry and pharmacology will not be included since these subjects are already well catered for in the literature.

The articles will be an appraisal of a subject rather than a mere factual abstraction of the literature, and may not refer to the most recent papers on a topic unless they are adjudged to be of significant importance. The authors are expert in their field and are encouraged to include the results of their experience so that their articles may contain hitherto unpublished information. Inevitably, this means inviting reviews from those who are already heavily committed and the success of the series will depend on their generous co-operation. This is particularly so as the intention is to explore a subject in both depth and breadth, but some reviews will focus attention on relatively narrow fields of current importance.

The Editors are indebted to the contributors to the present volume for the time and labour they have devoted to their reviews and to the publishers for their patience and meticulous presentation of the material.

Chelsea College of Science & Technology
June 1964

H. S. Bean
A. H. Beckett
J. E. Carless

CONTENTS

CONTEMPORARY TRENDS IN HEAT STERILIZATION

G. R. Wilkinson and *L. C. Baker*

RHEOLOGY

ALFRED N. MARTIN[1] AND GILBERT S. BANKER

School of Pharmacy and Pharmacal Sciences, Purdue University, Lafayette, Indiana, U.S.A.

and

A. H. C. CHUN

Research Division, Abbott Laboratories North Chicago, Illinois, U.S.A.

According to Fischer (1948) the term rheology was suggested in 1929 by Bingham and Crawford to describe that branch of science which deals with the deformation and flow of matter.

The flow characteristics of matter can be discussed in terms of a limited number of flow classes; and the complex materials of interest to the pharmaceutical chemist can be described with reference to these idealized types of deformation and flow. In the first section we shall consider Newtonian flow, plastic flow, pseudoplastic flow, dilatancy and thixotropy.

[1] 1962–1963 Gustavus A. Pfeiffer Research Fellow. The senior author wishes to thank the American Foundation for Pharmaceutical Education for the support which permitted him to complete part of the manuscript while studying and carrying out research in Paris, France.

The various instruments, both empirical and those founded on a theoretical basis, which have been designed for the measurement of rheological properties will be surveyed under Section II.

Finally, some applications of rheology to various pharmaceutical systems will be considered in Section III.

I. Theoretical Considerations

The isothermal flow of simple liquids can be described by a single value, the absolute viscosity. The rheological properties of heterogeneous dispersions are more complex and must be expressed by a quantity which depends on the time and on the speed at which the material is deformed. Most alarming, the rheological characteristics may also be a function of the previous treatment which the material has undergone.

A. Flow Characteristics of Newtonian Liquids

We begin with a review of the properties of those materials which follow Newton's law of viscous flow. This class includes liquids such as water, glycerin and chloroform; true solutions such as syrups; and very dilute colloidal systems. Most dispersions, including pharmaceutical emulsions, suspensions and semi-solids, fail to follow Newton's equation of flow; they will be considered in a later section.

Newton recognized that the higher was the flow-resistance or viscosity of a liquid, the greater was the force required to cause the liquid to flow. The force per unit area, F, imposed on the liquid is called the shearing stress. The velocity gradient of the liquid produced by this force is referred to as the rate of shear. It is ordinarily written in differential form as dv/dr, where dv is the infinitesimal velocity of the planes of liquid, and dr is the infinitesimal distance of separation of the planes. The symbol G is frequently used for the rate of shear.

The rate of shear is directly proportional to the shearing stress, and accordingly the relationship may be written:

$$F \propto \frac{dv}{dr} \tag{1}$$

Changing this proportionality to an equality by introducing a constant, η, equation (1) becomes:

$$F = \eta G \tag{2}$$

or

$$\eta = \frac{F}{G} \tag{3}$$

where F is the shearing stress, η is the coefficient of viscosity, ordinarily called by the shortened term, viscosity, and $G = dv/dr$ is the rate of shear.

The unit of viscosity is the poise or dyne sec/cm^2. A more convenient unit of viscosity is the centipoise, 100 centipoises being equal to one poise. The centipoise is abbreviated cP. Kinematic viscosity is sometimes used in industry. It is the viscosity defined in equation (3), divided by the density of the liquid, and is expressed in the units of stokes (s) or centistokes (cs).

1. *Analysis of Newtonian Materials*

The viscosity of Newtonian liquids is ordinarily determined by means of capillary viscometers and rotational viscometers, although a number of other types of instruments are also available.

a. *Capillary viscometers.* The viscosity of a Newtonian material is measured by noting the time required for the liquid to flow from one mark to another in a capillary tube suspended vertically in a constant temperature device. The technique and the apparatus are familiar to most workers in the pharmaceutical sciences; several capillary instruments are described in Section II of this chapter. A number of monographs are available which give detailed instruction in the use of capillary viscometers (Barr, 1931; Cannon and Fenske, 1938; Cannon, 1950; Markwood, 1951; A.S.T.M. Standards, 1952).

The capillary viscometer is not particularly useful for a detailed rheological study. The rheologist is in the habit of plotting the rate of shear G versus the shearing stress F, in the analysis of the flow of materials, because such a graph can provide valuable information. The simple capillary viscometer, unfortunately, cannot be used to obtain such a plot. It affords only one mean value of head pressure, corresponding to the shearing stress, and consequently yields only one point on a flow curve. For this reason the capillary viscometer is known as a "one-point instrument". Multiple-head capillary viscometers have been designed to provide data for several points on the flow curve (Krieger and Maron, 1951), but they require the use of complex equations and do not provide the precision and reproducibility of simple capillary viscometers (Hamlow, 1958).

b. *Rotational viscometers.* The rotational viscometer probably lends itself better than do the other apparatus to the theoretical treatment of both Newtonian and non-Newtonian materials. Although various types of rotational instruments will be discussed in the section on apparatus, a description of the Stormer viscometer will be introduced at this point to assist in discussing the flow curve of a Newtonian liquid.

Rotational viscometers may be classified broadly into several types, the revolving-cup or Couette type and the revolving-bob or Searle type being the most well known. The Couette instrument has been used extensively in industry in the form of the MacMichael viscometer (Fig. 31). A refinement of this apparatus was described by Green (1949) and a modification was reported by Samyn and Mattocks (1957).

The Searle type is represented by the commercially available Stormer viscometer (Fig. 27). It is simple in design and operation, inexpensive, and, when modified as suggested by Fischer (1950), it can be used for the

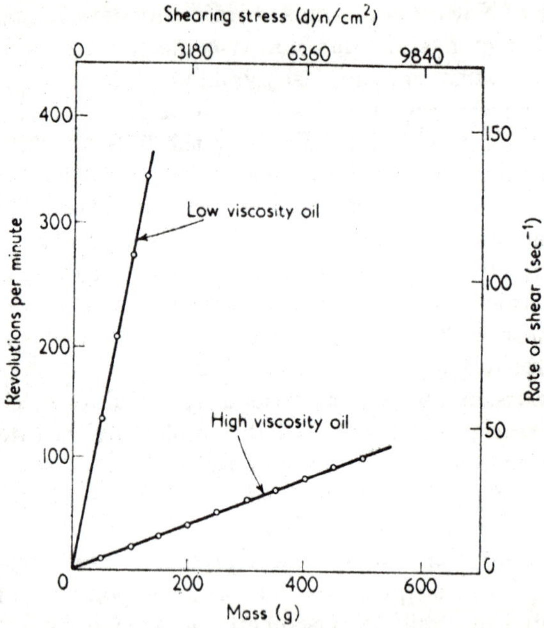

FIG. 1. Flow curves for Newtonian liquids analysed in a Stormer viscometer.

analysis of non-Newtonian as well as Newtonian materials. When a Newtonian liquid is placed in the cup of the viscometer and weights of increasing mass are successively added to the weight hanger, data are obtained which yield the curve shown in Fig. 1. This kind of graph is often referred to as a rheogram. When the Stormer viscometer is used to obtain the data for the rheogram the rate of shear is expressed in revolutions per minute (r.p.m.) and the shearing stress is given in terms of the mass in grams suspended from the weight hanger. The results may also be converted into shear-rate units of sec^{-1} and shear-stress units of dyn/cm^2 as seen in the figure.

The plot obtained when a Newtonian material is analysed is linear and passes through the origin of the graph. The slopes of the lines, shown in Fig. 1, are a measure of the reciprocal of viscosity. This is seen by rearranging equation (2) to:

$$G = \frac{1}{\eta} F \tag{4}$$

or

$$\frac{1}{\eta} = \frac{G}{F} \tag{5}$$

When a rotational viscometer is employed, equation (4) assumes the form:

$$\Omega = \frac{1}{\eta} \frac{T}{4\pi h} \left(\frac{1}{R_b^2} - \frac{1}{R_c^2} \right) \tag{6}$$

where T is the torque in dyn cm required to maintain an angular velocity of Ω radians/sec, R_b is the radius of the bob in cm, R_c is the inside radius of the cup and h is the depth to which the bob is immersed in the liquid. Equation (6) can be used to compute the viscosity when the angular velocity and the torque are known. However, a correction must be made for the "end-effect" which is due to the resistance produced by the liquid touching the bottom of the submerged bob. It is more convenient to combine the fixed quantities of equation (6), together with certain conversion factors, to arrive at an instrumental constant, K_v. Equation (6) then reduced to the simple formula,

$$\eta = K_v \frac{w}{v} \tag{7}$$

where η is the viscosity in poises, w is the driving weight in grams, and v is the velocity of rotation of the bob in r.p.m. The constant, K_v, may be determined by using a standardized liquid in the viscometer. Standardized oils may be obtained for this purpose from the National Bureau of Standards in Washington, D.C. In the United States the certified viscosity standards are specially prepared and are standardized against water at 20·0° C in a capillary viscometer (Swindells, 1947). The method of the National Bureau of Standards compares closely with the standardization procedure described by Cannon (Swindells *et al.*, 1954).

2. *Viscosity Coefficients of Dilute Colloidal Dispersions*

The particles in colloidal sols are widely separated and do not interact to any significant extent. They simply raise the viscosity in proportion to their concentration in the dispersion. However, when the concentration of the particles in suspension is high, the frequent collision and mutual interference of the particles lead to non-Newtonian behaviour such as plasticity, pseudoplasticity, and dilatancy. At this point we shall discuss the Newtonian viscosity of dilute colloidal dispersions, in which particle interaction may be disregarded.

Einstein (1906, 1911) derived an equation,

$$\eta = \eta_0(1+2{\cdot}5\phi) \tag{8}$$

relating the viscosity, η, of a dilute colloidal suspension to the volume fraction, ϕ, of the particles in the mixture. The volume fraction, ϕ, is the volume of the particles per unit volume of suspension. The volume of the particles is obtained from the mass and the true density of the particles. The quantity, η_0, is the viscosity of the dispersion medium or solvent. The equation is strictly applicable only to systems in which the particles are perfect spheres which do not interact with one another. It also may be used to describe dilute true solutions in which the particles are the molecules or ions of the solute. Broughton and Windebank (1938) and Eirich *et al.* (1936) have made experimental verification of the Einstein equation.

In order to employ equation (8) at higher concentrations various modifications must be made, one of which is applicable to suspensions of rigid spheres in moderate concentration showing no Brownian motion (Guth and Simha, 1936). The equation is written:

$$\eta = \eta_0(1+2{\cdot}5\phi+14{\cdot}1\phi^2) \tag{9}$$

where the symbols have the same meaning as those in equation (8). Vand (1948) and Robinson (1949) have also derived formulas which apply at higher concentrations. It will be observed that no terms defining the size, shape and interaction of the particles appear in these equations. In hydrophilic colloidal systems the swollen, flexible particles of irregular geometry make a greater contribution to the viscosity than is accounted for by their concentration alone. Interaction of lyophilic particles with one another and with the solvent molecules also contribute greatly to deviations from the simpler equations, and still more elaborate treatments are required to account for these effects. These complications will be considered in later sections of the chapter.

Beginning with the Einstein equation several viscosity coefficients, frequently encountered in the literature, may be defined.

a. *Relative viscosity*. This coefficient, abbreviated η_r, is defined as the ratio of the viscosity of the dispersion to that of the solvent. When relative viscosity is used, the Einstein equation is written as

$$\eta_r = \frac{\eta}{\eta_0} = 1+2{\cdot}5\phi \tag{10}$$

in which the ratio η/η_0 is, by definition, the relative viscosity.

b. *Specific viscosity*. This term is defined as the relative increase in viscosity of the dispersion over that of the solvent alone, or:

$$\eta_{sp} = \frac{\eta - \eta_0}{\eta_0} = \frac{\eta}{\eta_0} - 1 \tag{11}$$

Notice that the specific viscosity, η_{sp}, is equal to the relative viscosity minus unity. Using specific viscosity, the Einstein equation becomes:

$$\eta_{sp} = \frac{\eta}{\eta_0} - 1 = 2{\cdot}5\phi \tag{12}$$

Now, since volume fraction, ϕ, is directly proportional to concentration, equation (12) may be rewritten in the form:

$$\eta_{sp} = kc \tag{13}$$

in which k is a constant. The equation shows that specific viscosity is directly proportional to the particle concentration in a dilute colloidal dispersion. The concentration, c, is ordinarily expressed as grams of dispersed phase (particles) per 100 ml of total dispersion. For real systems at finite concentrations the equation is ordinarily written as a power series:

$$\eta_{sp} = \alpha c + \beta c^2 + \ldots \tag{14}$$

where α and β are constants that must be determined by experimentation.

c. *Reduced viscosity*. We now define a reduced viscosity, namely η_{sp}/c. It may be obtained from equation (14) by dividing both sides through by the concentration:

$$\frac{\eta_{sp}}{c} = \alpha + \beta c + \ldots \tag{15}$$

d. *Intrinsic viscosity*. When the reduced viscosity is determined at various concentrations and the results are plotted as shown in Fig. 2, the resulting line can be extrapolated to $c = 0$ to obtain the intercept, α. The intercept is known as the intrinsic viscosity and is given the symbol $[\eta]$. The intrinsic viscosity is an important quantity in polymer science, for it is used to obtain the average molecular weight of high polymers. The average molecular weight $\bar{M}$ is related to the intrinsic viscosity by the expression:

$$[\eta] = K\bar{M}^a \tag{16}$$

where K and a are constants for a series of polymers and must be obtained from separate experiments with the given polymer-solvent system. The constant, a, ordinarily has a value of unity or close to unity.

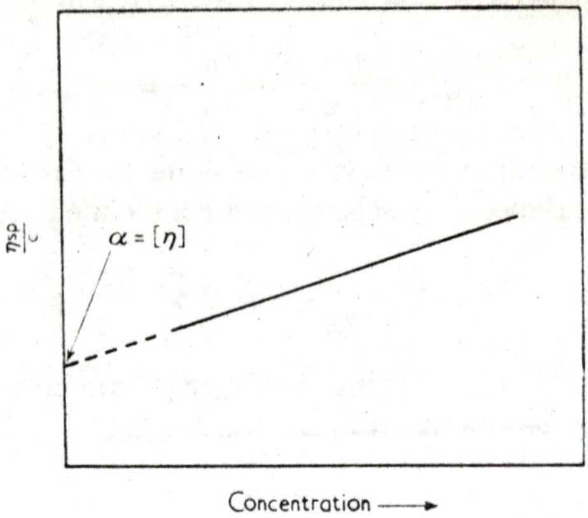

FIG. 2. Intrinsic viscosity of a high polymer.

B. FLOW CHARACTERISTICS OF NON-NEWTONIAN MATERIALS

Concentrated heterogeneous dispersions, including colloidal dispersions, emulsions, suspensions and ointments, comprise a class of systems whose flow do not follow the simple Newtonian relationship. Characteristic consistency curves or rheograms are obtained for the various types of flow, plastic, pseudoplastic and dilatant, when non-Newtonian materials are analysed in a suitable viscometer.

1. *Plastic Flow*

The characteristic properties of materials which exhibit plastic flow are depicted in the rheogram of Fig. 3. Such materials are called Bingham bodies in honour of E. C. Bingham who first studied their properties (Reiner, 1943). The curve is linear over most of its length, corresponding to that of a Newtonian fluid. However, the curve does not pass through the origin; instead, its linear portion intersects the horizontal axis at a point known as the yield value, f. Contrary to a Newtonian liquid that yields under the slightest force, a Bingham body fails to flow until a definite shearing stress, the yield value, is exceeded. The yield value is thought to result mainly from a network of floccules which is broken down as the material begins to flow.

Materials which show pure plastic flow are few. A suspension of zinc oxide in mineral oil serves as a simple example of a Bingham body. Certain paints, printing inks and firm jellies also fall in this class.

The equation describing plastic flow was first given by Bingham as:

$$(F-f) = UG \tag{17}$$

where F is the shearing stress, f is the yield value, G is the rate of shear, and U is the plastic viscosity. U may be defined as the shearing force in excess of the yield value, required to induce a unit rate of shear, G. It is not identical with the coefficient of viscosity used to describe a Newtonian liquid, as will be explained more clearly later.

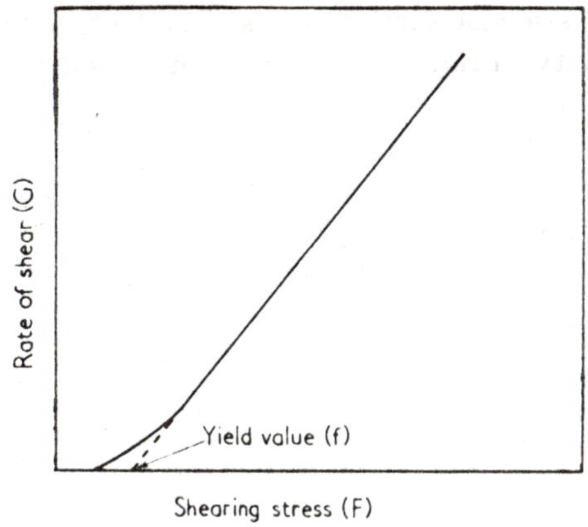

FIG. 3. Flow curve of a Bingham body.

a. *Plastic flow in a capillary.* Buckingham (1920) investigated the flow of plastic materials through capillary tubes and found that the flow curve so obtained was not linear. Buckingham then derived an equation describing the flow of a Bingham body in a capillary tube. He was able to separate the flow curve into two parts, one portion accounting for the flow of the material as a coherent plug, or the slippage-flow portion, and the other part of the curve representing laminar or streamlined flow.

b. *Plastic flow in a rotational viscometer.* The Buckingham equation shows that plug flow can never be entirely eliminated in a capillary viscometer, and the flow curve of a Bingham body can never become entirely linear. Consequently, when a capillary viscometer is used to analyse plastic flow, the flow curve cannot be extrapolated to the shearing stress axis in order to obtain the yield value.

Fortunately, the difficulty may be overcome by using a rotational viscometer. The geometry of the rotational viscometer makes it quite suitable for the analysis of Bingham bodies. Although plug flow does occur in a rotational viscometer at sufficiently low shearing stress, at stresses above this region only laminar flow occurs and the curve is linear.

Reiner and Riwlin (1927) derived an equation for the flow of a Bingham body in a rotational viscometer. The equation is a linear one, describing the portion of the rheogram (Fig. 3) that represents laminar flow. By extrapolation to the shearing stress axis it also provides an unambiguous definition of yield value.

The Reiner-Riwlin equation is:

$$U = \frac{T}{4\pi h\Omega}\left(\frac{1}{R_b^2} - \frac{1}{R_c^2}\right) - \frac{f}{\Omega}\ln\frac{R_c}{R_b} \tag{18}$$

where U is the plastic viscosity in poises, T is the torque in dyn cm, Ω is the angular velocity in rad/sec, h is the depth in cm to which the bob is immersed in the plastic material, R_b is the radius of the bob in cm, R_c is the inside radius of the cup, and f is the yield value in dyn/cm^2.

By the use of this fundamental expression, it is possible to derive practical equations for calculating the yield value and the plastic viscosity of a material. When using the Stormer viscometer (a Searle-type instrument) these expressions become:

$$f = K_f w_f \tag{19}$$

and

$$U = K_v \frac{w - w_f}{v} \tag{20}$$

The terms of equations (19) and (20) are defined as follows: f is the yield value, U is the plastic viscosity, w is the mass in grams on the weight hanger, w_f is the yield value intercept in grams, v is the velocity of the bob in r.p.m., and K_f and K_v are constants characteristic of the instrument. Martin (1960) has provided examples showing the use of these equations.

When the Couette-type rotational viscometer is used, the practical equations for yield value and plastic viscosity become:

$$f = K_f \theta_f \tag{21}$$

$$U = K_v \frac{\theta - \theta_f}{v} \tag{22}$$

where θ is the angle through which the torque wire is twisted, and θ_f is the corresponding value obtained when the line is extrapolated to the torque axis.

c. *An explanation of plasticity*. Plastic flow is considered to result from the contact of flocculated particles in a concentrated suspension. These particles are held together in a flocculated state continuous throughout the mass, and they must break contact before flow can occur. For the reader who is unfamiliar with the phenomenon of flocculation, it may be

at stresses below yield value substance acts as an elastic material described as a kind of structure in which the particles are aggregated in the dispersion medium in the form of fluffy soft clumps. The van der Waals force, which is no doubt responsible for this phenomenon, may be referred to as the force of flocculation. Friction between the moving particles as well as the force of flocculation contribute to the yield value. If the particles are wetted by a deflocculating agent the force of flocculation can be reduced considerably. However, it is possible that the frictional forces between the particles in a concentrated suspension are not affected by this means, and the yield value may remain large.

The form of the plastic flow curve of Fig. 3 is explained in the following manner. Below the yield value the shearing stress produced in the rotational viscometer is not sufficient to bring about flow; but when the stress exceeds that of the yield value the force of flocculation and the frictional resistance are no longer capable of holding the particles in position. The shearing stress in dyn/cm^2 required to overcome these forces is roughly the yield value of the material. When the yield value is exceeded and flow begins, the rate of shear, G, becomes directly proportional to $(F-f)$, the force in excess of the yield value, as already demonstrated in equation (17). Consequently, the flow curve becomes a straight line at a shear stress somewhat above the extrapolated yield-value intercept.

2. *Pseudoplastic Flow*

Unlike Bingham bodies, pseudoplastic materials exhibit no yield value, but instead are characterized by rheograms which approach the origin of the graph, as in the case of Newtonian liquids. However, unlike the curve for a Newtonian material, the pseudoplastic flow curve is non-linear, as seen in Fig. 4. Another way of expressing this fact is to say that the shear stress, F, does not increase linearly with the shear rate, G, hence the viscosity does not remain constant at different rates of shear.

Solutions of suspending agents such as tragacanth, gelatin, carboxymethylcellulose, and other water-soluble mucilages and gums exhibit pseudoplastic flow. These materials consist of long-chain molecules or other complex structures which are disarranged and matted together at rest and remain so at low shear rates, but which tend to become aligned at higher rates of shear. Some of the solvent associated with the molecules may also be excluded as the particles align, and the resistance of the effectively smaller particles to flow is reduced somewhat. Thus the material becomes less viscous as the shear rate is increased. Because of the decrease in viscosity with increasing shear rate, pseudoplasticity is sometimes called "shear rate thinning".

a. *Possible indices for pseudoplastic flow.* Several techniques have been used to analyse the flow curves of pseudoplastic materials. After a detailed study of the phenomenon, Green (1949a) concluded that the most satisfactory method of expressing the viscosity of a pseudoplastic material was to plot the rheogram and use the Newtonian viscosity, obtaining it as near to the origin of the graph as possible. In a like manner, other workers have obtained the reciprocal of the slope of a line joining a specified point along the pseudoplastic curve with the origin of the graph (corresponding to Newtonian viscosity), and have called it

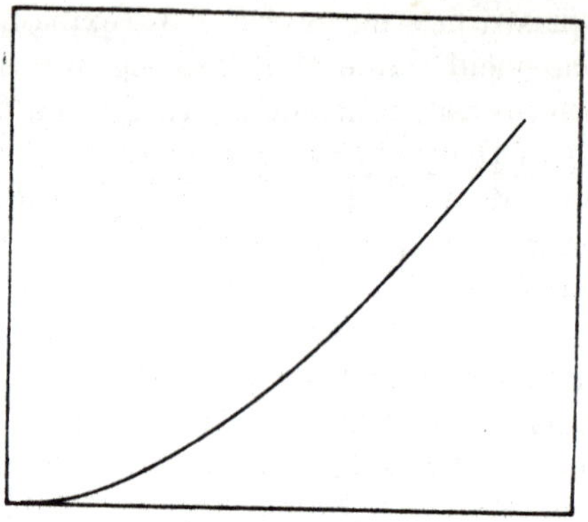

FIG. 4. Flow curve of a pseudoplastic material.

"apparent viscosity". Still others have suggested that the ratio of two viscosities be used. The reciprocal of the slope of the F versus G plot is obtained both at a low shear rate near the origin and at a high shear rate where the curve approaches linearity. A ratio of these differential viscosities, namely $\eta_{\text{low rate}}/\eta_{\text{high rate}}$ is then employed as an index of pseudoplasticity.

Rheologists have not yet been able to represent the pseudoplastic curve with a suitable equation founded on a theoretical basis. However, an exponential formula,

$$F^N = \eta' G \tag{23}$$

has often been used as an empirical approach to the problem (Farrow *et al.*, 1928; Porter and Rao, 1927; Krieger and Maron, 1951). In equation (23) F is the shearing stress and G is the rate of shear. The exponent, N, is indicative of non-Newtonian behaviour. When N assumes a value of unity we have the simple Newtonian equation of flow. The further the value of N rises above unity, the greater the pseudoplastic character of the material. The particular viscosity coefficient, η', defined in this equation, is a constant characteristic of a particular material, but, unlike Newtonian viscosity η and plastic viscosity U, it is difficult to assign to it any physical meaning.

Equation (23) is often written in logarithmic form,

$$\log G = N \log F - \log \eta' \tag{24}$$

and plotted to yield a straight line from which both N and η' can be obtained.

Pseudoplastic materials should be analysed in rotational viscometers capable of operating within a wide range of shearing rates so as to obtain a representative consistency curve. Capillary and falling-ball viscometers which operate at a single rate of shear are unsuited for the study of pseudoplastic flow. However, multihead capillaries can be designed to provide a sufficient number of points for analysis of the flow curves in terms of equations (23) or (24).

b. *Inadequacies of equation* (23). Hamlow (1958) found that the equation, $F^N = \eta' G$ was not particularly useful for describing the flow of many of the pseudoplastic suspending agents used in pharmacy. Although equation (24) suggests a linear relationship, non-linear log-log plots of G versus F were obtained with solutions of methylcellulose, sodium cellulose sulphate, and various algin derivatives. Thus equation (23) does not satisfactorily describe the flow characteristics of these systems. Krieger and Maron (1951) have encountered similar difficulties in the rheological analysis of latex emulsions. Shangraw *et al.* (1961) proposed an equation which may overcome some of the objections of previous formulations. The equation is written

$$F = f + \eta_\alpha S - b_v c^{-as}$$

where F is the shearing stress, S is the rate of shear, and f, η_α, b_v and a are constants characteristic of a particular system. The term f is the intercept on the stress axis of the asymtote to the flow curve at high rates of shear, and η_α is the slope of this line. The yield value is $f - b_v$; a is a constant found to have a value of 0·001 for the systems investigated. The equation is reported to represent flow data obtained with solutions of suspending agents, emulsions and suspensions of solids in various media. It can be used to calculate yield values from non-linear flow curves, and to obtain limiting viscosities at very low rates of shear.

3. *Dilatant Flow*

Dilatancy is a phenomenon, discovered by Reynolds (1885), in which the material exhibits an increase in resistance to flow with increasing rate of shear. The material returns to a state of fluidity when the shear is removed or the agitation is stopped. The phenomenon is sometimes referred to as "shear-rate thickening". Dilatant flow is shown in Fig. 5, where the curve is observed to be concave towards the shearing stress axis.

a. *An equation describing dilatancy.* As in the case of pseudoplastic flow, dilatant flow may be expressed by the exponential expression, equation (23)

$$F^N = \eta' G$$

Whereas in the case of pseudoplasticity N takes on values greater than one, in dilatancy N is always less than one. N approaches unity and the

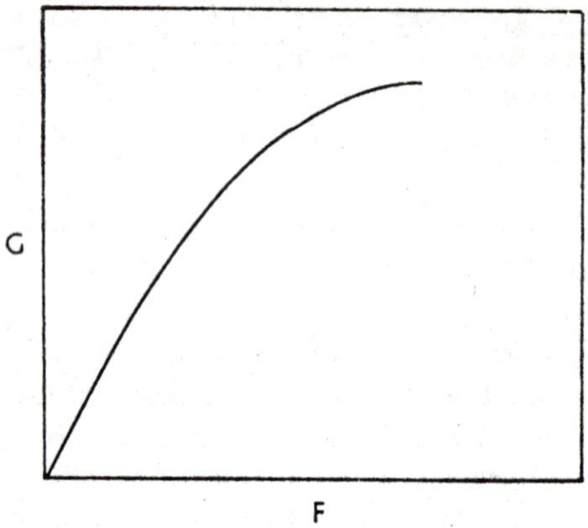

FIG. 5. Flow curve characteristic of dilatancy.

material approaches Newtonian behaviour as the line becomes more nearly linear. The consistency of a dilatant material, like a pseudoplastic body, may be expressed in terms of the viscosity coefficient, η', and a ratio of high-shear η' to low-shear η' could perhaps be used as a suitable measure of dilatant character.

b. *An explanation of dilatancy.* Dilatant flow is exhibited by suspensions containing a high concentration of very fine particles. The particles, although in close-packed arrangement, are in a state of deflocculation. Flocculated suspensions, on the other hand, tend to show plastic flow rather than dilatancy.

As a dilatant material is rapidly stirred or passed through a mill it becomes much thicker than it was before agitation. This is explained in a qualitative way as follows. When the deflocculated particles of a suspension settle, they pack into a mass of minimum volume. Only a small quantity of vehicle is needed to fill the voids between the particles, but it is sufficient to allow the suspension to flow like a liquid. When the undisturbed mass is vigorously agitated, the bulk is increased as the particles force past one another. This expansion results in a larger volume between the particles and an insufficiency of vehicle to fill the voids. Thus the unlubricated particles show an increased resistance to flow, and a rigid paste results.

Dilatancy does not occur in a dilute suspension where the vehicle is in great excess. It can, however, be demonstrated by mixing about 50 per cent by weight of potassium silicate or fine starch powder with cold water to which a deflocculating agent may be added if necessary. If the mass is stirred rapidly with a paddle, the material thickens to the point where the paddle will stand upright unassisted for a moment in the mass. However, as soon as the shearing action is stopped, the material loses its paste-like consistency, reverts to a fluid suspension, and the paddle soon topples over. Metzner and Whitlock (1958) have carried out experiments involving the dilatancy of concentrated titanium dioxide suspensions.

"Crazy putty", also called "silly putty" and "bouncing putty", which can be purchased in toy or novelty stores, represents an interesting example of dilatancy. It is a suspension of solid polymer particles in a silicone base and has the consistency of putty. When rolled into a sphere and allowed to fall it bounces like a ball. It can be drawn out slowly and moulded into various shapes like putty, but when pulled rapidly it breaks like a brittle solid.

Dilatancy is a particularly troublesome effect in the manufacture of paints, printing inks, and some pharmaceutical suspensions. When dispersions of high solid content are passed through a roller mill or a colloid mill, the material may tend to solidify. The motor of the mill can become overloaded and seriously damaged, therefore great care is demanded in the milling of dilatant products.

C. RHEOLOGICAL STRUCTURE

The basic types of flow, Newtonian, plastic, pseudoplastic and dilatant, are distinguished by their characteristic flow curves, as we have already seen. The shapes of these curves have been rationalized in terms of the kinds of flow exhibited by the molecules, particles and aggregates in the various materials. The three basic types of flow are further illustrated schematically in Figs. 6*a*, *b*, and *c*, which should be self-explanatory.

The structural features of these systems involve flocculation and gel formations, effects which become evident in the flow diagrams as yield value, thixotropy and spur value. The yield value has already been considered; it remains for us to discuss the other manifestations of structure associated with disperse systems.

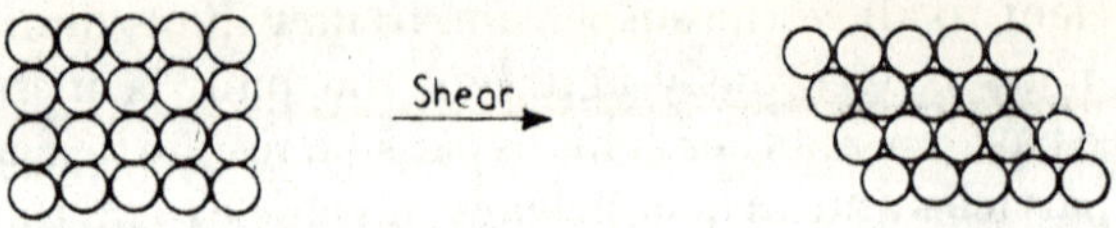

FIG. 6*a*. Bingham body. At rest the particles are held together by the force of flocculation. Particles are displaced with respect to one another during the shearing process.

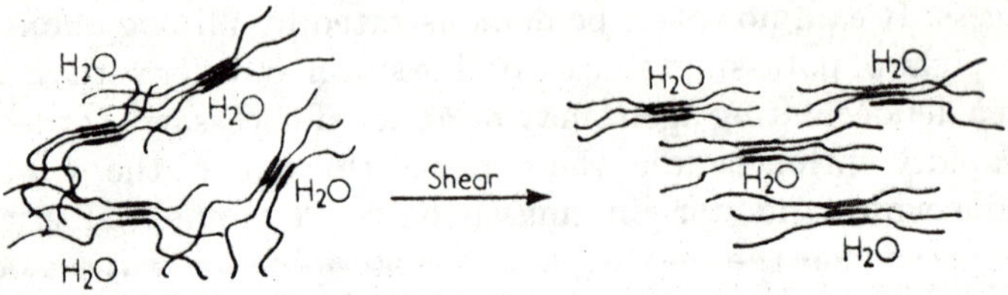

FIG. 6*b*. Pseudoplastic body. At rest the molecules lie in random arrangement, intertwined and bound to the solvent molecules. Polymer molecules such as carboxymethylcellulose are ordinarily depicted as shown here. Under shear the molecules align and squeeze out the bound water molecules. The viscosity of the system consequently decreases proportional to the increase in rate of shear.

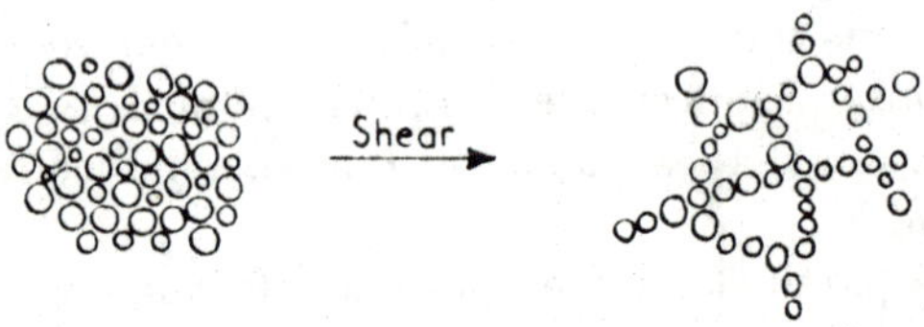

FIG. 6*c*. Dilatancy. Deflocculated close-packed sediment (dilatant system at rest). Sediment expands during shear, resulting in increased resistance to flow.

1. *Thixotropy*

Early in the development of rheology, investigators observed the break-down of concentrated non-Newtonian dispersions when stirred, and the resetting of the material to a semi-solid consistency when allowed to stand undisturbed. The term, thixotropy, was given to this phenomenon. It means "to change by touch", and may be described as a reversible isothermal sol-gel transformation (Freundlich, 1935).

Thixotropy arises from the break-down and build-up of floccules as found in a suspension of bentonite, or of aggregates of crystallites as found in a solution of carboxymethylcellulose.

a. *Thixotropy as a structural factor*. We shall consider thixotropy not as a separate type of non-Newtonian flow but rather as a structural break-down and reaggregation superimposed on the basic flow types. Thixotropy can occur in conjunction with simple plastic flow to produce materials which are referred to as Bingham bodies with thixotropy, or as thixotropic Bingham bodies. Thixotropy is also observed with pseudoplastic flow and with dilatancy.

Rheograms with thixotropy superimposed on the three fundamental non-Newtonian types are shown in Fig. 7. Figure 7*a* is characteristic of a Bingham body with thixotropy as shown by bentonite magma and by petrolatum; the curve of 7*b* demonstrates pseudoplasticity with thixotropy, often shown by dispersions of synthetic suspending agents; 7*c* is a flow diagram depicting dilatancy with thixotropy, a property of some quicksands.

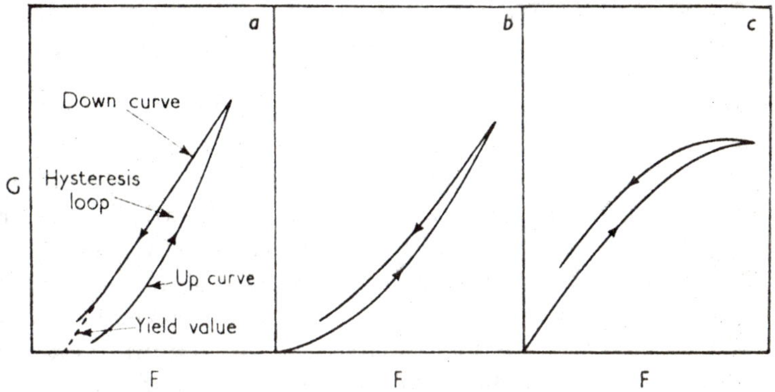

FIG. 7. Flow curves exhibiting thixotropy. *a*. Rheogram of a Bingham body with thixotropy; *b*. rheogram of a pseudoplastic material showing thixotropy; *c*. rheogram of a dilatant paste showing thixotropy.

b. *The hysteresis loop*. The criterion of thixotropy suggested by Green (1949b) and accepted by most rheologists today is the hysteresis loop in the flow diagram of a non-Newtonian material. In order to analyse such a material in a rotational viscometer, the shearing stress or the rate of shear is steadily increased to obtain points on what is called the upcurve. It is stopped at an arbitrarily chosen upper value and then the shear is steadily decreased to obtain data for what is called the downcurve.

If the material is a simple non-Newtonian without thixotropy, the up- and the downcurves coincide. If the curves do not coincide but instead form a hysteresis loop, then the material is thixotropic, and the area of the loop can be used as a measure of the thixotropic breakdown of the body. Thixotropic breakdown may also be given in the form of an analytical expression as described in a later section.

The loop formed by the up- and downcurves of thixotropic materials results from a gel-like structure which is broken down as the material is agitated. The process is a dynamic one. At any given shearing rate along the upcurve, the breakdown is in equilibrium with the build-up of structural units in the mass. As the shear rate is raised to a new value, the material breaks down still further until the rate of breakdown again equals the build-up of structure. Then, after an arbitrarily selected upper limit has been reached and the shear rate is reduced gradually, the material remains in the state of the structural breakdown which was attained at the highest shear rate. Consequently, the downcurve is linear. Since obviously the up- and downcurves do not coincide, a loop is formed with an area corresponding to the extent of thixotropic breakdown. As observed in Fig. 7*a* the lower portion of the downcurve may bow towards the shear rate axis rather than being linear, in the case of some materials. In this region of shear the structure is apparently in the process of reforming, just as it is when the material is allowed to stand undisturbed (Eyring *et al.*, 1959).

In an aqueous suspension of bentonite, repeated runs, producing both the up- and the downcurve, cause a reduction in the area of the loop. A loop of constant size is finally obtained, which can be reproduced on subsequent cycling. If, however, sufficient time is allowed for the structure to rebuild completely before the next run is made, the up- and downcurves produce a loop corresponding to the original loop obtained.

In the case of petrolatum or a lubricating grease, repeated runs in a rotational viscometer may reduce the hysteresis loop until it disappears completely to give a simple Bingham body. The original structure of such materials may not be reformed during the resting stage at ordinary temperatures.

c. *Quantitative expressions of thixotropy.* As described by Green and Weltmann (1946) thixotropic breakdown can be expressed quantitatively in a number of ways. The use of the hysteresis loop, already described, appears to be one of the most satisfactory methods of analysis to date (Price-Jones, J., 1936, 1941). Green and Weltmann (1943, 1944, 1946a) and Weltmann (1943) have studied the method extensively, and Green (1949c) devoted considerable space in his book to a discussion of thixotropy and hysteresis-loop measurements. These workers have proposed several coefficients of thixotropic breakdown, which will now be briefly described.

The most widely used coefficient of thixotropic breakdown of Bingham bodies is M, the loss in shearing stress per unit increase in shear rate. It is obtained by forming two separate loops in the curve. The plastic material is placed in a suitable rotational viscometer, and data for the upcurve is obtained. The instrument is stopped at an arbitrarily chosen top rate of shear, which we shall designate in Fig. 8 as v_1. The downcurve is now run and the plastic viscosity, U_1, is obtained from the slope of this line, using equation (22). Without disturbing the material in the cup, another cyclic run is performed and the data plotted as shown in Fig. 8. This time the upcurve is begun at an r.p.m. above v_1, and the upcurve is carried to a new top r.p.m., designated v_2. A downcurve is again obtained

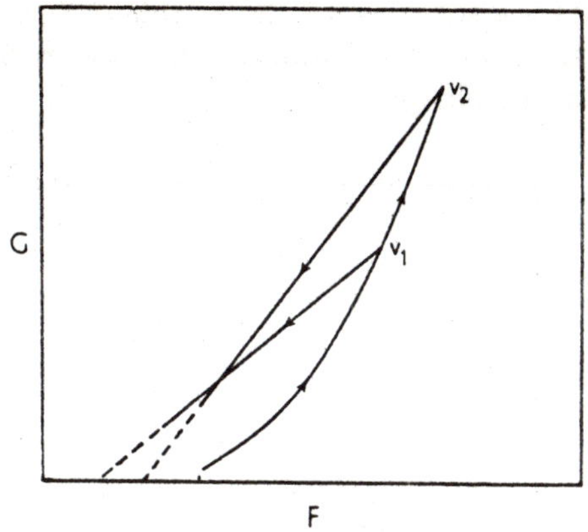

FIG. 8. Determination of M, one of the coefficients of thixotropic breakdown.

and the viscosity U_2 is computed. The coefficient of thixotropic breakdown, M, is then calculated, using the formula:

$$M = \frac{U_1 - U_2}{\ln \frac{v_2}{v_1}} \tag{25}$$

One of the criticisms of this method for measuring thixotropic breakdown is that the coefficient M depends on upper rates of shear chosen by the investigator. Consequently this coefficient is not a constant which may be recorded for each material, but rather a value which must be determined each time under carefully controlled conditions.

A second factor which influences the coefficient is that of the time of measurement, as can be seen in Fig. 9. If the material is held at a constant rate of shear, for example at point B, until the shearing stress falls off to, say, point C, one will obtain the downcurve, CA. However, if the material is held at the uppermost shear rate for an extended period of time before producing the downcurve, an equilibrium value, point D, is reached, and the downcurve DA is then obtained. (An analysis such as this is readily made using a Couette instrument; a Searle viscometer cannot be conveniently used for such an experiment.)

Thus we see that the area of the loop is influenced not only by the uppermost rate of shear employed, but also by the time that the material is held at any given rate of shear. The "breakdown by time", produced at a definite rate of shear, has actually been used by Weltmann and Green to define another coefficient of thixotropic breakdown, *B*. A third coefficient, *V*, has also been suggested. For a detailed discussion of this topic, the reader is referred to the book by Green (1949c).

Zettlemoyer and his associates (1953) have also proposed an expression for thixotropy, based on an equilibrium method rather than on the formation of a hysteresis loop.

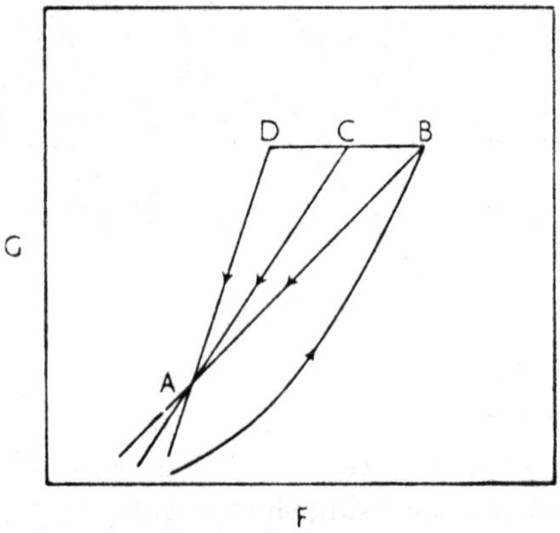

FIG. 9. Flow curves showing breakdown with time.

2. *Bulges and Spurs in the Hysteresis Loop*

A number of types of dispersions are characterized by thixotropic loops which are more complicated than the ones already mentioned. These include highly concentrated aqueous bentonite gels (Rehbinder, 1954; Peter and Stolle, 1957; Eyring *et al.*, 1960), colloidal dispersions of graphite in organic vehicles (McKennel, 1954), china in water (Moore, 1959) and gels of procaine penicillin for intramuscular injection (Ober *et al.*, 1958).

In Fig. 10 we see the flow diagram of a 12 per cent aqueous bentonite suspension showing a characteristic bulge in the upcurve. Figure 11 represents the curve of a 2 per cent solution of carboxymethylcellulose in water. Its upcurve is seen to be deformed so sharply as to yield a spur-like protrusion. These two materials are no doubt thixotropic bodies, but the bulge and the spur add complications to the non-Newtonian properties of these materials. Bulges and spurs in the upcurves are thought to result from a three-dimensional gel-like structure in thixotropic materials.

The spur value *Y* of Fig. 11 represents the high initial yield value characteristic of such a gel structure. The application of the spur value to the design of pharmaceutical gels is discussed later in the chapter.

An explanation for the bulge in the loop of bentonite gels has been suggested along the following lines. Michaels (1958) assumed that the

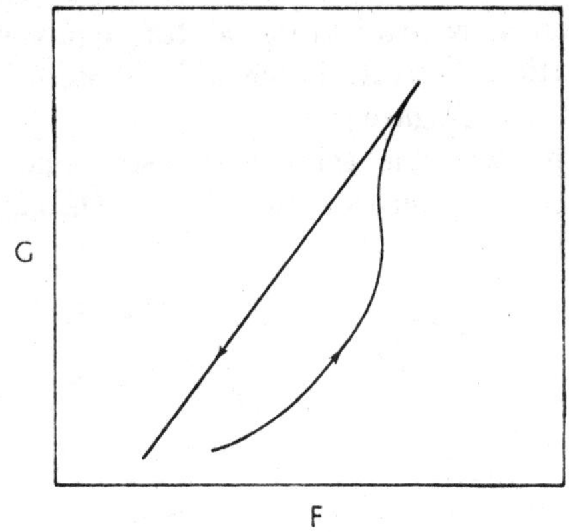

FIG. 10. Flow curve of a 12 per cent aqueous bentonite suspension.

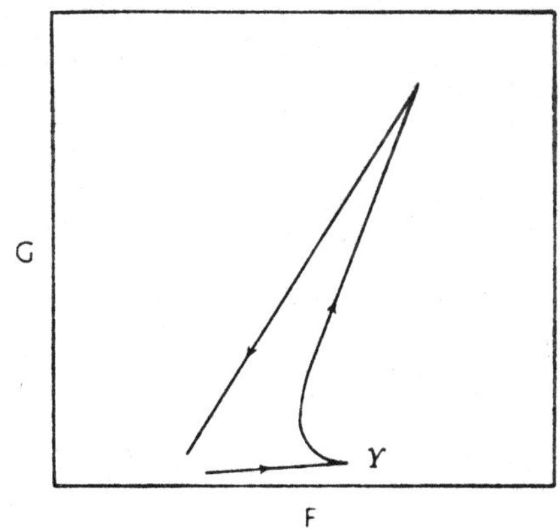

FIG. 11. Flow curve of a 2 per cent solution of carboxymethylcellulose.

crystalline plates of bentonite take on a "card-house" structure in a moderately dilute aqueous suspension; in a highly concentrated solution a "block-house" arrangement of plates prevails. These structures are shown in Fig. 12. It will be observed that the block-house structure consists of packs or blocks of cards adhering to one another. The bonding of these card packs is probably weaker than the attachment of the individual cards in the card-house aggregation. Bentonite swells in water and Eyring and his associates (1960) conclude that the bulge in the rheograms of moderately concentrated aqueous bentonite suspensions is due to the card-house structure. Bentonite does not swell in glycerin and a suspension of bentonite in glycerin shows no thixotropy at concentrations below 20 per cent. Above this concentration, bentonite in glycerin shows ordinary thixotropy without the bulge in the upcurve. The glycerin system is considered to be representative of the weaker bonding block-house aggregation. Thus the bulge in the hysteresis loop is probably due to the card-house aggregate.

It may be hypothesized that the card-house phenomenon is a three-dimensional branched structure, continuous throughout the mass,

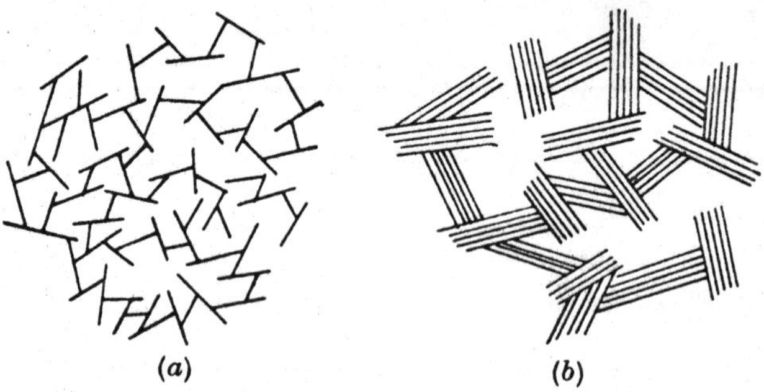

FIG. 12. Schematic diagrams of (*a*) card-house, and (*b*) block-house structures in thixotropic materials. (Reproduced with permission from Eyring *et al.*, 1960.)

whereas the block-house aggregation is localized and predominantly non-branching (Eyring *et al.*, 1960).

Although structural characteristics have been invoked to explain the flow properties of materials since the beginning of rheology, much remains to be learned about the relationships of structure and rheological properties. One may gain a better insight into the complications that the rheologist must face by referring to such reports as Ott and Elliott (1955) and Gabrysh *et al.* (1961).

D. A NEED FOR SOUND INSTRUMENTATION

1. *Multi-point versus One-point Measurements*

Measurements on Newtonian materials can be made satisfactorily using "one-point" instruments such as simple capillary viscometers. These provide a single shearing force and hence only one point on the flow curve. But with non-Newtonian materials such as emulsions, suspensions and solutions of suspending agents, ointments and pastes, the multi-point consistency curve must be plotted. This requires the use of instruments which can be operated at a number of shear-stress or shear-rate settings.

It is sometimes argued that although a one-point measurement cannot characterize the rheological properties of a system, it does provide a reproducible value with sufficient precision for industrial control purposes. As Green (1949) has insisted, this idea is spurious and should be confronted with convincing arguments whenever it is advanced.

Let us attempt to do this by reference to Fig. 13. Here we see the flow diagrams of four products having different rheological characteristics. *A* is a Newtonian liquid, *B* is pseudoplastic, *C* and *D* are two Bingham bodies with different yield values and different plastic viscosities. Suppose that a viscometer is operated at a single rate of shear, G_1, to

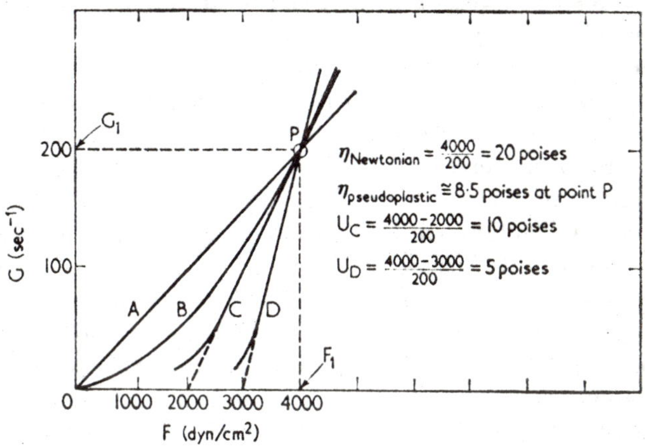

FIG. 13. Demonstration of multi-point versus one-point viscosity calculations. *A* Newtonian flow curve; *B* pseudoplastic flow curve; *C* and *D* plastic flow curves.

obtain a measure of consistency of these four materials. Since such a measurement defines but a single point on the rheogram, it expresses the properties of all four materials in terms of only a single parameter, namely the Newtonian viscosity:

$$\eta = \frac{F_1}{G_1} = \frac{4000\ \text{dyn/cm}^2}{200\ \text{sec}^{-1}} = \frac{20\ \text{dyn sec}}{\text{cm}^2}$$

Thus we would record the viscosity of the several products as 20 poises, whereas they actually have the viscosity coefficients shown in Fig. 13.

We might excuse ourselves for defining a pseudoplastic material and the two Bingham bodies in terms of a Newtonian parameter by referring to the results as "apparent viscosity". But no such apology can erase the fact that we are dealing with four materials which act differently in processing, flow at different rates through feeding lines, pour more or less readily from bottles and jars, feel different to the touch, and perform in different ways under various environmental conditions. When considered in this light, a one-point characterization of these rheologically-unlike materials provides an inaccurate and misleading viscosity parameter.

We might also admit that the one-point method is inadequate for widely different materials, but argue that it is still suitable for controlling the quality of successive batches of a product of a definite rheological class. But our findings do not allow us to accept even this conclusion. The plastic flow curves, *C* and *D*, of Fig. 13 represent such a material processed at different times in a particular laboratory. Our one-point method would categorize these batches as identical, both having the apparent viscosity of 20 poises. Yet the total flow curves clearly show that product *C* would feel softer to the touch than *D* because of its lower yield value. Conversely, product *D* would flow more readily once the yield value was exceeded, because its plastic viscosity is less than that of *C*. Thus a one-point method is unsatisfactory for the analysis or the quality control of materials other than Newtonian liquids.

In making a final plea for rheologically sound instrumentation, we mention here two factors which no doubt discourage some workers from using fundamentally designed viscometers in the analysis of non-Newtonian materials. The first of these is that instruments of different design (e.g. a cup and bob instrument and a cone and plate instrument) may produce significantly different flow diagrams. Secondly, the results may also show great variance if the batches of material under test have been subjected to different physical treatment before analysis.

However, once one has some knowledge of rheology, these apparent inconsistencies cause no difficulty; they can, in fact, be turned to good use. We have seen that viscosity coefficients can vary depending on the rate of shear or shearing stress that the material is subjected to and on the time required to carry out the measurement. These factors depend on the design of the particular instrument and on the geometry of the shearing surfaces. Furthermore, if the heating, milling and flow conditions under which samples of the material have been processed are dissimilar, it is not difficult to see, following our discussion of structural factors, that the rheological results may differ. These are facts of nature which should be welcomed by the investigator, for by their application he can often predict how certain materials will behave in processing and in practice.

2. *Fundamental Viscometers versus Empirical Instruments*

Only in very recent times have properly designed viscometers become commercially available for use in control and rheological analysis. Many devices have been suggested over the years for measuring the consistency of materials in an empirical way. These instruments are ordinarily incapable of providing rheological data in rational units, often because the bob and cup of a rotational viscometer is of unusual design, for example a bob consisting of a shaft and cross bars, or a cup with vanes attached to its inner surface. Instruments which operate on the principle of squeezing the material from an irregularly shaped tube, allowing a weighted object to fall on the surface of the mass, or drawing a plate across the material under test also belong to the class of empirical instruments. They do not ordinarily account for plug flow, end effects, turbulence, and other important design problems.

Although these devices cannot be recommended as basic rheological instruments, they are often used in pharmaceutical control and are frequently referred to in the current literature. For this reason we have included in this chapter a brief description of some of these devices.

II. Instrumentation

In describing various instruments which have been used in measuring rheological properties, representative types of instruments will be covered and grouped according to the principle of operation. Some of the instruments mentioned are empirical in nature, and the significance of the results thus obtained is not known. No attempt is made to cover all of the instruments which have been used, or are now available. Descriptions, procedures, and calculations for these are adequately treated in the original articles, instrument brochures, and several books (Hatschek, 1928; Barr, 1931; Scott-Blair, 1949; and Green, 1949). A compilation of various instruments is published in a book by Van Wazer *et al.* (1963). Addresses of the suppliers of a number of instruments are listed on page 51 following Table II.

The instruments can be classified as one-point and multi-point. The one-point or single point instruments are useful in measuring materials exhibiting Newtonian flow, and multi-point instruments can be used to measure materials exhibiting either Newtonian or non-Newtonian flow. Pharmaceutical preparations such as emulsions, suspensions, magmas, ointments and gels exhibit non-Newtonian flow and should be characterized by the use of multi-point instruments as previously discussed.

In the selection of an instrument to measure a pharmaceutical preparation, it may be desirable to determine the rheological properties of the preparation under the approximate conditions of treatment which it will undergo in practice. Henderson *et al.* (1961) have calculated the approximate rates of shear encountered in pharmaceutical processing such as milling, extrusion from orifices and pouring from bottles as shown in Table I.

TABLE I

Approximate Rates of Shear for Various Processes

Process	*Rate of shear*
Rubbing on ointment tile	150 sec^{-1}
Roller mill	1000 to 12,000 sec^{-1}
Colloid mill	Several thousand sec^{-1}
Hypodermic needle	Up to 10,000 sec^{-1}
Nasal spray (plastic squeeze bottle)	2000 sec^{-1}
Pouring from bottle	Less than 100 sec^{-1}

These values are given to indicate the approximate amount of shear the product will encounter. The rates of shear can easily be calculated by knowing the velocity at which the sample is being worked and the thickness of the sample. For example, the approximate rate of shear in spreading a layer of ointment 1–3 mm thick on the surface of the skin using a 6 cm stroke at 4 strokes/sec is given by Kostenbauder and Martin (1954) by the equation,

$$S = \frac{\Delta V}{\Delta r} \tag{26}$$

where S is the rate of shear, ΔV is the velocity the top layer moves in respect to the layer next to the skin, and Δr is the thickness of the layer.

By substituting the values into the equation, the rate of shear is found to be

$$S = \frac{24 \text{ cm/sec}}{0{\cdot}2 \text{ cm}} = 120 \text{ sec}^{-1} \tag{27}$$

As the ointment is spread into thinner layers using the same conditions of application, the rate of shear increases tremendously. If the layer were 20 μ in thickness, the rate of shear would be 12,000 sec^{-1}.

In the calibration of instruments, standard oils are usually used. The National Bureau of Standards (Miscellaneous Publication 241, 1962) have special oils as mentioned earlier for use in calibration of viscometers. These oils are calibrated at 20° C and 25° C for absolute viscosity and at 100° F and 200° F for kinematic viscosity. The viscosity range for the common oils are 0·020 to 14 poises and are designated as D, H, I, J, K, L, M, and N in the order of increasing viscosities. Higher viscosity oils OB and P are also available.

A. CAPILLARY INSTRUMENTS

1. *Capillary Constriction*

This type of instrument is very accurate for the measurement of Newtonian fluids of low viscosity. The flow data from this type of system are well defined as the mathematics have been worked out well. Hatschek (1928a) gives the historical development and description of these instruments. During measurement the time for the fluid to flow by gravity from one mark in a capillary column to the second mark is measured, and

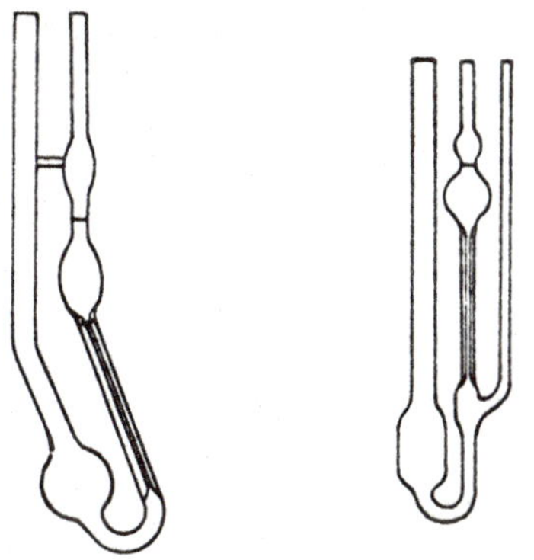

Cannon-Fenske. Ubbelohde.

FIG. 14. Capillary viscometers.

this value is substituted into an equation to obtain relative or absolute viscosity. Examples of the calculations are given by Martin (1960a). The magnitude of the kinetic energy correction necessary for highly accurate work is discussed by Cannon and co-workers (1960).

Viscometers with capillaries of varying diameters are commercially available for the measurement of fluids over a wide range of viscosity. The simplest viscometer of the capillary type was used by Ostwald. Other viscometers of this type are the Cannon-Fenske and the Ubbelohde which are shown in Fig. 14.

2. *Efflux Rheometers*

In the efflux instrument, the time for a specified volume of sample to flow out of a reservoir of varying sized orifices is measured. The head is continually changing as the liquid is discharged, thus changing the rate of shear through the orifice. One of the most popular instruments of this type is the Saybolt viscometer. The Engler, Scott and the Ford Cup are variations of the Saybolt viscometer. These viscometers are useful for simple comparison among Newtonian fluids and are used most extensively in the petroleum industry.

The Zahn cup is another type of efflux viscometer. Several different size orifices are available for different viscosity ranges. The cup shown in Fig. 15 is dipped into the fluid to fill it, the cup is removed, and the time for the column of fluid to flow from the orifice is measured. The viscosity obtained this way is for comparative purposes, as there is no general formula to convert the Zahn reading to other units. This is so because different materials with the same absolute viscosity do not have the same

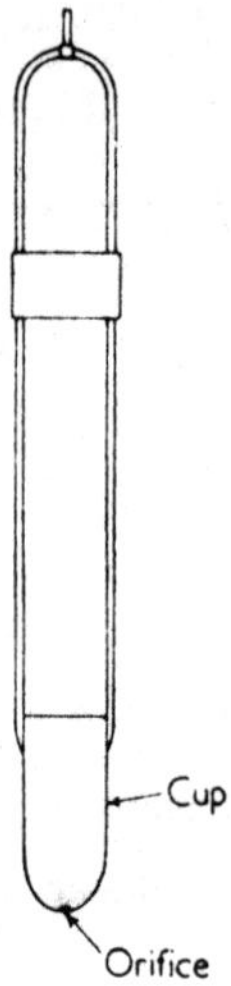

FIG. 15. Zahn cup viscometer.

flow characteristics with respect to the surface of the cup. Any conversion curves which are made will apply only to the specific liquid used.

3. *Extrusion Rheometers*

a. *Capillary extrusion.* Moness and Giesy (1926) early applied the science of rheology to the area of pharmacy. They designed a capillary apparatus in which various pressures were applied by means of a column of mercury to a reservoir filled with the sample to be tested. The degree of movement of the sample produced by the applied pressure was measured in a capillary tube. Buckingham's equation for plastic flow was used to obtain results in absolute units.

b. *Extrusion rheometer.* In the Burrell-Severs rheometer, samples are extruded through an orifice under various pressures into tared containers, and the rate of flow is calculated from the weight and the elapsed time of each extrusion. By substitution of these values into appropriate equations, the shear stress, rate of shear and viscosity can be calculated. A series of Burrell-Severs extrusion rheometers is available for measurement over a wide range of viscosity at low and high rates of shear.

Wood *et al.* (1962) modified an extrusion rheometer so that collapsible tubes containing thixotropic material could be used. The nozzle of the tube is screwed into an adapter plate. The sealed end of the tube is cut and the tube with adapter is assembled into the rheometer above the capillary

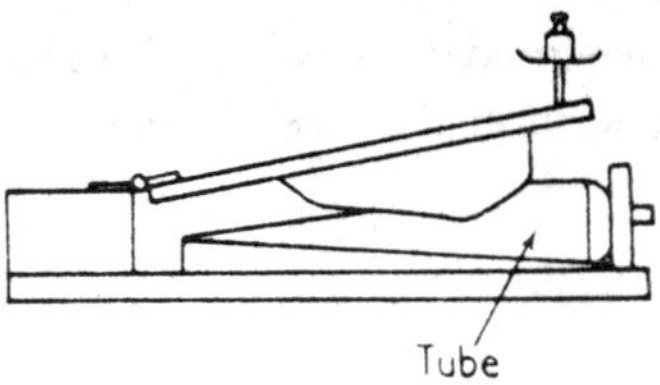

Fig. 16. Tube extrusion apparatus (Fiero).

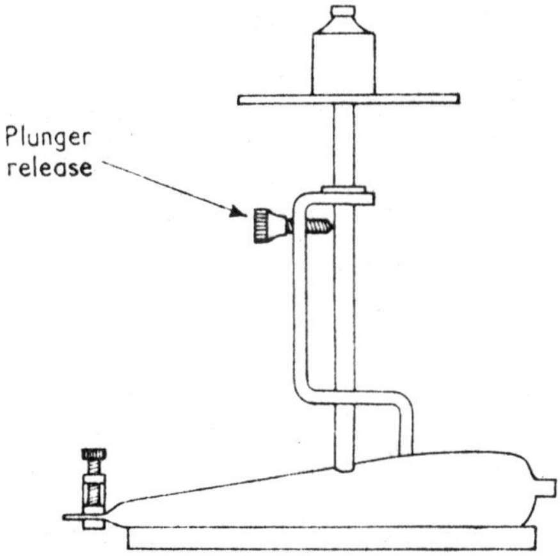

Fig. 17. Tube extrusion apparatus (Mutimer).

plate. The sample is extruded from the tube by the usual procedures. An advantage of measurement using this method is that the sample remains literally "undisturbed" before making the measurement. This is important in thixotropic materials, because the previous history of the sample affects the measurement. Using this extrusion instrument, comparisons among products can be made regarding the effect of filling under various shearing stress, upon storage under various conditions, and extrusion under different pressures. Two kinds of tube extrusion apparatus are shown in Fig. 16 (Fiero, 1940) and Fig. 17 (Mutimer *et al.*, 1956).

B. PARALLEL PLATE INSTRUMENTS

Parallel plate viscometers are used in testing very viscous substances. There are several ways in which the measurements can be conducted such as by pulling the plates apart, sliding the plates apart, compressing the plates, and rotating one plate relative to another. A description of these techniques follows.

1. *Tackmeter*

The instrument is designed to analyse the rheological factors which contribute to tack. Tack, or stickiness, is very important in the printing

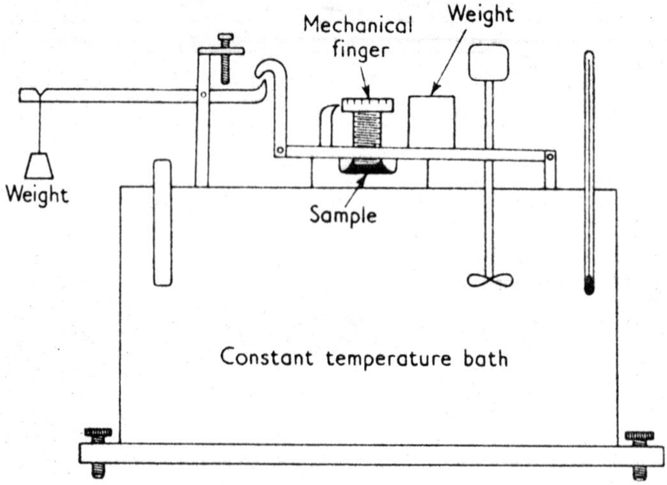

FIG. 18. Tackmeter.

industry and is usually measured by rubbing a drop of ink with a finger into a thin layer on glass or paper. The finger is then pressed firmly into the ink and quickly withdrawn. The resistance to pull can be felt. If the pull resistance is great, the tack is considered to be large; if the pull resistance is small, the tack is slight.

The tackmeter (Green, 1941) measures pull resistance by the following procedure. A mechanical finger, seen in Fig. 18, is pressed down on the sample on the plate. The thickness of the film is adjusted by the micrometer head. Weights are added to the lever arm connected to the mechanical finger, and the time for the lever to rise and touch the set screw is recorded. As the finger is raised, the material flows between the finger and the plate. The rate of flow is proportional to the reciprocal of time. By using various weights and recording the time for the end point, a consistency curve can be obtained by plotting weight against $1/t$ where t is the time. Knowing the film thickness, the radius of the finger, the weight and time, an empirical equation can be deduced from which viscosity and a function of the yield can be obtained.

2. *Sliding Plate Apparatus*

Havemeyer (1956) designed a sliding box apparatus, shown in Fig. 19, for measuring spreadability. The ointment is placed in a plastic box which has a narrow slit on the bottom and is covered with a lid. A piece

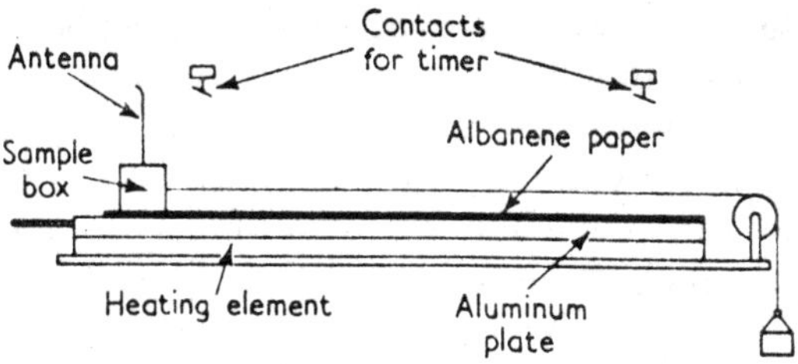

FIG. 19. Sliding box apparatus for measuring spreadability.

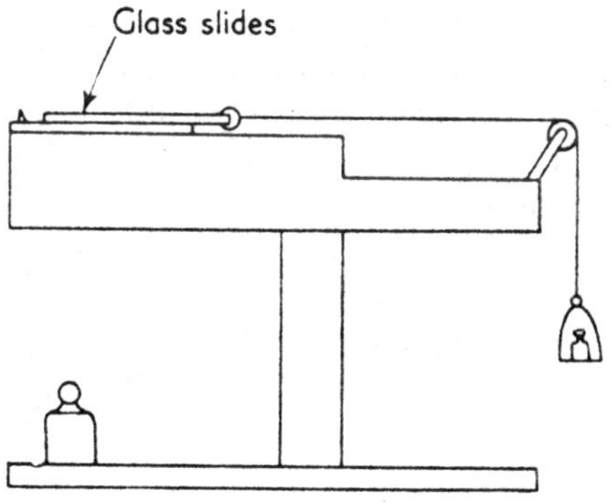

FIG. 20. Sliding plate apparatus for measuring spreadability.

of lead the size of the lid is then placed on top of the lid so that a downward pressure is exerted on the sample under test. The box is pulled across a sheet of albanene paper (non-absorbent smooth paper) on a temperature controlled plate by means of a pulley system. Weights are added to the pulley to increase the driving force. During measurement the antenna on the moving box makes contact with the first switch and activates an electric timer. The timer is turned off as the antenna contacts the second switch. The time interval for the sample to pass two reference points is thus measured automatically. A consistency curve can be made by plotting weights against time.

Mutimer *et al.* (1956) measured spreadability of ointments with the apparatus shown in Fig. 20. An excess of ointment is placed between two glass slides and a 1000-g weight is placed on the slides for 5 min to compress the sample to a uniform thickness. The bottom slide is anchored to the apparatus, and weights (80 g) are placed in the pan. The time in seconds needed to separate the two slides is taken as a measure of spreadability. A shorter time interval indicates better spreadability.

3. *Plate Plastometers*

Plate plastometers (Houwink and Heinze, 1938; Williams, 1924) are instruments used for testing synthetic resins or rubber. The sample is compressed by means of weights between two parallel plates. The height of the sample is noted after compression under specified conditions of temperature, time, weights, and sample size. Simple comparisons between samples can be made in this way, or the results can be substituted into empirical equations and related to viscosity.

4. *Rotating Plate Instruments*

The shearing disc viscometer (Mooney, 1934) is designed to measure unvulcanized rubber. The rotating plate is located in a stator, and the sample is placed on both sides of the rotating disc and compressed so that there is a firm contact between the disc and stator. The sample is heated to 100° C and sheared by the rotating disc at very low speeds. The torque exerted by the sample is measured and can be converted to viscosity units.

The cone-plate type instrument also appears to be essentially a parallel plate apparatus due to the very slight angle of the cone in relation to the plate, but it will be discussed under rotational instruments rather than here.

C. FALLING AND RISING BODY APPARATUS

1. *Rolling Sphere Viscometer*

The Hoeppler viscometer, a rolling ball instrument, is shown in Fig. 21. The viscometer uses a short, nearly vertical glass tube of large diameter and a closely fitting ball of either steel or glass. A wider range of viscosities can be measured with this instrument than with the falling sphere apparatus described in British Standard 188: 1957, where the sphere is small in proportion to the bore of the tube. The sample and a ball are loaded into the inner cylinder and brought to the temperature of measurement by means of the constant-temperature outer jacket. The locking pin is released and the apparatus inverted to place the ball in the initial starting position. The time for the ball to traverse the distance between two marks is measured. A minimum falling time of 30 sec is used for best results.

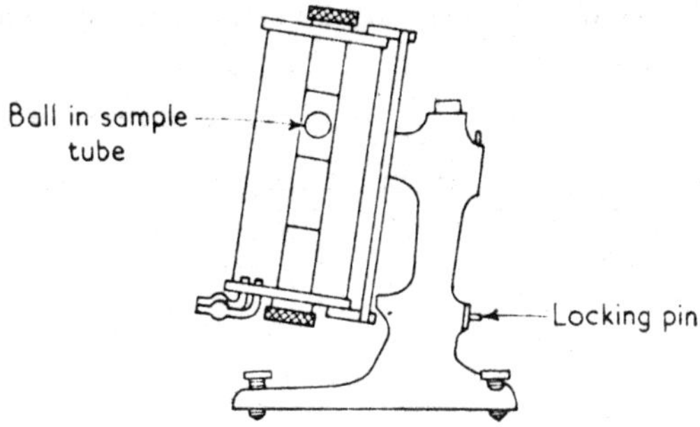

FIG. 21. Hoeppler precision viscometer.

The viscosity in centipoises is given by the following equation:

$$\eta = t \times (S_b - S_f) \times B \tag{28}$$

where η is the viscosity, t is the time interval in seconds for the ball to pass between two points, S_b is the specific gravity of the ball, S_f is the specific gravity of the fluid at the temperature of measurement, and B is the ball constant. Kinematic viscosity in centistokes, the unit used in the petroleum industry, can be obtained by dividing the viscosity in centipoises by the specific gravity. This viscometer is useful for Newtonian fluids.

Balls with different diameters, different specific gravity, and different ball constants are used to give a range of viscosities from 0·5 to over 200,000 poises. Glass balls are used for less viscous materials and metal balls for more viscous bodies. For highly viscous fluids a tungsten ball is used. The ball constants can be obtained by measurement of a standard of known viscosity and specific gravity, placing these values in equation (28), and solving for the ball constant, B.

2. *Rising Sphere Rheometer*

McVean and Mattocks (1961) designed a rising sphere instrument which appears to have promise as a tool for the study of yield value. This instrument is shown in Fig. 22. A 1·9-cm diameter stainless-steel sphere connected to a strain gauge via a platinum-rhodium wire is lifted through the material under test at a very slow rate by a motor driven arm. The shearing stress caused by the strain in the gel structure is recorded continuously. Stokes' equation for a falling sphere is used in calculating the rate of shear or rate of strain. Eight different rates of strain are possible with this instrument.

Only substances possessing structure showed shearing stress with this instrument. This shearing stress may be considered to be due only to the

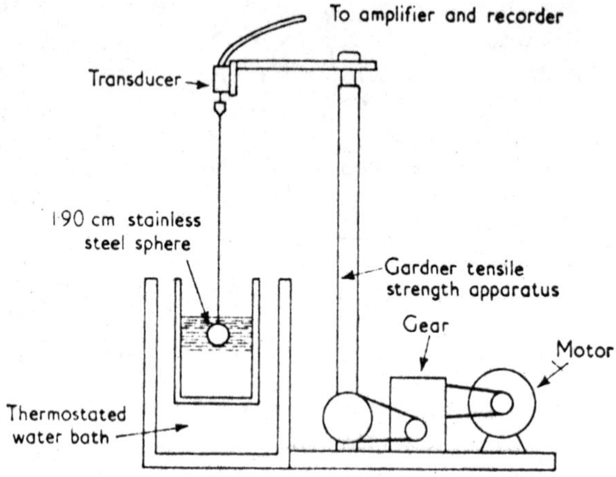

FIG. 22. Rising sphere rheometer.

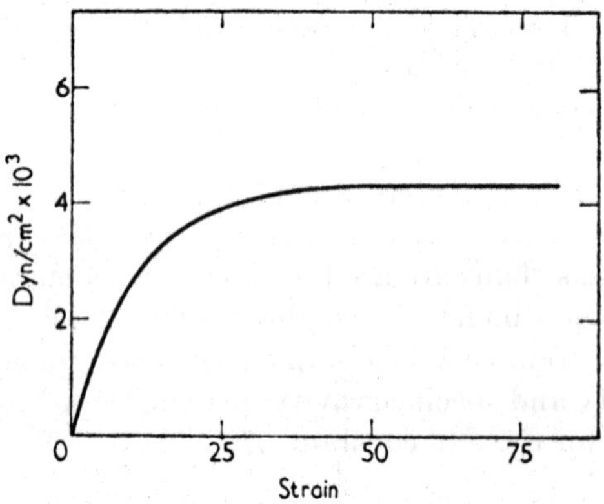

FIG. 23. Typical upcurve with the rising sphere rheometer. Flow starts at the horizontal portion of the curve.

gel structure and not to viscous flow, since no measurement is recorded when glycerin or syrup is used. An example of a typical curve of a substance which has yield value is shown in Fig. 23. Calculation and examples of measurement of yield value and structural relaxation are given for several substances in the original article.

3. *Penetrometer*

The penetrometer has been used for measuring relative hardness of materials such as petrolatum, lubricating greases, wax, and asphalt. Penetration is defined as the consistency of a material expressed as the distance that a standard cone or needle penetrates a sample under known conditions of loading, time and temperature. Penetration tests are usually made at 25° C for 5 sec. The unit of penetration is expressed in

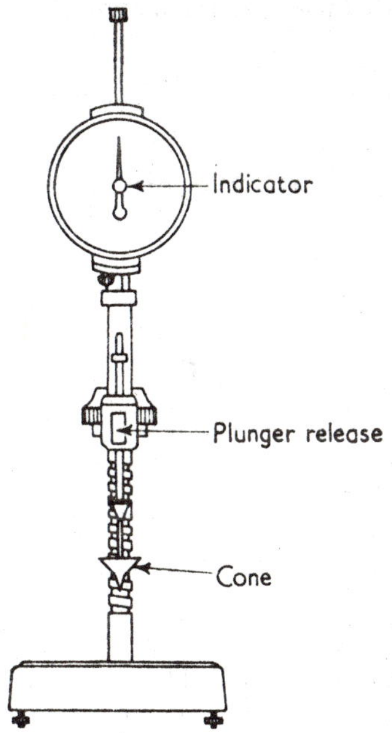

FIG. 24. Universal penetrometer.

tenths of a millimeter. The container sizes are also specified as follows: A 3-oz jar, 55 mm (2·17 in) in diameter and 35 mm (1·38 in) in depth, should be used for penetrations of 200 and less. For penetrations over 200, a 6-oz jar with dimensions of 70 mm (2·75 in) in diameter and a depth of 45 mm (1·77 in) should be used (ASTM Designation D5-61).

a. *Universal penetrometer.* A Universal penetrometer is shown in Fig. 24. Other American Society for Testing Materials (ASTM Standards, 1961) penetrometers differ slightly in design but operate on the same principle. The apparatus is shown with a double cone of 30 and 90°. To make a measurement the jar is placed in position with the apex of the cone resting on the surface of the sample. The plunger is released for

5 sec allowing the cone to penetrate into the sample. The penetration, in tenths of a millimeter, is read off from the indicator scale. An automatic timer with a pre-set 5-sec cycle cam and a reset switch for zero start can be attached to this instrument to reduce operator error in timing.

b. *Miniature penetrometer.* This apparatus (Kaufman *et al.*, 1939), shown in Fig. 25, is designed for small samples of 3 to 5 g. A split cylinder is used to hold the sample. Each half is loaded separately, and then brought together, thus preventing entrainment of air. The modified cylinder, cone and plunger is used in the ordinary ASTM penetrometer. Weights can be added to the apparatus when harder greases are being tested.

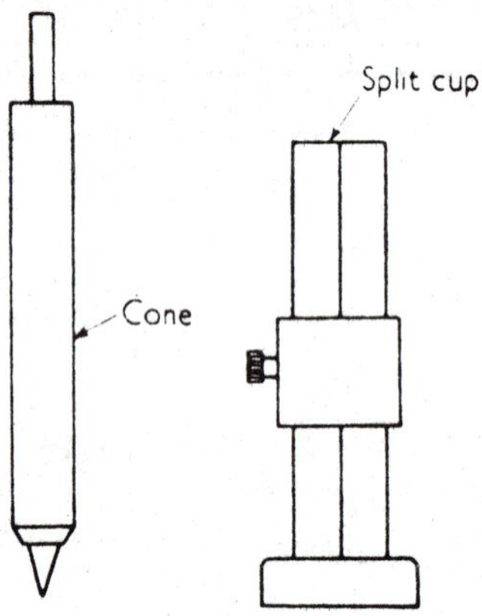

FIG. 25. The cone and cup for the miniature penetrometer.

c. *Tapered hole disc penetrometer.* The tapered hole disc penetrometer (Birdsall and Hooten, 1952) is designed for product control of the consistency of semi-fluid greases. These soft greases are non-Newtonian with a fragile structure so that the measurements must be made at low rates of shear if the consistency of the thickened oil rather than the viscosity of the base oil is to be measured. The disc is $\frac{1}{2}$ in in thickness and $2\frac{3}{4}$ in in diameter and has nine tapered holes. The disc is used with the penetrometer.

4. *Mobilometer*

The Gardner Mobilometer is a falling plunger apparatus which is used to determine consistency of fluid and semi-fluid materials. The apparatus consists of a cylinder which is attached to a base plate, a plunger and plunger support and a weight pan. In making a measurement the cylinder is filled with sample. The disc end of the plunger is placed in the cylinder, and the plunger rod is connected to the bracket. When the plunger is released, the time for two marks 10 cm apart on the plunger rod to pass a reference point is measured. Additional weights can be placed on the plunger, and the results can be recorded as a load-time curve.

D. ROTATIONAL INSTRUMENTS

There are many rotational instruments available commercially. The measuring unit of some of the instruments are supplied with prongs, paddles, vanes and discs, and the geometry of such systems are difficult to describe. Hence these viscometers cannot be used to obtain rheological data in absolute units for non-Newtonian systems. For absolute measurements, the annular space between the rotating and stationary portions must be small to allow the flow to be laminar; and the measuring system must be geometrically describable, since the equations for non-Newtonian flow are based on these dimensions as discussed earlier in the chapter.

The differences among the various rotational instruments are in the measuring and sensing system, rotation of the bob, cup or cone, recording of the rheogram, measuring range, temperature control, ease of operation, ease of data reduction, portability and cost. It is desirable to have the instrument designed so that the speeds of the rotating elements can be changed without interruption, and the resulting rheogram plotted automatically. This is important in the measurement of thixotropic materials, as structural build-up can take place in a short interval of time. There should also be efficient temperature regulation to prevent temperature rise due to frictional heating.

1. *Cone Plate Viscometer*

The Ferranti-Shirley viscometer (McKennel, 1954), a sketch of which is shown in Fig. 26, is a cone-plate instrument suitable for measurement of both Newtonian and non-Newtonian flow. The indicator unit and speed control amplifier are not shown in the figure. To make a measurement, a sample is placed on the plate which is then raised until it contacts the cone. The cone is driven by a variable-speed motor, and the sample between the rotating cone and stationary plate is sheared. The revolutions per minute or rate of shear is increased and decreased continuously by a speed selector. The resulting torque or shearing stress caused by the viscous traction on the cone is transferred to an electromechanical dynamometer and displayed on the indicator unit. The cone speed can be operated manually, and the torque readings for each speed written down at the time it is obtained; or the apparatus can be instrumented so that the speed is programmed and the resulting rheograms are automatically plotted on an x–y recorder.

The viscosity of a Newtonian fluid in poises as measured in this viscometer can be calculated by the equation:

$$\eta = C\frac{T}{v} \tag{29}$$

where η is the viscosity in poises, C is an instrument constant, T is the torque or meter reading and v is the cone speed in revolutions per minute.

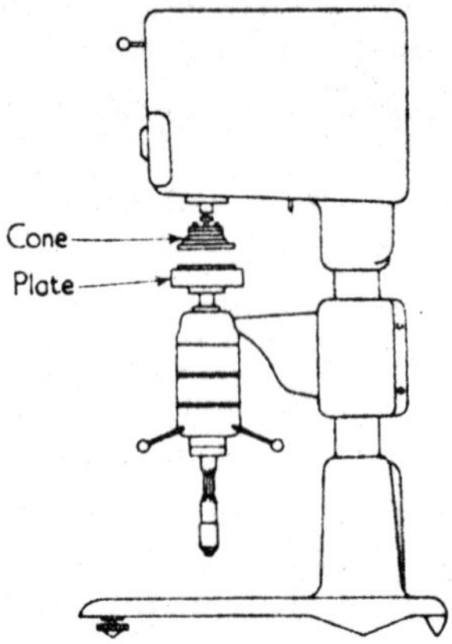

FIG. 26. The measuring unit of the Ferranti-Shirley cone-plate viscometer.

For Bingham bodies, the plastic viscosity U can be found by using the equation:

$$U = C\frac{T - T_f}{v} \tag{30}$$

where T is the meter reading at v r.p.m. and T_f is the torque where the extrapolated linear portion of the curve crosses the shearing stress axis. The yield value f is given by the expression:

$$f = C_f \times T_f \tag{31}$$

where C_f is an instrument constant.

A temperature bath is installed underneath the plate with thermocouples in contact with the sample. Since the sample size is small (less than 1 g), temperature equilibrium is quickly reached.

The cone is designed so that there is uniform shearing throughout the sample. The angle of the cone is also very small so that edge effects are negligible. A wide range of rate of shear is possible with this instrument by combinations of different cones and two speed ranges. The standard cones are suitable for suspensions provided that the particle size does not exceed about 30 μ.

2. *The Stormer Viscometer*

The Stormer viscometer is an instrument in which the bob rotates and the cup is stationary. Relative viscosities can be obtained by comparing the revolutions per minute with one fluid in regard to a standard fluid using the same driving weights and temperature.

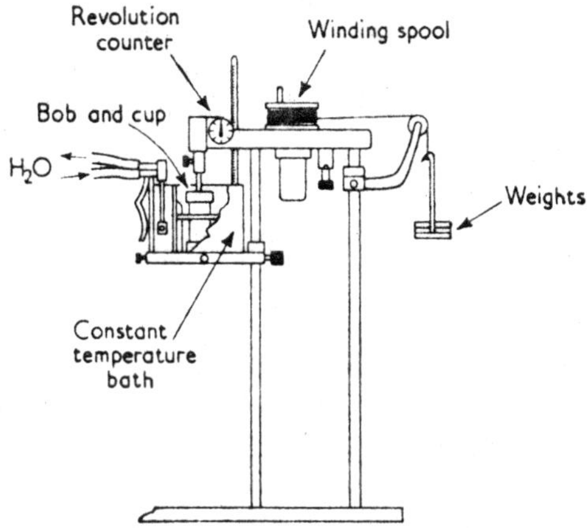

FIG. 27. Modified Stormer viscometer.

The Stormer viscometer as ordinarily supplied is not suitable for measurement of non-Newtonian systems; however, it can be used to obtain fundamental rheological properties such as yield value, plastic viscosity, and thixotropic index when modified by using a bob and cup of known dimensions, and a weight hanger to which various weights can be added or removed. The modified instrument is shown in Fig. 27.

The method of obtaining a consistency curve is as follows. Upcurves are made by placing weights on the weight hanger in increasing amounts. The least amount of weight causing the bob to rotate is used as the starting shearing stress. The weight is released and the time for the bob to rotate 100 revolutions is measured and converted to r.p.m. The cord is rewound on the drum, additional weights are added, and the procedure is repeated until a predetermined speed is reached. The downcurve is then started by repeating the procedure for the upcurve except that weights are now successively removed. Typical curves for Newtonian and non-Newtonian materials, obtained with the Stormer viscometer, are found in Figs. 1, 3, 4, 5 and 7.

To transpose the measurements to absolute units, the revolutions per minute and the driving weights can be converted to the rate of shear in reciprocal seconds and shearing stress in dynes per square centimeter respectively by multiplication by appropriate factors. The means of obtaining these factors are discussed by Fischer (1948) and Martin (1960).

The modified Stormer instrument is very useful for obtaining fundamental rheological data, but is time consuming compared to other methods in which part of the process is automated. Also there is a difficulty in obtaining the same top rate of shear for samples since the r.p.m. is controlled by the driving weights, and it is difficult to predict the exact weight needed to give a particular speed for non-Newtonians. Thus the top rate of shear must be obtained through trial and error. Also there is a lapse of time between measurements as the weights are added and removed, and this may be a disadvantage in the analysis of thixotropic materials.

3. *Rotovisko Viscometer*

The Rotovisko is a rotating viscometer in which either bob and cup or cone and plate attachments can be used. The rotor rotates at various rates and the torque created by the viscous drag of the fluid is measured by a torsion dynamometer. The measurement is read off the control panel or can be recorded.

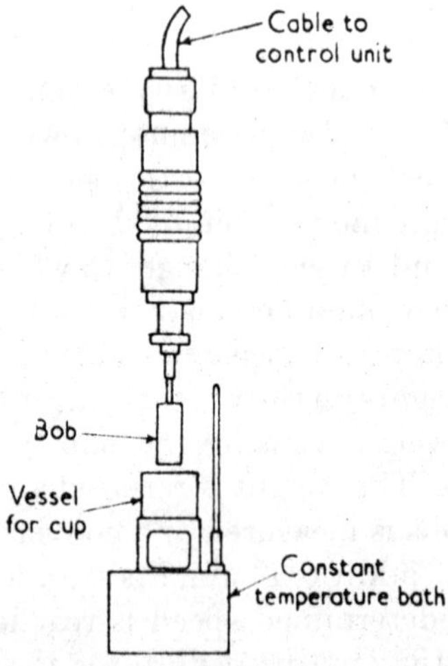

FIG. 28. The measuring unit of the Rotovisko viscometer.

A synchronous motor connected to a gearbox provides ten speeds from 3 to 486 r.p.m. By use of interchangeable gears, the speed can be reduced by a factor of 10 or 100. Thus a total of thirty speeds from 0·03 to 486 r.p.m. is possible with this instrument. The speeds can be changed without stopping the instrument.

The Rotovisko, Fig. 28, is suitable for many applications as there are six different measuring systems available. A wide range of viscosity can be measured with this instrument by interchanging bobs and cups, cone and plates, gears and torsion springs in the measuring head. A shear stress range of 10 to 10^6 dyn/cm^2 and a rate of shear of 10^{-2} to 10^4 sec^{-1} are possible. The sample varies from less than 1 ml for the cone-plate attachment to about 70 ml for one of the larger attachments.

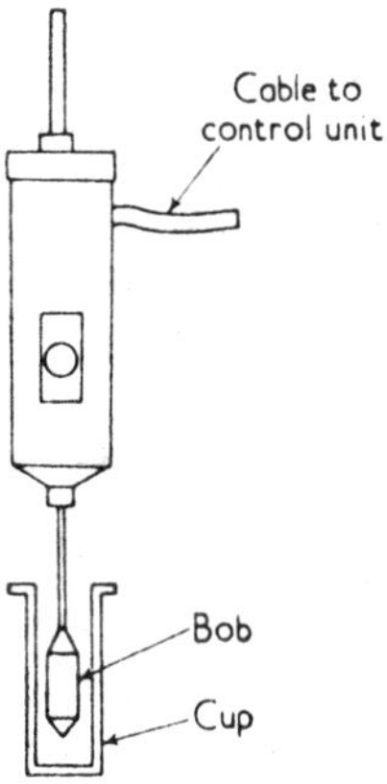

FIG. 29. The measuring unit of the Epprecht viscometer.

4. *Epprecht*

The Epprecht rotational viscometers are Swiss made, and are available in several models. The Rheomat-15, Fig. 29, is suitable for measurement of both Newtonian and non-Newtonian materials and operates at fifteen speeds which are manually selected. The bob is rotated in a cup and the torque exerted by the sample can be seen on the visual readout or can be recorded. The range of shear is 1 to 2000 sec^{-1} and the shearing force is from 2 to 200,000 dyn/cm^2. This range is obtained by a combination of bobs and cups, and the addition of reduction sleeves to the cup to change the annular space.

5. *Hercules High Shear Viscometer*

The Hercules High Shear Viscometer, a bob and cup instrument, is shown in Fig. 30. The recording drum is driven so that 1 cm of graph paper is equivalent to 50 r.p.m. of the bob. The springs are calibrated to give a deflection of 1 cm per 100,000 dyn cm of torque. Other torque springs are available which increase the sensitivity of the instrument.

In making a measurement, the bob is lowered into the cup and the starting position on the graph paper on the recording drum is marked with the pen which is attached to the cord connected to the springs. The speed control wheel is turned manually to increase the r.p.m. As the bob rotates, the viscous drag caused by the sample on the cup is transferred to the torque spring and recorded on the drum. When a predetermined upper r.p.m. is reached, the wheel is reversed and returned to the starting position to complete the rheogram in a very short period of time. The

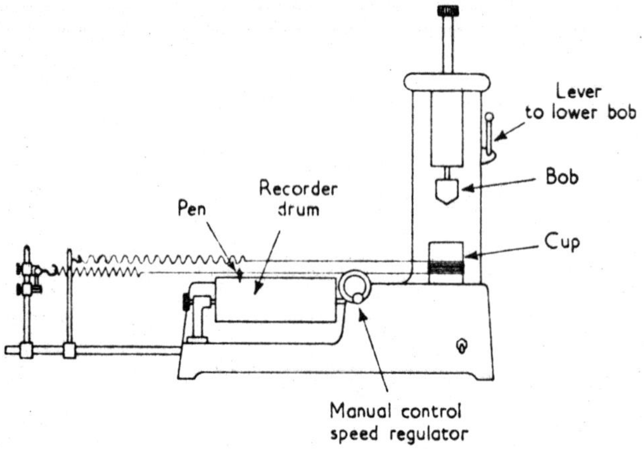

FIG. 30. Hercules high shear viscometer.

results are converted to absolute units by multiplying by the instrument constants.

Four bobs are supplied with this instrument. Three of the bobs have the same radius (1·95 cm) differing only in their heights and thus their end effects. The fourth bob is of a smaller radius (1·5 cm). The clearance between the large bobs and cup is 0·05 cm and for the small bob 0·5 cm. Due to the design of the instrument, there are no provisions for temperature control.

6. *MacMichael Viscometer*

The MacMichael viscometer is a rotating cup instrument. One end of a calibrated torsion wire is connected to the top of the instrument and the other end to a spindle as shown in Fig. 31. A plunger is connected to the spindle and suspended in the sample. As the cup rotates, the viscous drag on the plunger imparted by the sample causes the wire to twist. The amount of deflection is measured on a calibrated disc attached to the spindle. The disc is divided into 300 equal units and is referred to as MacMichael degrees. These units can be converted to absolute units by standardizing the instrument against fluids of known viscosities or by using wires with various torque constants.

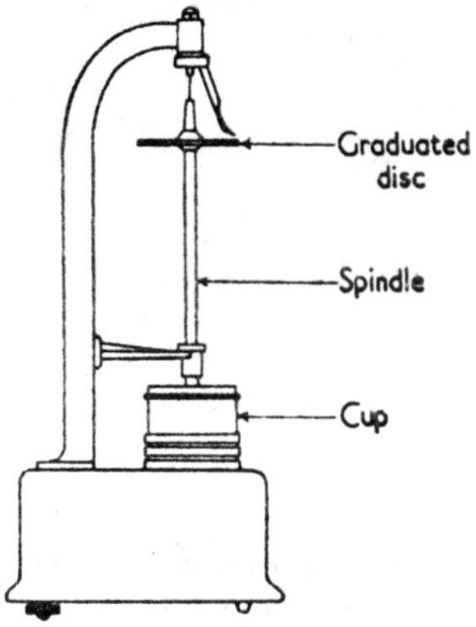

FIG. 31. MacMichael viscometer.

A wide range of viscosities can be covered with this instrument by interchange of torsion wires of different torque, and the use of different cups and plungers, and various speeds; however, it is not well suited for the analysis of non-Newtonian materials.

7. *Interchemical Viscometer*

The Interchemical viscometer (Green, 1942) is a Couette type instrument. The bob is suspended from a torsion wire attached to the instrument, and the cup is driven by a variable-speed transmission. During measurement the viscous drag of the sample on the bob produces a torque which can be read as degrees on a scale disc as in the MacMichael viscometer, and the torque for the particular speed is recorded.

The consistency curve is constructed by plotting the torque against the increasing speeds for the upcurve and the decreasing speeds for the downcurve. The instrument is useful for measuring both Newtonian and non-Newtonian substances.

The modified viscometer of Samyn and Mattocks (1957) is shown in Fig. 32. The design of the speed control unit allows it to be operated either manually or automatically. The torque wire is replaced by a strain gauge which is connected to a recorder so that rheograms can be continuously recorded. Combinations of bobs and lever arms are used to extend the range of measurement using a single strain gauge, and other strain gauges can also be used.

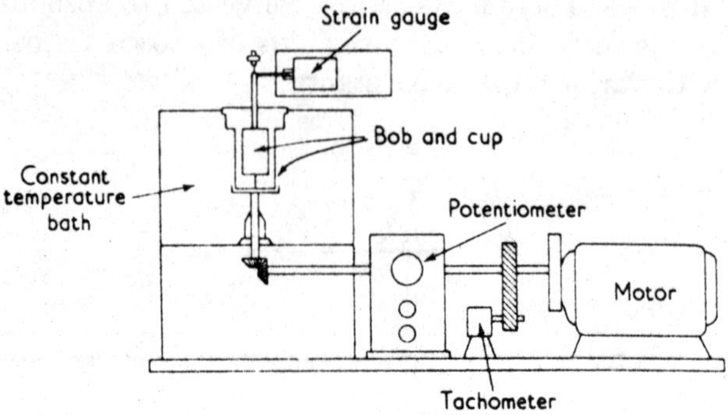

FIG. 32. Modified Interchemical viscometer.

8. *Low Shear Viscometer (Squibb)*

The Squibb viscometer (Myers and Zettlemoyer, 1955) was designed for structural studies of dispersions at low shears, since at moderate and higher shear rates much of the structure of pharmaceutical dispersions is broken down.

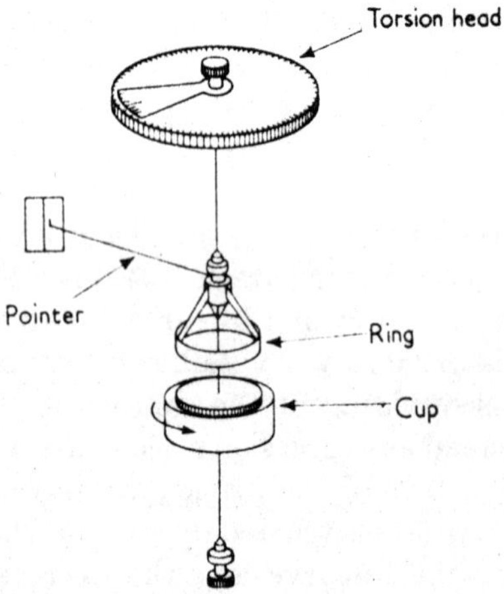

FIG. 33. Low shear (Squibb) viscometer.

This is a rotational type viscometer in which a ring is suspended in a cup as shown in Fig. 33. The ring is attached to the midpoint of a calibrated wire, the top end of which is connected to a torsion head and the lower end anchored to the instrument. The stainless-steel ring suspended on the wire can be rotated or oscillated without friction since the only attachment is on the wire.

The double-walled cup is rotated by a variable-speed d.c. motor. The tangential force acting on the ring is calculated by use of the instrument constants and the angle which the torsion head vernier must be turned to bring the pointer back to the zero mark.

Cups of various dimensions and wires with different torsion constants can be used to cover a wide range of viscosity. Viscosities of 0·01 to 200 poises have been studied at rates of shear of 1 to 100 sec^{-1} and higher.

The long torque arm and the shearing action on both sides of the ring increases the sensitivity of the instrument. End effects are negligible as they occur only at the edge of the ring. In conventional rotational viscometers, end effects are operative over the entire cross-section of the bob and must be taken into account.

9. *Brookfield Synchro-lectric Viscometer*

The Brookfield viscometer is a rotating spindle instrument in which the spindle is rotated by a synchronous motor through gears and a calibrated beryllium-copper spring. As the motor rotates the viscous drag of the sample on the spindle is shown as a deflection on the dial. When analysing Newtonian fluids, the dial readings for each combination of spindle and speed can be converted to absolute units by the use of certain constants furnished by the manufacturer.

Figure 34 shows the Brookfield viscometer with the bar-type spindle attachment. The attachment or coupling is used to ensure that the spindle is kept vertical as it goes through the material. The bar-type spindle and a suitable model of the viscometer is used in conjunction with the Helipath stand for the measurement of viscous materials such as gels, printing ink, toothpastes, shaving cream, etc. The viscometer is placed on the Helipath stand and the viscometer with the spindle is lowered into the sample by a chain driven by a synchronous motor in the base of the unit. The path traced by the spindle is a helix, and readings on the dial can be made as the spindle continues to rotate in new material. These readings can only be expressed in relative units.

The ordinary Brookfield viscometer has been used for measuring viscosities of Newtonian and non-Newtonian fluids. However, in the case of non-Newtonian materials, the results are only of comparative value, and the conditions of the test such as the speed, the spindle, and the temperature should be indicated.

Wood *et al.* (1960) have modified the Brookfield LVT and RVT viscometers, by use of a bob and cup system, into an absolute rheometer which can measure non-Newtonian flow. A low shear range of 0·1 to 15 sec^{-1} was possible with this modified instrument.

The models of the Brookfield viscometer are designated by letters such as LVF, LVT, RVF, RVT, HAT, and HBT. The first two letters indicate the spring tension and spindles and the last letter the speeds. The F series have four speeds and the T series eight speeds. The LV series are used for low viscosity work, RV are used for medium viscosities such as gums, food products and paints, and the HA and HB series are used for high viscosity materials such as tars and asphalt.

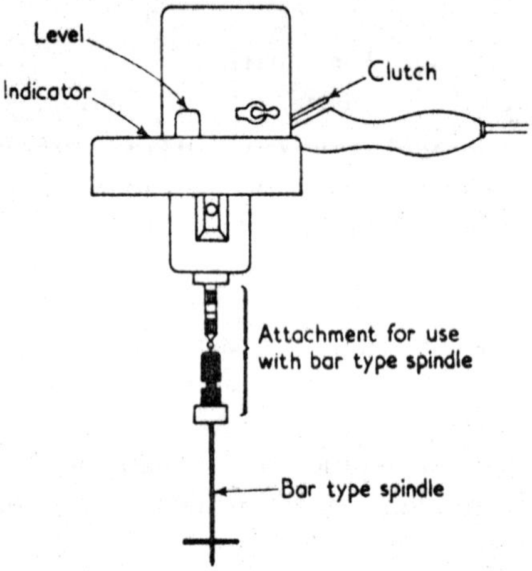

FIG. 34. Brookfield viscometer.

10. *Brabender Viscograph*

The Viscograph is an instrument in which a stainless-steel cup containing 400 to 450 ml of sample is rotated. The viscous traction imparted to a spindle or feeler with prongs is transferred to a highly sensitive balance system. The amount of deflection is continuously recorded. Preloading weights can be attached to the measuring system to extend the range.

This instrument allows for continuous measurement of viscosity under physical and chemical changes in the system. For example, viscosity can be measured as the temperature is continually being changed. The results of such changes due to various conditions can be used to estimate in advance what may be expected of a product during manufacture.

11. *Rheogoniometer*

The Rheogoniometer is a rotating cone and plate instrument in which rotational and oscillatory measurements can be made. In the rotational measurements, the viscous behaviour of the material under test, and any normal forces produced, are measured. The coefficient of viscosity and elastic modulus can be calculated from the values obtained. In the oscillatory measurements, the sample is oscillated about the vertical axis. The input strain and resultant stress is in phase for completely elastic substances and out of phase to different degrees for viscous and visco-elastic materials. This type of instrument represents a new principle of measurement in rheology.

E. INDUSTRIAL VISCOMETERS

A compilation (Bates, 1960) of various commercially available viscometers are listed in Table II. Data are given for the various instruments such as the viscosity range in centipoises or in other units; the units of measurement in arbitrary numbers, in time, torque, or directly in centipoises; the type of operation of the instrument, whether, for example, it is multipoint or single point, and whether or not measurements can be made continuously; and, finally, the major areas of application. The addresses of the suppliers are given at the end of the table.

III. APPLICATIONS AND PRACTICE

The applications of rheology are numerous and significant to the pharmaceutical scientist, whether he is engaged primarily as a product formulator, manufacturer, or physical scientist. Just as the flavour, odour and appearance of food affects a person's psychological response to food, so does the appearance and rheology of most fluid and semi-solid drug or cosmetic products affect the users' psychological response toward that product. Harper (1953) has termed these phenomena psychorheology, and treats in detail the important psychological responses of individuals to product consistency. In the pharmaceutical product not only may the product consistency be critical to its acceptance by the ultimate user, but the consistency and total rheology may be related to the therapeutic effectiveness and stability of the product. It is the responsibility of the product formulator to achieve product rheology best meeting the demands of the user while achieving maximum stability and greatest therapeutic effectiveness. The responsibility of the manufacturing pharmacist is then to retain these rheological properties under the conditions of scale-up and large-scale manufacture.

A. INTRODUCTION

Some of the notable areas in which rheology is pharmaceutically significant are listed below, together with the factors which may be affected by rheology. Unusual or exceptional effects are not included.

TABLE II[a]

Industrial Viscometers: Types, Ranges and Applications

	Viscometer	*Viscosity range (centipoises)*[b]	*Viscosity*[c] *units*	*Multi-shear*[d]	*Batch*	*Contin-uous*	*Major area of application*
Capillary (Time)	Atlantic	0·6 to 5000	Seconds		X		Petroleum products
	Cannon-Fenske	0·3 to 20,000	Seconds		X		Petroleum products
	Fitz Simons	0·6 to 5000	Seconds		X		Petroleum products
	Hellige	0 to 28	Relative		X		Blood, plasma
	Ostwald	0·4 to 16,000	Seconds		X		Petroleum products
	Ostwald-Fenske	0·4 to 16,000	Seconds		X		Petroleum products
	Ubbelohde	2 to 10,000	Seconds		X		Petroleum products
Orifice (Time)	Barbey (Fr.)	1 to 4000	cc/h		X		Petroleum products
	Demmler	4 to 20,000	Seconds		X		Varnish
	Engler (Ger.)	1 to 1500	Sec/200 cc or relative deg[e]		X		Tar, petroleum products
	Ford cup	1 to 1200	Seconds		X		Paint, varnish
	Gardner One-Shot	—[f]	Seconds		X		Paint, varnish
	Marsh Funnel	—[f]	Sec/946 cc		X		Drilling mud
	Redwood (Eng.)	1 to 5000	Sec/50 cc		X		Petroleum products
	Saybolt	1 to 4000	Sec/60 cc		X		Petroleum products
	Scott	—[f]	Sec/50 cc		X		Oils, varnish, glue
	Zahn	20 to 1200	Seconds		X		Varnish, lacquer
Capillary (Pressure)	Apex pressure	100 to 6×10^6	Lb/in^2, seconds	X	X		Grease
	Cox	0·5 to 30	Centistokes		X		—
	Hallikainen-Shell	—[f]	—			X	Petroleum products, refinery
	Instron[h]	—[f]	Lb/in^2, seconds	X	X	X	Polymers
	McKee Consistometer	100 to 6×10^6	Pressure drop	X	X		Rubber, greases
	Severs Extrusion	1 to 10^7	Lb/in^2, seconds	X	X		Plastisols, polymers

Falling Ball (Velocity)	Gerin Comparator	—[f]	Relative		X		Engine oil
	Hoeppler	0·01 to 10^6	Seconds		X		Gases, petroleum products
	Ruska Pressure	—[f]	Seconds		X		High pressure (to 12,000 lb/in^2)
	Visgage	40 to 450	Saybolt U sec		X		Lube oil
Rising bubble (Velocity)	ASTM Timer Tube	400 to 100,000	Seconds		X		Paint, varnish, lacquer
	Gardner Bubble	50 to 106,000	Relative		X		Varnish, oils, resins
	Gardner Vertical	1000 to 200,000	Stokes		X		Oils
	Inter-Chemical	60 to 15,000	Stokes		X		Oils
Piston (Velocity)	Gardner Mobilo-meter	— to ASTM 360[e]	Seconds		X		Pastes, greases
	Norcross	0·2 to 10^6	Centipoises			X	Solvent, starch, petroleum products
	SIL Mobilometer	65 to ASTM 380[e]	Arbitrary number		X		Oils, greases
Float Position	F and P Viscorator	0·5 to 550	Saybolt U sec			X	Petroleum products, food
Disk or Paddle (Torque)	Brabender Visco-graph	1 to 20,000	Centipoises		X		Food, coatings, paint
	Brookfield Synchro-lectric	0 to $1{\cdot}6 \times 10^8$	Centipoises	X	X		General
	Brookfield Visco-metran	0 to 10,000	Centipoises			X	Starch cooking, paper coatings, food
	Hallikainen Dow	— to 500,000	—			X	Polymers
	MacMichael	50 to 300,000	Arbitrary deg.	X	X		General
	Mooney Plastometer	—to 10^8	Deflection		X		Rubber
	Precision	100 to 250,000	—	X	X		Greases, paints, plastics
	Stormer (also cyl.)	1 to 100,000	g/arb. r.p.m. or sec/arb. rev.	X	X		General

TABLE II[a]—*cont.*

	Viscometer	*Viscosity range (centipoises)*[b]	*Viscosity*[c] *units*	*Multi-shear*[d]	*Batch*	*Continuous*	*Major area of application*
Concentric Cylinders (Torque)	Baroid Rotary	5 to 269	Centipoises		X		Drilling mud, ceramic slips
	Corn Industries	—[f]	g-cm		X		Starch pastes
	Epprecht[h]	0·2 to 10^6	Centipoises	X	X		General
	Fann VG	1 to 300,000	Centipoises	X	X		Drilling mud, adhesives, ceramics
	Ferranti Portable	1 to 2×10^7	Centipoises	X	X		General
	Fisher Electro-viscometer	0 to 50,000	Centipoises		X		General
	Hagan High Shear	10 to 2000	Dyn-cm	X	X		Paper coatings, pigments
	Hercules High Shear[h]	200 to 60,000	Dyn-cm	X	X	X	Paper coatings, pharmaceuticals
	Polarad RV-2	— to 800	Volts	X	X		Polymers, low shear
	Rao Birefringence	1 to 100	—	X	X		Molecular studies
	Rotovisko	1 to 10^8	Centipoises	X	X	X	General
	Sherwin-Williams	—[f]	g	X	X		Paint brushability
Parallel Plates	Ferranti-Shirley	0 to 3×10^6	Arbitrary Scale	X	X	X	Starches, gums, ointments, suspensions
	Shell Sliding Plate	10^4 to 10^{13}	Microns	X	X		Asphalt
	Weissenberg Rheo-goniometer	0·5 to 10^{10}	Centipoises	X	X		Polymers, bitumen, visco-elastic materials

Vibrating Reed (Dampening Rate)	Bendix Ultra-Viscoson	0 to 50,000	Centipoises × g/cc		X	Coatings, Petroleum products, inks
	Ultrasonic Engr.	0 to 30,000	Centipoises × g/cc	X	X	Petroleum products, paint, food

[a] This table was adapted from Bates (1960). Most of the instruments listed are distributed by laboratory equipment suppliers. Only the suppliers of instruments not commonly found in general catalogues are listed. The addresses are as follows:

Hellige (Hellige, Inc., Garden City, N.Y.); Demmler (Westinghouse Electric); Marsh (Baroid Div., National Lead Co., Houston, Tex.); Zahn (General Electric, West Lynn, Mass.); Apex (Apex Scientific, Orinda, California); Cox (G. L. Nankervis Co., Detroit, Mich.); Hallikainen-Shell (Hallikainen Instruments, Berkeley, Calif.); Instron (Instron Engineering Corp., Canton, Mass.); Severs (Burrell Corp., Pittsburg, Pa.); Gerin (Gerin Corp., Avon, N.J.); Ruska (Ruska Instrument Corp., Houston, Tex.); Visgage (L. C. Eitzen, N.Y.C.); Gardner (Gardner Laboratories, Inc., Bethesda, Md.); Norcross (Norcross Corp., Newton, Mass.); Brabender (C. W. Brabender Instruments, Inc., Hackensack, N.J.); Brookfield (Brookfield Engineering Laboratories, Inc., Stoughton, Mass.); Corn Industries (Gaertner Scientific Corp., Chicago, Ill.); Epprecht, also Drage and Contraves (J. W. Fecker Div., American Optical Co., Pittsburg, Pa., Drage Products, Union City, N.J., and Contraves AG, Zurich, Switzerland); Hercules (Martinson Machine Co., Kalamazoo, Mich.); Rao (Rao Instrument Co., Brooklyn, N.Y.); Rotovisko (Brinkman Instruments Inc., Great Neck, L.I., N.Y.); Bendix (Bendix Corp., Cincinnati, Ohio); Ferranti-Shirley (Ferranti Ltd., Manchester, England); Weissenberg Rheogoniometer (Farol Research Engineers Ltd., Bognor Regis, England).

[b] In many cases, requires several sizes to achieve full range.

[c] Units are arbitrary in some cases and absolute in others.

[d] Indicates usefulness for non-Newtonian liquids.

[e] Cone penetration for semi-solids.

[f] — notation means data not available.

[g] Use of the term "relative" means the viscosity is stated as a ratio relative to a reference fluid.

[h] Added to original table.

1. Fluids
   a. Mixing.
   b. Particle size reduction of disperse systems with shear.
   c. Passage through orifices, including pouring, packaging in bottles, and passage through hypodermic needles.
   d. Fluid transfer, including pumping and flow through pipes.
   e. Physical stability of disperse systems.
2. Quasi-solids
   a. Spreading and adherence on the skin.
   b. Removal from jars or extrusion from tubes.
   c. Capacity to take up solids or miscible liquids.
   d. Release of the drug from the base.
3. Solids
   a. Flow of powders from hoppers and into die cavities in tabletting or into capsules during encapsulation.
   b. Packagability of powdered or granular solids.
4. Processing
   a. Production capacity of the equipment.
   b. Processing efficiency.

Flow properties of fluids and semi-solids, and in particular the flow properties of disperse systems and colloidal solutions, change appreciably with a change in composition or concentration, according to the manufacturing processes (mechanical work), with the degree of dispersion of the system, with the physical environment (most notably temperature), and with time. Rheological problems would be greatly simplified if these factors operated, and could be treated, independently, but as Lin (1962) points out the various factors affecting rheology of a system work in consort and are usually beyond absolute resolution. Many other more subtle factors may also affect the rheology of a system. Heinrich and Clements (1960), for example, have shown by the use of rheograms the very real effects on emulsion rheology of shaking, varying the source of the raw materials, ageing, temperature cycling, and other factors.

Regardless of the many factors which affect rheology, careful measurement of product rheology permits the control of product quality and is necessary to achieve reproducibility between batches of many liquid and semi-solid pharmaceuticals.

Where available, knowledge of appropriate mathematical relationships (concentration vs. viscosity, processing variables vs. viscosity, or other rheological parameters) may be employed to achieve the desired viscosity. However, with our present state of knowledge, it is quite unlikely that the pharmaceutical scientist can retire to his desk and by computation alone develop or predict the total rheology of a given new system, or develop the system to a given set of rheological specifications. For the most part it is still necessary to go to the laboratory and vary the ingredients, the proportions and the manufacturing procedure in a systematic and ordered way, until flow properties are obtained in the system which are in an acceptable range. It is worthwhile to review the effects of formulation (variation in ingredients and their concentration), manufacturing variables, or alterations in physical conditions, on product rheology.

B. FACTORS AFFECTING RHEOLOGICAL PROPERTIES

1. *Chemical Factors*

a. *Degree of polymerization and depolymerization.* Suspending agents and emulsion stabilizers act in low concentration to produce viscous solutions by virtue of their high molecular weight or high molecular weight fractions. Indeed, the hydrophilic natural and modified gums are all polymeric in nature (with the polymeric fraction nearly always being a polysaccharide), as are the synthetic viscosity imparting agents. The molecular weight of the polymeric fraction of the natural gums is usually much higher than the average molecular weight of the synthetic polymers commonly used. For example, Basu *et al.* (1955) determined the molecular weight of the free acid or its sodium salt in tragacanth to be 80,000 to 100,000, and Oakley (1936, 1937) calculated the molecular weight of the polymeric fraction of gum arabic and found it to be 200,000 to 245,000, all determinations being made osmometrically. The reason that more natural gum is required to produce a given viscosity than is required using a synthetic polymer, is that the natural gum contains the polymeric fraction in low concentration. The very high molecular weight fraction of the natural gums probably accounts in part for their rheological instability and susceptability to depolymerization.

The mathematical relationship between the viscosity and the molecular weight of polymers is elusive, based on the fact that such a relationship is affected by secondary factors such as hydration and coiling of the molecules. The relationship between intrinsic viscosity $[\eta]$, and polymer molecular weight, $\bar{M}$, was given in equation (16).

The higher molecular weight grades of synthetic and modified natural gums are more economical since lower concentrations may be used to obtain the desired viscosity. However, the longer polymer molecules may be too prone to shear depolymerization or to depolymerization by chemical degradation for practical use. Levy (1961) found that low molecular weight sodium alginate solutions exhibit a decrease in viscosity that was four to five times slower than that of the high molecular weight sodium alginate solutions. Levy also made a stereochemical analysis of the structural features of the polysaccharide polymers in relation to their rheological stability. He theorized that hydroxyl groups in the axial position were less available to hydrogen bonding thereby permitting less intermolecular association of the polysaccharide molecules. This resulted in instability since the glycosidic linkages were not then shielded from hydrolysis. Asbeck and Baxter (1959) found that the degree of depolymerization of polyethylene oxide in aqueous solution was proportional to the intensity of shear and the original molecular weight of the polymer. Ultrasonic energy, owing to the high shear intensity of the cavitation effect, produces depolymerization and viscosity decreases in various natural and modified gums according to Head and Lauter (1957), Akiya *et al.* (1949) and Freundlich and Gillings (1938), and in synthetic polymers according to Jellinek and White (1951). Schmidt (1940) and Sobue and Ishikawa (1941) have actually offered equations to attempt to quantify the rate of polymer depolymerization and the viscosity decrease brought about by ultrasonic processing. Other high-shear processing such as colloid milling or high-shear mixing is also capable of producing depolymerization.

The apparent high incidence of polymer depolymerization by ultrasonic or other high-shear processing may frequently be avoided by redesigning the processing sequences, i.e. by processing the disperse system under high shear in the presence of the minimum amount of colloid used to impart the viscosity. Then the remaining polymer vehicle or stabilizer can be added. In other cases a selection of lower molecular weight grades of polymer may result in improved rheological stability.

b. *Extent of polymer hydration.* Whistler (1959) presents one of the more complete discussions of the effect of polymer hydration on viscosity and defines hydration of hydrophilic molecules as an immobilization of the water molecules near the polymer molecule. In aqueous solution the hydrophilic polymer molecules may be regarded as completely surrounded by an "atmosphere" of partially immobilized water molecules. The associated water molecules are held primarily by hydrogen bonds, with other secondary forces such as ionic charges. Dipole and induced dipole interactions are also possibly involved. If the bonding forces are strong, the water molecules tend to hold the polymer molecules in an extended linear form and prevent their coiling. The extended molecules will have a relatively large space requirement thereby producing a maximum viscosity effect. The fully hydrated polymer molecules will also have the greatest resistance to viscosity change caused by alterations in pH or addition of salts in low concentration (provided a complex is not formed), due to the presence of the adsorbed water molecules. The tendency of aqueous polymer solutions to increase in viscosity with time or with low or moderate shear processing is widely reported and is due undoubtedly in part to increased hydration. This effect of continuing or increased hydration is especially to be noted with colloidal earth products and natural gums.

c. *Impurities, trace ions and electrolytes.* Natural gums may be expected to contain impurities; those which are grossly visible such as plant or insect fragments or mineral matter, as well as chemical impurities such as the residual calcium ion reported (Levy and Schwarz, 1958) to be contained in the alginates. From a rheological standpoint only the chemical impurities are of importance, and these may lead to considerable rheological variability on ageing or under such effects as freezing and thawing. Very marked viscosity increases, even to the point of gelling, have been noted with sodium alginate solutions, and these are attributed to conditions which lead to an increase in effective calcium ion concentration and hence the formation of calcium alginate.

Ordinarily, electrolytes do not greatly affect the viscosity of neutral colloids in aqueous solution. At high concentrations, however, the salts compete for the adsorbed water molecules surrounding the hydrated polymer or clay molecules, due to the affinity of the salt ions for water. As the polymer or clay molecules become dehydrated, their dispersions decrease in viscosity, and ultimately the polymer or clay will precipitate from solution. In the case of the linear hydrophilic polymers, a decrease in the layer of adsorbed solvent molecules may permit the polymer chain to coil, in which case it will have a smaller space requirement and viscosity will decrease. Batdorf (1959) attributes the relative insensitivity of the cellulose derivatives to viscosity change to the result of ionic effects which prevent the stiff, rod-like cellulose molecules from coiling as much as other synthetic and natural polymers.

The effect of various salts on the viscosity of aqueous polymer solutions varies with the concentration of the salt, its valency, the pH of the solution, and the degree of substitution of the polymer. As a general rule the polymer solutions have a much lower tolerance to polyvalent cations than to monovalent cations, from the standpoint of both the concentration which will produce a substantial viscosity change, and that which will produce gelation or precipitation. The more highly substituted polymers will generally have a greater tolerance for salts. This effect may be attributed to the greater degree of association and protective hydration of the more highly substituted products. The salt tolerance of a number of clays and of the natural and synthetic polymers and gums is indicated in Table III, pp. 72, 73. It should be remembered, though, that these concentrations are not absolute, and may be altered by many factors such as those described above. For further discussion of the stability of polymeric agents, and such effects as caused by added electrolytes and non-solvents, the reader is referred to a textbook of colloidal chemistry dealing with the stability of hydrophilic colloids.

d. *Effect of pH*. pH greatly affects the viscosity and stability of the hydrophilic natural and synthetic gums. The natural gums usually have a relatively stable viscosity plateau extending over three or four pH units, with the pH range covering, if not centered at, neutrality. Above and below this stable pH range, viscosity decreases sharply. The synthetic gums generally have the advantage of a stable viscosity plateau extending over a wide pH range. Methyl cellulose is one of the most exemplary with a reported stable viscosity plateau over the pH range of 3 to 12. Other gums, both natural and synthetic, which exist as sodium salts, are stable over a narrower pH range, and are precipitated by any appreciable quantity of mineral acid. The fact that a polymer exists as a sodium salt is no guarantee that it will be stable in more than mild alkaline media. Bolliger and Munzel (1958), for example, found that sodium alginate solutions were quite unstable above a pH of 8. It should also be noted that the range over which gums produce rheologically stable solutions may vary with time. While Schon and Fuerst (1941) reported that the maximum viscosity of freshly prepared tragacanth solutions was obtained at pH 8, Schwarz *et al.* (1958) found that maximum long term viscosity was obtained at pH 5. The stable pH ranges of a number of viscosity imparting agents are reported in Table III.

Not only do gums have an optimum pH for rheological stability, but many gums apparently also have an optimum pH for preservation with given preservatives. Taub *et al.* (1958) found that while the optimum pH for viscosity stability of tragacanth solutions or jellies was at 5 or above, the optimum pH for preservation was below 5. In such cases Taub recommended that the gum solution be prepared at the pH corresponding to the maximum viscosity stability, and preservatives be properly selected and used which were effective at that pH.

e. *Interaction with polyhydroxy compounds*. Polyhydroxy compounds such as sorbitol, glycerin, propylene glycol and the polyethylene glycols are reported to affect the gel point, viscosity and other rheological characteristics of a number of gums with which they are mixed. The addition of a polyol to an aqueous solution of a hydrophilic gum usually produces a viscosity increase. Segur *et al.* (1956) have tabulated the effect of an addition of glycerol on a large number of gums, and found an increase in viscosity or gel strength in most cases. Levy and Schwarz (1957, 1958) found that both glycerin and propylene glycol produced an increase in the initial viscosity of sodium alginate solutions, and they attributed the effect to a partial association of the sodium alginate by the presence of the hydrophilic polyols. Certain polymers and polyols may apparently also interact with each other to produce a viscosity increase. Storz *et al.* (1963) found that the lower molecular weight polyethylene glycols produced a very substantial viscosity increase with the development of thixotropy in sodium carboxymethylhydroxyethylcelluloses. Dialysis studies indicated that the molecules were bound by some type of association. High concentrations of polyols (above 20 to 25 per cent), may be expected to interfere with the hydration of gums, and a viscosity decrease may become apparent. Bolliger and Munzel (1958) also noted that high concentrations of polyol caused a normally pseudoplastic gum solution to become thixotropic.

f. *Sequestering agents and buffers*. The effect of calcium ions in increasing the viscosity of sodium alginate solutions has been previously mentioned. As might be expected, removal of these ions by sequestering agents such as EDTA or hexametaphosphate will cause a viscosity decrease in sodium alginate solutions. Tragacanth solutions also suffer a rapid loss in viscosity, regardless of the pH, in systems which bind calcium ion, such as citrate buffers (Schwarz *et al.*, 1958). Sequestering agents may have a stabilizing effect on viscosity in polymer gum solutions where trace elements cause instability. Addition of a sequestering agent to the carboxyvinyl polymer, Carbopol (B. F. Goodrich Chem. Co.), is reported to retard decomposition of its solutions when subjected to daylight. This effect is due to the fact that the sequestering agent combines with the trace metals thought to catalyze decomposition (Schwarz and Levy, 1958).

2. *Physical Factors*

a. *Temperature*. Temperature changes produce a pronounced change (usually approaching a first order rate relationship) in the viscosity of hydrophilic gum solutions. A temperature increase usually produces a rapid viscosity decrease, with the exception of certain synthetic polymers such as methyl cellulose, whose aqueous solutions gel with a temperature increase. In the latter cases the temperature at which gelation occurs depends on the polymer concentration, degree of polymerization and nature of substitution (Davies and Rowson, 1957). Two examples are cited to illustrate the drastic viscosity decrease which occurs with a temperature increase in most gum solutions. Osborne and Lee (1951) reported that the apparent viscosity of a 35 per cent acacia mucilage decreased in viscosity from 220 cP at 20° C to 63 cP at 60° C, and the viscosity of a 2 per cent solution of medium viscosity grade sodium carboxymethylcellulose decreased from about 700 cP at 20° C to less than 200 cP at 60° C.

Elevated temperatures may be useful in preparing vegetable gum and other polymer solutions. Middleton (1936) was one of the first workers to recognize that the heating of gum solutions to 100° C, if applied for relatively brief periods of time (2 to 15 min) during solution preparation, caused an increase in viscosity. The increase might be attributed to increased hydration of the system. If the solutions are subjected to continued heating at temperatures of 100° C for periods of longer than 15 min enhanced viscosity is not obtained, due to polymer decomposition (Schwarz and Levy, 1957). Temperature of manufacture, temperature of storage and temperature cycling also affect the viscosity of disperse systems. These effects are discussed under the headings of suspensions and emulsions.

b. *Aeration.* Aerated products usually result from high shear mixing or milling. Due to their high viscosity, gum solutions are prone to aeration and produce very stable aerated systems from which it is difficult to remove the air. Aerated solution of proteinaceous agents such as gelatin or zein may be very prone to denaturation and should not be aerated if prolonged stability is sought.

Aeration is a serious problem with disperse systems, particularly emulsions having a high yield value (Lin, 1962). Aerated samples may appear to be more viscous or have a more viscous creamed layer than non-aerated samples. Some aerated emulsions will be less viscous and less stable than unaerated samples, due to concentration of the surfactant or emulsion stabilizer at the air–liquid interface and thus depletion of the stabilizer at the oil–water interface. All aerated samples are less dense than non-aerated samples, and density can serve as a standard measure of the degree of aeration. Deaeration may be brought about in some cases mechanically by roll milling, which in effect squeezes out the air; however, a more practical approach may be to heat the aerated system. The best approach to an aeration problem is, of course, prevention, which can usually be achieved by improved process design.

c. *Light.* Various hydrocolloids in aqueous solution are reported to be sensitive to light. These colloids include Carbopol (Schwarz and Levy, 1958), sodium carboxymethylcellulose (Davies and Rowson, 1957), and sodium alginate (Bolliger and Munzel, 1958). To protect photosensitive hydrocolloids from decomposition and resultant rheological change, some possible approaches are the use of light-resistant containers, screening agents, antioxidants or, in the case of Carbopol, the use of sequestering agents.

d. *Degree of dispersion and flocculation.* The viscosity of disperse systems may be expected to vary according to their degree of dispersion, particularly for dispersions of solids in liquids. In concentrated suspensions (3 per cent solids and higher according to the definition of Ward and Kammermeyer, 1940), a decrease in particle size or an increase in the surface area of the solid phase, is reported to produce an increase in viscosity of the system (Sweeney and Geckler, 1956; Zettlemoyer and Lower, 1955). The viscosity increase in concentrated systems has been attributed to immobilization of the vehicle with an increase in the fraction of the suspension volume effectively occupied by the solid. Some workers (e.g. Zettlemoyer and Lower, 1955) report that slight changes in the range of the particle size distribution (0·1 to 0·4 μ) had no effect on suspension viscosity. However, other workers have found that suspensions with a narrow particle size distribution are substantially more viscous than suspensions of approximately equal average particle size but wider particle size range (Sweeney and Geckler, 1956; Williams, 1953). The explanation of this effect is that particles having a narrow particle size range will occupy a larger effective volume than the same weight of particles having a wider particle size range. Where there is a wide particle size range, the smaller particles can fill the void spaces between the larger particles, resulting in a more closely packed system with a smaller effective volume.

In addition to affecting viscosity, the particle size of the dispersed solids in concentrated suspensions is reported to affect the total rheology of the system. It is well known that the addition of insoluble solids to a Newtonian vehicle is capable of producing non-Newtonian flow properties in the system. Zettlemoyer and Lower (1955) found that the smaller the particle size of the dispersed solid phase the lower the concentration of solids required to produce non-Newtonian flow and thixotropy.

In very dilute suspensions and in suspensions in which the particle size of the dispersed phase is in the colloidal range, the repulsive (electrical) and attractive (physical-chemical) forces may play a very significant role in acting on the particles in suspension (DeWaele and Mardles, 1949). The effect on viscosity of a change in particle size in these systems is usually the same as with concentrated suspensions, though the mechanism may be different. In dilute suspensions at a given volume ratio of solids to liquid, Brownian movement increases as the particle size decreases, thus increasing the rate of agglomeration and, in effect, restricting the flow of the continuous phase. Accordingly, the viscosity increases (Broughton and Windebank, 1938).

Flocculation of a suspension system produces very pronounced effects on rheology. Indeed, the increase in viscosity and especially the great increase in thixotropy of a system are strong evidence for flocculation. The flocs or clustered particles are held weakly together as aggregates, and are capable of forming extended networks which give the flocculated suspension its structural properties (Michaels and Bolger, 1962, 1962a). Immobilization of a portion of the dispersing media in the network and between the flocs is thought to be the mechanism accounting for the viscosity increase (Sherman, 1963).

In discussions of the effect of the degree of dispersion of emulsions on emulsion viscosity, some workers (e.g. Mullins and Becker, 1956) find that in the systems studied, viscosity is not influenced by the degree of dispersion of the discontinuous phase. Other workers such as Richardson (1953) report that the apparent viscosity of emulsions which have the same concentration and size distribution about a mean globule diameter, is inversely proportional to this diameter. Whether a change in emulsion globule size results in a viscosity change probably depends on several factors, including the presence of any unemulsified fraction, changes in the oil or water concentration due to the partial separation of a phase, and the composition of the system. The concentration of the dispersed phase may also be a factor: Sibree (1941) and Leviton and Leighton (1936) reported that changes in the globule size from 3 to 0·7 μ did not substantially alter emulsion viscosity, below concentrations corresponding to close packing. The effect of close packing was also used by Lyttleton and Traxler (1948) to explain why emulsions with globules of approximately equal size are much more stable and more viscous than emulsions having a wide particle size distribution. Sumner (1954) explained the effect of globule size range on emulsion viscosity on the basis that the more uniform the globule size the lower the volume ratio necessary to achieve close packing, with the close-packed system offering more resistance to flow by the continuous phase at any volume concentration.

While quantitative relationships cannot yet be completely and accurately drawn between viscosity and the effects of the degree of dispersion of suspensions and emulsions, progress is being made along these lines.

C. RHEOLOGY AND PRODUCT DESIGN

1. *Emulsions, Lotions and Creams*

a. *General rheology of emulsions.* Emulsions are systems composed of at least two immiscible liquids, one of which is dispersed in the other as minute globules. Fluid pharmaceutical emulsions intended for topical application are termed lotions, while semi-solid emulsions intended for topical application are called creams. Lotions differ from simple oil and water emulsions in that they commonly contain waxes or aliphatic acids, alcohols or esters. These compounds are normally solids at room temperature, and are primarily responsible for the body or consistency typical of lotion products. Creams are an important class of pharmaceutical products, since the majority of the ointment bases in use today are creams.

All emulsion systems, with the exception of those which are very dilute and thus contain a low concentration of dispersed phase, may be expected to be non-Newtonian. Heinrich and Clements (1960) found that most cosmetic emulsions which they studied were pseudoplastic, with some of the more concentrated and viscous lotions being truly plastic. Most creams demonstrate plastic flow properties. Weltmann (1956) reported that many emulsions, even simple mineral oil–water emulsions, exhibited plastic viscosity and yield values.

Of the pharmaceutical emulsions which have been rheologically described, the great majority can be regarded as shear thinning. A shear thinning product is one which becomes more fluid when subjected to shear, such as thixotropic materials. The majority of the emulsions which exhibit plastic flow are thixotropic, have a substantial yield value, or have a spur value which for practical purposes may be described as an exaggerated yield value. Most pseudoplastic emulsions which have been observed also appear to be thixotropic when measured at room temperature. However, simple emulsions of oil in water, not containing an appreciable quantity of plastic or pseudoplastic stabilizers, do not develop an appreciable gel structure and do not show strong thixotropic characteristics.

The fact that most emulsions are shear thinning may be of some significance in the physical stability of the systems. A shear-thinning emulsion is definitely the best type of product from the consumer's standpoint, particularly if the emulsion is intended for topical use. A pharmaceutical emulsion should have considerable consistency and body, and yet the product must pour readily from the bottle, be administered conveniently on a spoon, or be easily applied and spread on the skin. The shear-thinning product has these properties and is also readily adapted to topical absorption.

b. *Viscosity and emulsion stability.* There are several types of instability which emulsions may undergo. Viscosity in some cases is a related factor, while in other cases viscosity and emulsion stability are unrelated. Martin (1960b) classifies the instability of pharmaceutical emulsions into three categories as follows:

(*a*) flocculation and creaming,
(*b*) coalescence and breaking, and
(*c*) miscellaneous physical and chemical changes, including changes in rheological properties.

The effect of viscosity and other physical factors on the rate of creaming of emulsions may be expressed by Stokes' law,

$$v = \frac{d^2(\rho - \rho_0)g}{18\eta_0} \tag{32}$$

in which v is the rate of sedimentation or creaming, d is the mean diameter of the dispersed globules, ρ is the density of the dispersed phase, ρ_0 is the density of the continuous phase, η_0 is the viscosity of the continuous phase, and g is the acceleration due to gravity. While an expression such as this is completely valid only in very dilute systems in which the particles do not interfere with one another, analysis of the expression is of interest and indicates the relative significance of the various physical factors to emulsion creaming. For example, decreasing the average globule size to one-half the original size should decrease the creaming rate to one-fourth the original rate, other factors remaining constant. If the viscosity of the continuous phase is doubled, as by the addition of a hydrophilic colloid to the system, the creaming rate should be one-half that of the original rate. The adjustment of densities has not proven to be a practical method of retarding emulsion creaming, but milling of samples to produce fine globules (several microns to a tenth of a micron or less is typical of many pharmaceutical emulsions) and the addition of polymeric viscosity-imparting agents can retard creaming in these systems.

Emulsion coalescence and breaking is not significantly affected by the viscosity of the continuous phase, but is primarily a function of the volume concentration of the phases and the character of the adsorbed film at the oil–water interface. Mardles and DeWaele (1951) regard the character of the adsorbed surface film of emulsifier at the interface to be of primary importance in determining emulsion stability. Serrallach *et al.* (1933) measured the strength of the interfacial films of emulsions and concluded that the interfacial tension of the film is related to emulsion stability. More recently Davies and Mayers (1960) have measured the interfacial viscosity of monolayers, and have experimentally substantiated the premise that emulsion stability is enhanced by a high interfacial viscosity.

Variations in the viscosity of emulsions with time is a kind of physical instability which has plagued pharmaceutical formulators for many years. Lauffer *et al.* (1958) concluded that the point of greatest interest in liquid cosmetic emulsions is the viscosity of the system after a long period of rest, rather than its viscosity immediately after manufacture. The authors suggested a method of predicting ultimate product viscosity by preparing a viscosity vs. time curve, taking readings over several months, after which extrapolation to ultimate or equilibrium viscosity is made. Barnett (1957) also recommended continued viscosity surveillance of newly formulated lotion-type emulsions. He suggested that viscosity measurements be made at 25° C and the data plotted daily for the first 2 weeks, weekly for the next 3 months, and monthly thereafter for a total of 12 months. A lotion emulsion having adequate viscosity stability is described as one which levels off at the desired viscosity range within 5 to 10 days, and shows a minimal viscosity change thereafter. Ideally, rheologically stable emulsion systems are sought, systems which vary but little not only in viscosity, but which maintain their degree of structure and thixotropy with time. Rheological stability is probably best promoted by the presence of a stable adsorbed emulsifier film at the interface.

c. *The effect of formulation on emulsion rheology.* General factors affecting emulsion stability are relative oil–water concentration, choice of the oil in oil–water emulsions, and the choice of the emulsifying agent. The relative concentration ratio of oil to water, or dispersed phase to continuous phase, usually has a pronounced effect on the viscosity of an emulsion. An increase in the concentration of the dispersed phase up to some critical value, corresponding perhaps to close packing, causes only a moderate or slight increase in viscosity. But above this critical concentration a very rapid rise to a maximum viscosity is observed, after which the emulsion may invert or break (Broughton and Squires, 1938; Bredee and deBooys, 1940; Sherman, 1950). Weltmann (1956) reported that the relative concentration of phases also affects the yield value.

The necessity to select the proper emulsifying agent for a given oil–water emulsion system is, of course, critical to the preparation of a stable system. Less well known is the fact that for a given emulsion system with a constant phase ratio, different emulsifying agents, all of which will form an emulsion, produce products with very different viscosities (Toms, 1941; Gabriel, 1935; Sumner, 1940; Axon, 1956). This effect is not surprising since different emulsifiers, though they may all produce stable emulsions, could be expected to form quite different interfacial emulsifier films, according to the physical–chemical properties of the emulsifiers.

While the viscosity of the oil in an emulsion system has little or no effect on emulsion viscosity (Shotton and White, 1960; Sibree, 1931; Broughton and Squires, 1938), different oils may produce systems with widely different viscosities. Shotton and White (1960) found that the physical–chemical nature of the oil, as well as the properties of the emulsifier, produce a great effect on emulsion viscosities by influencing the interfacial film surrounding the oil droplets.

Considerable information is available on specific formulation problems regarding the rheology of lotions. Some specific findings relating the formulation of lotions and their viscosity are reported by Strianse (1957) as follows. Stearate type lotions, usually containing 3 to 5 per cent stearic acid and emulsified with triethanolamine, are the most sensitive to gelation. The viscosity of these systems increases with time—up to several months or years—until the emulsion may actually appear to be a solid or semi-solid. Strianse indicates certain formulation methods which may prevent or retard the gelation of stearate lotions, and his paper should be consulted for the details.

While gelation appears to be the greatest problem with anionic lotions such as stearate products, the phenomena may also occur with non-ionic or cationic lotions but to a lesser degree. It can usually be corrected by simple reformulation, possibly involving no more than changing relative concentration of ingredients. Lehne (1957) reports that the viscosity of lotions may be varied effectively by modifying the concentration of partially sulphated alcohols in the product. Of the alcohols commonly used, stearyl alcohol is said to produce the most body. Janowitz (1950) found that less viscous emulsions are obtained using triethanolamine lauryl sulphate rather than the sodium salt.

The waxes, aliphatic acids, esters and alcohols not only give lotions their viscosity but also their body and gel structure, which is reflected in their thixotropy. Although thixotropic lotions are very prone to shear thinning, these products are unlikely to be subjected to sufficient shear in the hands of the consumer to produce much shear thinning until the product is actually applied to the skin. However, when these products are milled, they may undergo substantial shear thinning, and the product may require many months to recover its original viscosity.

2. *Suspensions*

a. *Rheology of suspensions*. Simple suspensions of dispersed solids in a liquid, unmodified by the presence of any suspending agent, commonly show thixotropic plastic flow behaviour. The Einstein equation (see equation 8) first related the viscosity of dilute colloidal suspensions to the volume fraction of dispersed particles; and numerous modifications of this equation have since appeared in an effort to approximate conditions in more concentrated systems. In the common pharmaceutical suspension which contains both an insoluble powder and a viscosity-imparting agent, the plastic viscosity of the suspended solids is usually overshadowed by the pseudoplastic character of the polymeric suspending agent.

Frisch and Simha (1956) have classified the factors found experimentally to affect suspension viscosity as follows:

(*a*) the shape, size and mass of the suspended particles,
(*b*) the size distribution of the particles,
(*c*) the relative volume fraction of the particles,
(*d*) the internal flexibility and ease of deformation of the particles,
(*e*) the thermodynamic condition of the system,
(*f*) The presence of electric charges in the system, and
(*g*) the concentration of the system.

These factors and their effect on suspension viscosity have been previously referred to under physical factors affecting dispersed systems, with the exception of thermodynamic considerations. Martin (1960c) discusses the thermodynamics of suspensions. The system becomes more thermodynamically stable as the surface free energy is reduced by particle aggregation or by a lowering of interfacial tension through the addition of a surface active agent.

b. *Rheology and suspension stability.* The viscosity of suspension systems is related to the rate of sedimentation of the dispersed particles according to the following Stokes' law expression:

$$v = K\frac{d^2(\rho-\rho_0)}{\eta_0} \tag{33}$$

in which K is a constant determined by experimentation, and takes into account effects of irregular particle shape plus the gravitation constant, with the other expressions in the equation corresponding to those of equation (32). The above equation would prove quite useful in dilute suspensions, but in the typical pharmaceutical suspension the particles exhibit hindered settling, in which case such equations can provide only gross approximations and have thus limited practical usefulness.

In addition to viscosity, other rheological properties such as thixotropy and yield value can be related to suspension stability. Foernzler *et al.* (1960) studied the effect of the thixotropy of two clays on suspension stability, and a centrifugation technique was used to evaluate stability. Figure 35 shows the relationship that was found between the thixotropic suspending agents and the rate of separation that occurred in the 10 per cent w/v zinc oxide suspensions. In both suspension systems the sedimentation velocity was directly proportional to the reciprocal of the thixotropic area. No such relationship was found between other rheological parameters and the sedimentation velocity in the systems studied, indicating the predominant effect thixotropy can play in suspension stability in some products.

Meyer and Cohen (1959) have reported an approach to the preparation of permanent suspensions involving the rheological parameter, yield

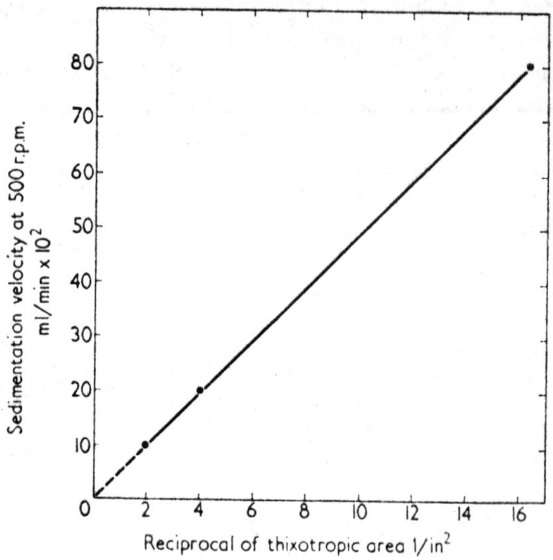

FIG. 35. Stability-thixotropy relationship for 10 per cent zinc oxide suspended in an activated attapulgite aqueous suspension vehicle.

value. Employing a carboxyvinyl polymer (Carbopol 934, B. F. Goodrich Chemical Co.) which exhibits plastic flow properties, suspensions of powdered drug, sand, and other materials were prepared. The suspensions were observed to be permanent when the medium exhibited a critical minimum yield value, irrespective of the apparent viscosity.

Martin (1960d) has suggested another approach to the preparation of stable suspensions involving the use of a combination of plastic and pseudoplastic viscosity imparting agents, and this possibility has been tested by Samyn (1961). The advantage of the combination is that the system will remain pourable based on its pseudoplastic character, and produce permanent stable suspensions of the dispersed solid particles based on the thixotropy and yield value of the plastic material. Samyn found that the best formulation could easily be determined for a new suspension product by preparing a series of preparations, varying the concentration of plastic and pseudoplastic materials, to determine the optimum flow properties for permanent particle suspension.

Martin (1961) and Haines and Martin (1961) depart somewhat from the rheological approach for the preparation of stable suspensions when they treat the insoluble particles so that they are kept in a state of controlled flocculation. The suspended material is thus uniform in composition and readily provides an accurate dosage of the dispersed drug. The flocculated character of the system prevents caking and allows easy redispersion of any settled matter. Flocculated systems may, of course, be further stabilized by viscosity-imparting agents, a minimal concentration of the agent effectively preventing floccule separation.

Flocculation and rheological control represent separate approaches to the preparation of stable suspensions. The methods may be used alone or together and both present problems of formulation. Before being flocculated the particles must often be coated to alter their charge, and suitable coating agents are not always readily available. The rheological formulation of suspension vehicles must be balanced to achieve satisfactory particle suspension, while maintaining the system in an adequately fluid condition to permit pouring and accurate volumetric measurement. Thixotropic suspensions must flow freely, and must have a sufficiently slow recovery after shaking so as to remain fluid long enough to be dispensed, yet set-up quickly enough to maintain the particles in a suspended state. Levy (1962) has recently studied the kinetics of the structural recovery of thixotropic dispersions. The addition of a viscosity-imparting agent to a suspension vehicle may retard the sedimentation of particles which cake on settling. However, once the particles have caked, a viscous suspension vehicle may prohibit rather than assist their redistribution on shaking. Thus, it is apparent that while rheological control is a most important aspect of suspensions formulation, the total suspension system must also be analysed, including the physical–chemical properties of the insoluble material, the presence of electrolytes and surface-active agents in the system, and all other factors affecting the stability of the dispersion.

3. *Ointments and Gels*

No class of pharmaceutical product is subjected to a closer or more critical evaluation by the consumer in the course of their use than are ointments, creams, pastes and gels. The pharmaceutical elegance of all topical semi-solid preparations is most directly related to consistency. The consistency of the ointment or cream directly affects product spreadability, extrudability from tubes or, to a lesser degree, ease of removal from jars. Consistency is also related to the capacity of a semi-solid to take up solids or liquids, to the adherence of an ointment to the skin, and in some cases to drug release. Marriott (1961) has discussed the consistency of cosmetic and semi-solid pharmaceuticals, and in addition to the factors already mentioned he relates smoothness and stickiness or tackiness of these products to their consistency. He has reviewed the methods of measuring some of these elusive and empirical properties.

The majority of topical semi-solids appear to have plastic flow properties. Kostenbauder and Martin (1954) found that hydrocarbon bases such as petrolatum exhibited plastic flow with varying degrees of thixotropy. Some pastes exhibit dilatancy when subjected to shear, whereas others demonstrate typical pseudoplastic flow with thixotropy (Bechtel and Fischer, 1949). Scott-Blair (1960) found that pharmaceutical pastes, tooth pastes, and some ophthalmic ointments move through tubes according to four distinct classes of flow behaviour, from plug flow to complete streamline flow. Mardles and DeWaele (1951) found that in ointments, pastes, and creams containing a high solids content, the effects of friction and adhesion between the particles outweighed the viscosity effect of the semi-solid vehicle in determining the rheological character of the total dispersion. The outstanding rheological property of gels or jellies is their thixotropic character (Scott-Blair, 1945; Martin, 1960e), which accounts for the fact that they may become solids on standing and liquids on agitation.

Another outstanding feature of gels is their great resistance to changes in consistency with a change in temperature (Chun, 1956). Foster *et al.* (1951) found that while a mineral oil–polyethylene gel showed a consistency change of less than 20 per cent in penetrometer values between 10° and 30° C, petrolatum showed a consistency change of about 40 per cent. The waxy matrix of petrolatum or wax-containing hydrocarbon bases is evidently broken down with temperature increase, resulting in their considerable consistency or viscosity loss (Chun, 1956). Creams are appreciably more stable rheologically to changes in temperature normally encountered in pharmaceutical use than are the hydrocarbon bases. However, creams will undergo consistency increases and hardening due to drying and water loss unless they are carefully stored and are stabilized against dehydration by the incorporation of humectants.

Kostenbauder and Martin (1954) have studied various factors which affect the viscosity of semi-solid pharmaceuticals. They reported that thermal and previous mechanical history affect the rheology of these products. Other findings apparent in their work were:

1. Addition of wax to a hydrocarbon base greatly increased thixotropy and yield value as well as plastic viscosity.

2. The addition of as little as 10 per cent insoluble powder to a petrolatum–mineral oil base had very similar effects to that of adding white wax to petrolatum, i.e. it greatly increased thixotropy, yield value and plastic viscosity.

3. Addition of water to a water-miscible base (Hydrophilic Petrolatum U.S.P.) caused a decrease in yield value and an increase in thixotropy and plastic viscosity.

4. Emulsified ointment bases became soft if stirred or subjected to mechanical work while cooled during manufacture, and hard and unacceptable if not stirred during cooling. The effect of packaging and other mechanical treatment on the rheology of these semi-solids may be critical factors in the preparation of an acceptable product.

4. *Powders and Granular Solids*

Powders and granular solids have properties of flow as do fluids, although the factors affecting flow in the two states differ markedly. The flow of powders and granular solids has become a matter of greatly increased interest to the pharmaceutical scientist in recent years with the adoption of high-speed tabletting, encapsulation, and filling equipment. The factor frequently limiting the production rate is not one of equipment but rather of the drug mixture being processed.

Increasingly rigid specifications of pharmaceutical manufacturers regarding permissible weight variation of tablets and capsules have resulted in an increased interest in powder rheology. The most important single factor affecting the flow properties of particulate solids is the surface characteristics of the particles (Crosby, 1960). Increased rate of flow of powders can be achieved by reducing the surface roughness of the particles or alleviating "stickiness" between the particles. Surface roughness may be reduced by the presence of fines in a powder or granular material; the fines may serve to fill in the depressions or irregularities in the particle surfaces. Stickiness of the particles may be reduced by the addition of lubricants such as soaps, talc, starch, mineral oil, or other agents capable of producing slippage between particles. The lubricants are more effective in producing flow if they are in a fine state of subdivision. Limitations of space permit only an enumeration of some of the other factors affecting the flow properties of particulate solids. These include:

1. Particle size and particle size distribution.
2. Particle shape and gross shape differences.
3. Particle orientation of heterogeneous multi-component systems.
4. Density.

5. Relative size and geometry of the hopper.
6. Bed depth in the hopper.
7. Manner of packing in the hopper.
8. Effect of turbulence, natural or induced in the powder.

5. *Viscosity-Imparting Agents:—Natural Gums, Modified Natural Gums, and Artificial Gums*

a. *Rheology of gums.* The majority of the materials used in pharmaceutical formulations as suspending agents, emulsion stabilizers, and bodying agents are colloidal aqueous dispersions which exhibit pseudoplastic flow properties. Figure 36 shows the relationship between the

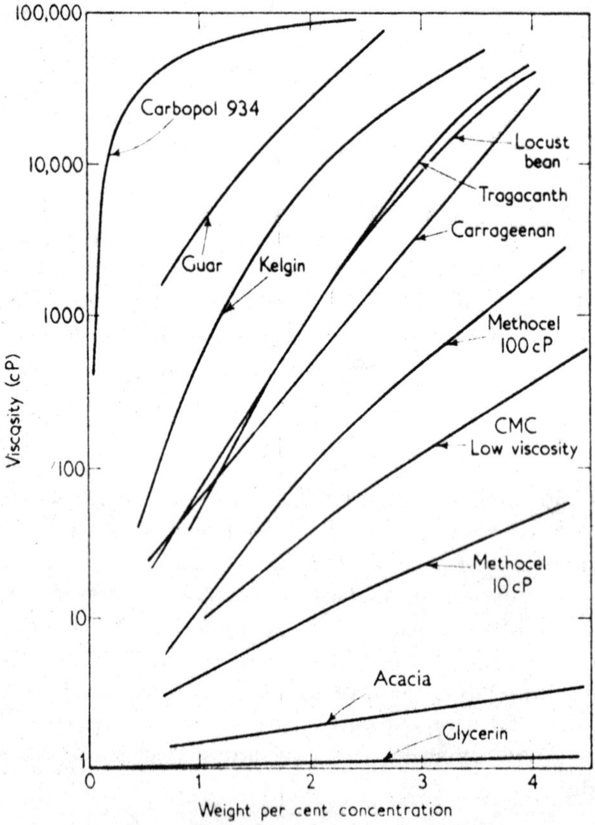

FIG. 36. Viscosity of hydrophilic natural and synthetic polymeric agents (and glycerin) as related to their concentration in water. The curve for Kelgin was obtained from "Algins at Work", Kelco Co., Clark, New Jersey. The data for the curve of Carbopol were obtained from the "Carbopol Service Bulletin GC-36", B. F. Goodrich Chemical Co., Cleveland, Ohio.

concentration of a number of hydrophilic polymeric agents and their viscosity (glycerin is included for comparison). The majority of the data used in preparing the curves of concentration versus apparent viscosity is from the work of Osborne and Lee (1951), who made their measurement with a Brookfield viscometer. An almost exponential relationship between apparent viscosity and concentration was observed for the pseudoplastic polymeric agents, with some deviation apparent for sodium alginate (Kelgin). This simple relationship did not hold for the plastic material, Carbopol.

Kabre *et al.* (1962) also studied the viscosity of a number of pseudoplastic gums, and they were able to relate viscosity to concentration for five algins, sodium carboxymethylcellulose, methyl cellulose and tragacanth. The relationship between the apparent pseudoplastic viscosity η' of the agents and their concentration C, was expressed as:

$$\eta' = e^{KC+B} \tag{34}$$

where K and B are material constants. Employing the concentration-viscosity relationship, the suspending action of the gums was compared at fixed viscosities of 1, 5, 10 and 20. An apparent viscosity of 10 was found to be adequate for the stabilization of insoluble drugs in combination with compatible suspending agents.

The fact that the great majority of the suspending agents and emulsion stabilizers are chosen from the group of pseudoplastic agents is undoubtedly the result of certain rheological advantages of the pseudoplastics. Pseudoplastic materials are usually composed of long molecules which are randomly oriented when the solution is at rest. These molecules tend to become oriented when they are subjected to shear. The system becomes more fluid and easy to pour, but the insoluble particles may more readily undergo sedimentation. The degree of sedimentation which occurs is directly dependent on the time required for the polymer-molecules to reach the disordered state in which they existed prior to shear. The recovery is very rapid in most pseudoplastic materials, resulting in minimal sedimentation after shaking.

Vegetable gums are subject to bacterial decomposition and should always be preserved to prevent a viscosity decrease due to decomposition. Most manufacturers of modified natural and synthetic gums also recommend preservation of their products. There have been numerous reports of the binding of preservatives by polymeric viscosity-imparting agents, including binding by methylcellulose (Tillman and Kuramoto, 1957), tragacanth (Eisman *et al.*, 1957), methylcellulose, Carbopol, and polyvinylpyrrolidone (deNavarre, 1959), gelatin, polyvinylpyrrolidone, polyethylene glycol 4000, and methylcellulose (Miyawaki *et al.*, 1959),

TABLE III[a]

Pharmaceutical Viscosity Imparting Agents

Viscosity imparting agents and type flow	*Composition*	*Stable pH range*	*Common incompatibilities*	*Appearance in water*	*% w/v for 800 cP apparent viscosity at 20° C*
I. Gums					
Acacia (Pseudoplastic)					
Tragacanth, U.S.P. (Pseudoplastic)	Dried gum tragacanth	2·5–9	Bi subnitrate; over 40% alcohol	Translucent off-white	2·75
Pectin, N. F.	Citrus or apple pectin	2–9	ZnO; over 10% of alcohol	Hazy, incompletely clear	3·2
Kelgin (Med. Visc.)[b]	Granular sodium alginate (Kelgin, Kelgin LV, Kelgin XL)	4–11·5	Ca ion, heavy metal salts, over 10% of alcohol	Clear straw coloured	1·15
Kelgin LV (Low Visc.)		4–11·5			2·05
Kelgin XL (Extra Low Visc.)		4–11·5			3·05
Kelcosol (Hi Visc.)	Fibrous algin	4–11·5			0·75
Kelcoloid HV (Hi Visc.)	Propylene glycol alginate (Kelcoloid HV, Kelcoloid LVF)	2·5–7			0·94
Kelcoloid LVF (Low Visc.) (Pseudoplastic)		2·5–7			1·55
Kraystay Type A (Low Visc.)[c]	Extract of Irish moss (*Chondrus*)	4–10	Cations: esp. K, NH_4, Ca and Mg, over 10% of alcohol	Translucent straw coloured	1·80[i]
Kraystay Type E (Med. Visc.)					1·38
Kraystay Type H (Hi Visc.) (Pseudoplastic)					1·23[i]
Jaguar[d] (Pseudoplastic)	Guar	6–10·5	Gels readily with some ions-borate	Clear to translucent straw coloured	0·2–0·3[k]

II. Cellulosics[e]					
Methylcellulose 15 cP	Methyl ether of cellulose	2–12	Tannins, fairly concentrated salt solutions	Clear	7·7
Methylcellulose 25 cP					6·2
Methylcellulose 100 cP					3·5
Methylcellulose 400 cP					2·4
Methylcellulose 1500 cP					1·7
Methylcellulose 4000 cP (Pseudoplastic)					1·35
CMC (Low Visc.)[f]	Sodium carboxy methyl ether of cellulose	3–11·5	Tannins, cations, fairly concentrated salt solutions	Clear	
CMC (Med. Visc.)					4·1
CMC (Hi Visc.)					1·9
(Pseudoplastic)					0·7
CMHEC 43 (Low Visc.)[f]	Sodium carboxymethyl hydroxymethyl cellulose (non-ionic and ionic combination)	3–11·5	Excellent resistance to electrolytes	Clear	3[k]
CMHEC 37 (Low Visc.)					4[k]
CMHEC 37 (Med. Visc.) (Pseudoplastic)					0·3[k]
III. Clays					
Bentonite (Plastic)	Colloidal Al silicate	3–10	Ca ions, di- and trivalent electrolytes	Light tan	6·3
Veegum[g]	Colloidal Mg Al silicate	3–11	Ca ions	Opaque White	6·0
Veegum HV (Plastic)					4·8
IV. Synthetic High Polymers					
Carbopol[h] (Plastic)	Carboxy vinyl polymer	6–10	Low tolerance to electrolytes	Clear	0·17

[a] Taken from Gerding & Sperandio (1954).
[b] Kelco Co., New York.
[c] Phenix Pabst-ett Co., Chicago.
[d] Stein, Hall & Co., New York.
[e] Dow Chemical Co., Midland, Mich.
[f] Hercules Chemical Co., Wilmington, Del.
[g] R. T. Vanderbilt Co., New York.
[h] B. F. Goodrich Chemical Co., Cleveland.
[i] Measurements made at 98° F.
[k] Measurements made at 25° C.

polyoxizolidones, polyvinylpyrrolidone, and methylcellulose (Deluca and Kostenbauder, 1960), and agar (Quisno *et al.*, 1946). The interaction between a gum and a preservative in aqueous solution does not necessarily mean the solution cannot be preserved. A somewhat higher concentration of preservative may afford an adequate concentration of free unbound preservative. Substituting another preservative may prove effective. There is also evidence to indicate that bound or complexed preservative can exert some antibacterial action.

Both the natural gums and the synthetic polymers have advantages and disadvantages as viscosity-imparting agents. However, the only major disadvantage which the synthetic agents have is their greater interaction with common preservatives, making them more difficult on occasion to protect from decomposition. Disadvantages of the natural hydrophilic gums, include gross impurities such as plant parts, insect or mineral contamination; variations in rheological properties of different lots due to climatic and other geographical factors during growth; rheological variability with time; susceptibility to bacterial growth; and rheological changes with temperature. The increasing use of synthetic polymeric viscosity-imparting agents is thus the result of the many advantages of these products over the more variable natural gums. The literature on the subject of natural and synthetic water-soluble gums is very extensive, and numbers of excellent books are available in the field (Mantell, 1947; Beach, 1954; Whistler and BeMiller, 1959; Eirich, 1958; and Davidson and Sittig, 1962). Some of the compatibility, stability and viscosity properties of the gums, colloidal earths and other viscosity-imparting agents used pharmaceutically are tabulated and shown in Table III (Gerding and Sperandio, 1954).

b. *Miscellaneous viscosity-imparting agents.* There are at least two classes of viscosity-imparting agents which are separate from all previously discussed materials, namely the antithixotropic materials and emulsion vehicles.

Chong *et al.* (1960) report that magnesia magma demonstrates the rheological behaviour known as antithixotropy. Antithixotropy differs from dilatancy and rheopexy in that it is dependent upon the duration as well as the rate of shear. The antithixotropic material is reported to possess good suspending ability while retaining easy pourability. While magnesia magma leaves something to be desired as a palatable suspension or other vehicle, other antithixotropic materials may be found among such synthetic polymers as the polymethacrylic acid esters. However, these may not be acceptable for pharmaceutical use.

Emulsions have been used as suspension vehicles, but have not found wide acceptance for this purpose. Emulsions so used are generally restricted to topical preparations, since emulsions frequently leave an oily feeling in the mouth. It is simpler to prepare a palatable gum solution than a palatable emulsion. However, emulsions can produce very elegant and cosmetic topical suspension vehicles, which may be made as viscous and thixotropic as desired. The emulsion vehicle can furthermore be formulated so as to be substantially non-ionic and compatible with virtually any insoluble material. In topical suspensions which do not contain a high concentration of soluble electrolytes, and in which the oil in the system would not be dermatologically contra-indicated, an emulsion may prove to be a very satisfactory vehicle.

D. RHEOLOGY AND PHARMACEUTICAL PROCESSING

1. *Effects of Rheology on Processing*

A knowledge of the rheology of liquid and semi-solid products can be of considerable importance in selecting the best type of processing equipment to achieve a processing goal or in predicting product quality following machine processing.

a. *Fluids.* The primary objective of fluid mixing is to achieve complete transfer by both horizontal and vertical flow throughout the body of the fluid being processed. In mixing Newtonian or pseudoplastic fluids possessing little structure, no particular problem is ordinarily encountered. In the mixing of pseudoplastic fluids which have considerable thixotropy, or plastics which are shear thinning with high yield values, a large impeller operating at a low shear rate is indicated. A smaller impeller operating at a high shear rate in thixotropic systems will not produce complete liquid turnover and effective mixing. There are a number of excellent discussions of the mixing theory of fluids and the effects of viscosity (Bates, 1959; Sellers and Wilkinson, 1959).

b. *Fluid dispersions.* Oldshue (1959) has suggested the use of two types of impellers in processing disperse systems. To achieve emulsification or dispersion, high shear is needed and is best supplied by a small impeller operating at high speed, providing an intense local zone of action. Once the dispersion has been produced, a high rate of flow with low shear provides the most desirable conditions if continued mixing is required. The lower rate of shear may also be important for secondary processing to prevent undue viscosity breakdown through depolymerization. The high flow–low shear mixing may be achieved at the same power input by simply using a larger impeller operated at lower speed. Oldshue (1961) has presented a recent review of the mixing of solid–liquid dispersions, in which the relationship of viscosity to impeller power consumption is discussed. The power consumption of propellers is reported to be greatly increased above a viscosity of about 500 cP, while the power drawn by a turbine impeller decreases slightly and then returns to the power drawn in water as viscosities increase from 1 to about 10,000 cP.

In the processing of dispersions it has frequently been noted that shear thinning products cause difficulties in homogenizers, especially when the equipment is operated intermittently. The dispersion becomes thicker and eventually "sets up" in the equipment to prevent its proper operation. The same effect may be observed in pumps and in filling equipment when the equipment is used intermittently.

The rheology of suspensions is reported to affect the ease of processing dispersions by ultrasonic equipment (Misek and Skauen, 1958; Araujo and Belcastro, 1958). At a constant acoustical energy the extent of cavitation in a liquid decreases as the viscosity of the liquid increases, which hinders the reduction in size of the dispersed particles. The solution to the problem may be to process the dispersion in the ultrasonic apparatus in the absence of the viscosity-imparting agent, after which the gum may be added.

c. *Semi-solids.* In the mixing of semi-solid materials all dilatant products should be processed with a low shear mixer to prevent a consistency build-up during processing. Thixotropic materials and those with a high yield value become thinner when mixed at high rates of shear, and may be processed at a low energy requirement.

Fischer and Gans (1946) have described the relationships between the rheology of semi-solids and their output from roll or ointment mills. An empirical equation is offered for the relationship between mill characteristics, output and plastic viscosity. Yield value was found to have a negligible effect on the rate of milling, provided the yield value was not so high as to prevent the material from entering the nip of the feed rolls. All dilatant materials adhered well to the rolls and gave a high output corresponding to the high equivalent plastic viscosity of the product at the shearing stress of the mill.

2. *Effects of Processing on Rheology*

a. *Gums in aqueous solution.* It is ordinarily found that the effects of processing on the rheology of aqueous gum solutions are negligible. But sometimes processing operations result in a viscosity decrease brought about by depolymerization, or a viscosity increase caused by increased hydration. These effects have already been discussed under Section III-B-1. Prolonged mechanical shear has been reported to produce a permanent viscosity decrease of 50 per cent or more in sodium alginate solutions (Schwarz and Levy, 1957). On the other hand, the homogenization of tragacanth solutions may increase the initial viscosity of the solutions up to ten-fold (Chambers, 1948; Middleton, 1936; Levy and Schwarz, 1958a) over non-homogenized samples. Meyer and Cohen (1959) have also reported that homogenized tragacanth solutions showed high yield values and produced permanent suspensions while non-homogenized samples demonstrated no appreciable yield values and had poor suspending ability. deButts *et al.* (1957) report a similar effect with solutions of sodium carboxymethylcellulose. Weak gel strength was produced by low shear processing, while good gel strength

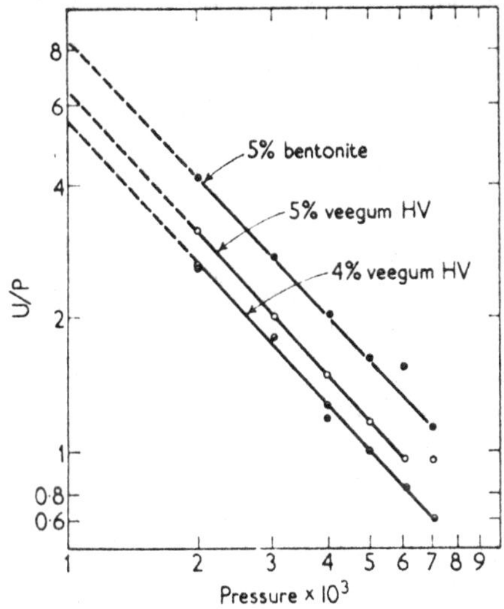

FIG. 37. The relationship between the plastic viscosity of two hydrated colloidal earth products in water, and homogenization pressure (Manton Gaulin two-stage homogenizer with second stage at 500 lb/in²). U is plastic viscosity; P is pressure.

followed high shear milling. However, the use of high shear processing of vegetable gum solutions for the production of greater initial viscosity may not always be a desirable manufacturing technique. Meyer and Cohen (1959) found that after 24 days the viscosity of processed and non-processed tragacanth solutions was equal, whereas the processed sample was initially twice as viscous. After 31 days the unprocessed sample was nearly twice as viscous as the processed sample.

b. *Dispersed systems.* Simon *et al.* (1961) have studied the effect of processing on the rheology of colloidal earth products. Their findings showed that processing substantially increased the yield value and spur value of the hydrated clay dispersions. Processing also affected the plastic viscosity of the dispersions. At higher shear levels the relationship between the plastic viscosity and the operating variable of the equipment is shown in Fig. 37, where U is the plastic viscosity in centipoise, and P is the operating variable in lb/in^2 for homogenizers or r.p.m. for colloid mills and high shear mixers.

Boylan *et al.* (1962) have investigated the temperature-induced rheological changes of an o/w emulsion system containing 8 per cent white wax and 25 per cent oil. They found that emulsions, prepared at 80° C or less and cooled slowly after preparation, were the least thixotropic initially and on ageing. These products also had the most consistent plastic viscosity on ageing. The emulsions which were prepared at the same temperature and cooled at a rapid rate were found by microscopic observation to contain smaller globules. But these globules were highly aggregated, which probably accounted for the greater degree of thixotropy, rheological instability, and rapid separation of water from these systems.

E. BIOLOGICAL APPLICATIONS

Rheology is of some interest in the administration of drugs and in the study of biological fluids, and these topics are briefly discussed in this section.

In at least one case the rheological properties of a system have been used to promote prolonged drug action. Ober *et al.* (1958) report that concentrated (40 to 70 per cent w/v) aqueous procaine penicillin G suspensions are highly thixotropic and possess exaggerated yield values or "T values". Ober's T value corresponds to Levy's (1962b) static yield value or to what other workers term spur value, and is the maximum torque or shearing stress on the initial upcurve. It represents a sharp breakdown point in the structure at a very low rate of shear, and appears on the rheogram as a sharp and fleeting spur (see Y of Fig. 11). The T value was the key to the sustained action of the injectable products of Ober *et al.* Suspensions possessing high T values were very thixotropic, and the authors found that these suspensions first became fluid as they passed through the hypodermic needle, then quickly recovered their structure to form a compact depot in the muscle, thereby providing prolonged therapeutic blood levels. The structural breakdown points or T values were found to be directly related to the specific surface of the powdered penicillin used in the suspensions.

The rate of structural recovery was found by Ober *et al.* to be important and, in fact, is of significance in all suspensions where thixotropy is employed to achieve stability. The rate of structural recovery has recently been studied from a kinetic standpoint (Levy, 1962a).

The viscosity of creams and lotions may affect the rate of absorption of the products by the skin, and their flow properties may be related to the ability of the agents to exert their therapeutic effect. Skauen *et al.* (1949) furthermore report that the consistency of semi-solid vehicles may influence the release of drugs which they contain. A greater release of active ingredients is generally possible from the softer, less viscous bases. The absorption of materials through the skin has been related to diffusion rates (Higuchi, 1960), which in turn are partly influenced by rheological factors (Lin, 1962). Consequently, the viscosity of semi-solid products may affect absorption of these topical products through the intermediate effect of viscosity on diffusion.

Kostenbauder and Martin (1954) attempted to establish ranges of consistency for dermatological ointment bases. In consultation with several dermatologists, they established three classes of ointments having various degrees of hardness and stiffness. Class I consists of ophthalmic ointments which are the softest type; Class II include the common medicated ointments such as boric acid ointment which is soft and unctuous yet stiff enough to remain in place; and Class III consists of the protective ointments such as zinc oxide paste which must be hard and stiff enough to remain in place when applied to moist, ulcerated areas.

The results of the study for Class I and II bases are presented in Table IV. Class III bases were not investigated adequately to provide entries for the table.

TABLE IV

Ranges of Yield Values, f, and Plastic Viscosities, U, for Dermatological Bases

	f, *dyn/cm*^{2}	U, *poises*
Class I Bases	2000–2500	14–18
Class II Bases	5000–12,000	20–26

An extension of this work might prove useful for the classification of official and nonofficial bases. The results would allow the physician to chose a semi-solid base for dermatological application according to desired ranges of consistency.

The majority of the body fluids and secretions have been subjected to rheological study (Frey-Wyssling, 1952). These studies have involved investigations of the relationship between the rheology of body fluids and the diagnosis of disease, determination of fertility, investigations of drug action mechanisms and toxicity at the cellular level, determinations of blood composition, and blood flow through normal and constricted arteries. The fluids which have been studied in greatest detail are protoplasm, blood and cervical secretions. The effects of drug activity (stimulants, anaesthetics, narcotics and smooth muscle relaxants), temperature changes, and mechanical and electrical shock on the flow properties of protoplasm have been studied (Seifriz and Pollack, 1949, 1949a; Seifriz, 1951). The rheology of blood is of considerable interest in studies of normal and abnormal blood and vascular states (Bayliss, 1952; Copley, 1948; Haynes, 1961). The viscosity changes of the cervical fluid appear to be related to ovulation in women (Clift, 1945; Clift *et al.* 1950) and to oestrus in cows. The rheology of milk has been extensively studied, but primarily in terms of a dairy application rather than from a biological viewpoint. Other biological systems studied for their deformation under stress include bone and nerve fibre (Scott-Blair, 1945).

References

Akiya, S., Nomoto, O., and Okui, S. (1949). *J. pharm. Soc. Japan* **69**, 133.

Araujo, O. E., and Belcastro, P. F. (1958). *J. Amer. pharm. Ass., Sci. Ed.* **47**, 307.

Asbeck, W. K., and Baxter, M. K. (1959). *J. Soc. cosmet. Chem.* **10**, 395.

A.S.T.M. Standards (1952). "Tentative Methods of Test for Kinematic Viscosity", A.S.T.M. Designation D445-52T, Part 5, p. 187.

A.S.T.M. Standards (1961). "Method for Penetration of Bituminous Materials", A.S.T.M. Designation D5-61, Part 4, p. 1144, American Society for Testing and Materials, Philadelphia.

Axon, A. (1956). *J. Pharm., Lond.* **8**, 762.

Barnett, G. (1957). *In* "Cosmetics, Science and Technology" (E. Sagarin, Ed.), p. 862. Interscience Publishers, New York.

Barr, G. (1931). "A Monograph of Viscometry", Oxford University Press, London.

Basu, S., Dasgupta, P., and Sincar, A. K. (1955). *J. Colloid Sci.* **10**, 263.

Batdorf, J. B. (1959). *In* "Industrial Gums, Polysaccharides and their Derivatives" (R. L. Whistler and J. N. BeMiller, Eds.), pp. 664–665. Academic Press, New York.

Bates, R. L. (1959). *Industr. Engng. Chem.* **51**, 1245.

Bates, R. L. (1960). *Chem. Eng.* **4**, 145.

Bayliss, L. E. (1952). *In* "Deformation and Flow in Biological Systems" (A. Frey-Wyssling, Ed.), pp. 355–418. Interscience Publishers, New York.

Beach, D. C. (1954). "Natural Plant Hydrocolloids", American Chemical Society, Washington, D.C.

Bechtel, W. G., and Fischer, E. (1949). *J. Colloid Sci.* **4**, 265.

Birdsall, D. H., and Hooten, B. W. (1952). *Industr. Engng. Chem.* (*Anal.*) **24**, 892.

Bolliger, R., and Munzel, K. (1958). *Pharm. Acta Helvet.* **33**, 141.

Boylan, J. C., DeKay, H. G., and Banker, G. S. (1962). *J. pharm. Sci.* **51**, 742.

Bredee, H. L., and deBooys, J. (1940). *Kolloidzschr.* **91**, 1939.

Broughton, G., and Windebank, C. S. (1938). *Industr. Engng. Chem.* **30**, 407.

Broughton, J., and Squires, L. (1938). *J. phys. Chem.* **42**, 253.

Buckingham, E. (1920). *Proc. Amer. Soc. Test. Mater.* **20**, 451.

Cannon, R. M. (1950). "Derivation of the Viscosity Equation and Sources of Error in Viscometry". A private report to the A.S.T.M. Sub-Committee on Viscosity.

Cannon, R. M., and Fenske, M. R. (1938). *Industr. Engng. Chem.* (*Anal.*) **10**, 297.
Cannon, R. M., Manning, R. E., and Bell, J. D. (1960). *Anal. Chem.* **32**, 355.
Chambers, W. P. (1948). *Quart. J. Pharm.* **21**, 44.
Chong, C. W., Eriksen, S. P., and Swintosky, J. V. (1960). *J. Amer. pharm. Ass., Sci. Ed.* **49**, 547.
Chun, A. H. C. (1956). M.S. Thesis, Purdue University; Martin, A. N. (1960). "Physical Pharmacy", pp. 635–636. Lea & Febiger, Philadelphia.
Clift, A. F. (1945). *Proc. roy. Soc. Med.* **39**, 1.
Clift, A. F., Glover, F. A., and Scott-Blair, G. W. (1950). *Lancet* **258**, 1154.
Copley, A. L. (1948). "Proceedings of the International Congress on Rheology", pp. 1–54. North Holland Publishing Co., Amsterdam.
Crosby, E. J. (1960). *Am. Perfumer Arom.*, 1960, **75**, 43.
Davidson, R. L., and Sittig, M. (1962). "Water Soluble Resins", Reinhold Publishing Co., New York.
Davies, R. E. M., and Rowson, J. M. (1957). *J. Pharm., Lond.* **9**, 672.
Davies, J. T., and Mayers, G. R. A. (1960). *Trans. Faraday Soc.* **56**, 691.
deButts, E. H., Hudy, J. A., and Elliott, J. H. (1957). *Industr. Engng. Chem.* **49**, 94.
Deluca, P. P., and Kostenbauder, H. B. (1960). *J. Amer. pharm. Ass., Sci. Ed.* **49**, 430.
deNavarre, M. G. (1959). *Am. Perfumer Arom.*, **73**, 31.
DeWaele, A., and Mardles, E. E. J. (1949). "Proceeding of the International Congress of Rheology", p. 166. North Holland Publishing Co., Amsterdam.
Einstein, A. (1906). *Ann. Physik.* **19**, 289.
Einstein, A. (1911). *Ann. Physik.* **34**, 591.
Eirich, F. (1958). "Rheology, Theory and Applications", Vol. II, Academic Press, New York.
Eirich, F., Bunzl, M., and Margaretha, H. (1936). *Kolloidzschr.* **74**, 276.
Eisman, P. C., Cooper, J., and Jaconia, D. (1957). *J. Amer. pharm. Ass., Sci. Ed.* **46**, 144.
Eyring, H., Hahn, S. J., and Ree, T. (1959). *Industr. Engng. Chem.* **51**, 856; *Spokesman* (Natl. Lubr. Grease Inst. J.) **23**, 129.
Eyring, H., Etsugi, H., Gabrysh, A., Cutler, I. B., and Ree, T. (1960). Paper presented at the 137th Annual Meeting of the American Chemical Society, Cleveland, Ohio, April 6.
Farrow, F., Lowe, G., and Neale, S. (1928). *J. Text. Inst.* **19**, T18.
Fiero, S. W. (1940). *J. Amer. pharm. Ass., Sci. Ed.* **29**, 18.
Fischer, E. K. (1948). *J. Colloid Sci.* **3**, 73.
Fischer, E. K. (1950). "Colloidal Dispersions", Chapter 5., John Wiley and Sons, New York.
Fischer, E. K., and Gans, D. M. (1946). *In* "Colloid Chemistry" (J. Alexander, Ed.), Vol. 6. Reinhold Publishing Co., New York.
Foernzler, E. C., Martin, A. N., and Banker, G. S. (1960). *J. Amer. pharm. Ass., Sci. Ed.* **49**, 249.
Foster, S., Wurster, D., Higuchi, T., and Busse, L. (1951). *J. Amer. pharm. Ass., Sci. Ed.* **40**, 123.
Freundlich, H. (1935). "Thixotropy", Actualités Scientifiques et Industrielles, No. 267, Hermann et Cie., Paris.
Freundlich, H., and Gillings, D. W. (1938). *Trans. Faraday Soc.* **34**, 649.
Frey-Wyssling, A. (1952). "Deformation and Flow in Biological Systems", Interscience Publishers, New York.

Frisch, H. L., and Simha, R. (1956). *In* "Rheology, Theory and Applications" (F. R. Eirich, Ed.), Vol. I, p. 532. Academic Press, New York.

Gabriel, L. (1935). "Technical Aspects of Emulsions", Harvey Publishing Co., London.

Gabrysh, A. F., Ree, T., Erying, H., McKee, N., and Cutler, I. (1961). *Trans. Soc. Rheology* **5**, 67.

Gerding, P. W., and Sperandio, G. J. (1954). *J. Amer. pharm. Ass., Pract. Ed.* **15**, 356.

Green, H. (1941). *Industr. Engng. Chem.* (*Anal.*) **13**, 632.

Green, H. (1942). *Industr. Engng. Chem.* (*Anal.*) **14**, 576.

Green, H. (1949). "Industrial Rheology and Rheological Structures", John Wiley and Sons Inc., New York.

Green, H. (1949a). "Industrial Rheology and Rheological Structures", pp. 80–83, 94, 210–214. John Wiley and Sons Inc., New York.

Green, H. (1949b). "Industrial Rheology and Rheological Structures", p. 47. John Wiley and Sons Inc., New York.

Green, H. (1949c). "Industrial Rheology and Rheological Structures", Chaps. 4 and 5. John Wiley and Sons Inc., New York.

Green, H., and Weltmann, R. N. (1943). *Industr. Engng. Chem.* (*Anal.*) **15**, 201.

Green, H., and Weltmann, R. N. (1944). *J. appl. Phys.* **15**, 414.

Green, H., and Weltmann, R. N. (1946). *Industr. Engng. Chem.* (*Anal.*) **18**, 167.

Green, H., and Weltmann, R. N. (1946a). *In* "Colloid Chemistry" (J. Alexander, Ed.), Vol. VI, p. 328. Reinhold Publishing Co., New York.

Guth, E., and Simha, R. (1936). *Kolloidzschr.* **74**, 266.

Haines, B. A., and Martin, A. N. (1961). *J. pharm. Sci.* **50**, 228, 753, 756.

Hamlow, E. E. (1958). "The Correlation of Several Rheological Methods for Measuring Newtonian and Non-Newtonian Materials", Ph.D. Thesis, Purdue University.

Harper, R. (1953). *In* "Foodstuffs, their Plasticity, Fluidity and Consistency" (G. W. Scott-Blair, Ed.), p. 201. Interscience Publishers Inc., New York.

Hatschek, E. (1928). "Viscosity of Liquids", Bell and Sons, London.

Hatschek, E. (1928a). "Viscosity of Liquids", pp. 239–240, Bell and Sons, London.

Havemeyer, R. N. (1956). *J. Amer. pharm. Ass., Sci. Ed.* **45**, 121.

Haynes, R. H. (1961). *Trans. Soc. Rheology* **5**, 85.

Head, W. F. and Lauter, W. M. (1957). *J. Amer. pharm. Ass., Sci. Ed.* **46**, 617.

Heinrich, H., and Clements, J. E. (1960). *Proc. Sci. Sect., Toilet Goods Assoc.* **33**, 16.

Henderson, N. L., Meer, P. M., and Kostenbauder, H. B. (1961). *J. pharm. Sci.* **50**, 788.

"Hercules Cellulose Gum, Properties and Uses" (1951). p. 6. Hercules Chemical Co., Wilmington, Del.

Higuchi, T. (1960). *J. Soc. cosmet. Chem.* **11**, 85

Houwink, R. and Heinze, P. N. (1938). *Industr. Engng. Chem.* (*Anal.*) **10**, 680.

Janowitz, H. (1950). *Seifen-Öle* **76**, 166.

Jellinek, H. H. G., and White, G. (1951). *J. Polym. Sci.* **6**, 745, 757.

Kabre, S., DeKay, H. G., and Banker, G. S. (1963). "Quantification of the Pseudoplastic Rheology of Pharmaceutical Sols", M.S. Thesis, Purdue University.

Kaufman, G., Finn, W. J., and Harrington, R. J. (1939). *Industr. Engng. Chem.* (*Anal.*) **11**, 108.

Kostenbauder, H. B., and Martin, A. N. (1954). *J, Amer. pharm. Ass. Sci. Ed.*, **43**, 401.

Krieger, I. M., and Maron, S. H. (1951). *J. Colloid Sci.* **6**, 528.
Lauffer, P. G., Barnett, G., Bell, S., Conrad, L. I. and Strianse, S. J. (1958). *J. Soc. cosmet. Chem.* **9**, 111.
Lehne, R. K. (1957). *In* "Cosmetics, Science and Technology" (E. Sagarin, Ed.), p. 573. Interscience Publishers, New York.
Leviton, A., and Leighton, A. (1936). *J. phys. Chem.* **40**, 71.
Levy, G. (1961). *J. pharm. Sci.* **50**, 429.
Levy, G. (1962a). *J. pharm. Sci.* **51**, 952.
Levy, G. (1962b). *J. pharm. Sci.* **51**, 947.
Levy, G., and Schwarz, T. W. (1957). *J. Amer. pharm. Ass., Sci. Ed.* **46**, 562.
Levy, G., and Schwarz, T. W. (1958). *J. Amer. pharm. Ass., Sci. Ed.* **47**, 455.
Levy, G., and Schwarz, T. W. (1958a). *J. Amer. pharm. Ass., Sci. Ed.* **47**, 451.
Lin, T. J. (1962). *In* "The Chemistry and Manufacture of Cosmetics" (M. G. DeNavarre, Ed.), Vol. I, pp. 315–338. VanNostrand Publishing Co., New York.
Lyttleton, D. V., and Traxler, R. N. (1948). *Industr. Engng. Chem.* **40**, 2119.
McKennel, R. (1954). "Proceedings of the Second International Congress of Rheology", p. 356. Butterworth Scientific Publications, London.
McVean, D. E., and Mattocks, A. M. (1961). *J. pharm. Sci.* **50**, 785.
Mantell, C. L. (1947). "Water Soluble Gums", Reinhold Publishing Co., New York.
Mardles, E. W. J., and deWaele, A. (1951). *J. Colloid Sci.* **6**, 42.
Markwood, W. G., Jr. (1951). *Proc. Am. Soc. Test. Mater.* **51**, 441.
Marriott, R. H. (1961). *J. Soc. cosmet Chem.* **12**, 89.
Martin, A. N. (1960). "Physical Pharmacy", p. 602. Lea and Febiger, Philadelphia.
Martin, A. N. (1960a). "Physical Pharmacy", pp. 532–534. Lea and Febiger, Philadelphia.
Martin, A. N. (1960b). "Physical Pharmacy", p. 609. Lea and Febiger, Philadelphia.
Martin, A. N. (1960c). "Physical Pharmacy", p. 615. Lea and Febiger, Philadelphia.
Martin, A. N. (1960d). "Physical Pharmacy", p. 621. Lea and Febiger, Philadelphia.
Martin, A. N. (1960e). "Physical Pharmacy", p. 624. Lea and Febiger, Philadelphia.
Martin, A. N. (1961). *J. pharm. Sci.* **50**, 513.
Metzner, A. B., and Whitlock, M. (1958). *Trans. Soc. Rheology* **2**, 239.
Meyer, R. J., and Cohen, L. (1959). *J. Soc. cosmet. Chem.* **10**, 143.
Michaels, A. S. (1958). *In* "Ceramic Fabrication Process" (W. D. Kingery, Ed.), p. 23. John Wiley and Sons Inc., New York.
Michaels, A. S., and Bolger, J. C. (1962). *Industr. Engng. Chem. Fundamentals* **1**, 24.
Michaels, A. S., and Bolger, J. C. (1962a). *Industr. Engng. Chem. Fundamentals* **1**, 153.
Middleton, G. (1936). *Quart. J. Pharm.* **9**, 493.
Misek, B., and Skauen, D. M. (1958). *J. Amer. pharm. Ass., Sci. Ed.* **47**, 36.
Miyawaki, G. M., Patel, N. K., and Kostenbauder, H. (1959). *J. Amer. pharm. Ass., Sci. Ed.* **48**, 315.
Moness, E., and Giesy, P. M. (1926). *J. Amer. pharm. Ass., Sci. Ed.* **15**, 94.
Mooney, M. (1934). *Industr. Engng. Chem. (Anal.)* **6**, 147.
Moore, F. (1959). *Trans. Brit. Ceram. Soc.* **58**, 470.
Mullins, J. D., and Becker, C. H. (1956). *J. Amer. pharm. Ass., Sci. Ed.* **45**, 105.

Mutimer, M. N., Hill, J. A., Glickman, M. E., and Cyr, G. N. (1956). *J. Amer. pharm. Ass., Sci. Ed.* **45**, 212.

Myers, R. R., and Zettlemoyer, A. C. (1955). *SPE Journal* **11**, 43.

Oakley, H. B. (1936). *Trans. Faraday Soc.* **32**, 1360.

Oakley, H. B. (1937). *Trans. Faraday Soc.* **33**, 372.

Ober, S. S., Vincent, H. C., Simon, D. E., and Frederick, K. J. (1958). *J. Amer. pharm. Ass., Sci. Ed.* **48**, 667.

Oldshue, J. Y. (1959). *J. Soc. cosmet. Chem.* **10**, 332.

Oldshue, J. Y. (1961). *J. pharm. Sci.* **50**, 523.

Osborne, G. E., and Lee, C. O. (1951). *Bull. nat. Formul. Comm.* **19**, 13.

Ott, E., and Elliott, J. H. (1955). *Macromolec. Chemie* **18–19**, 352.

Peter, S., and Stolle, I. (1957). *Z. Physik. chem.* **11**, 251.

Porter, A. W., and Rao, P. A. M. (1927). *Trans. Faraday Soc.* **23**, 311.

Price-Jones, J. (1936). *J. Oil Col. Chem. Ass.* **19**, 295.

Price-Jones, J. (1941). *J. Soc. Instruments* **18**, 39.

Quisno, R. A., Gibby, I. W., and Foter, M. J. (1946). *J. Amer. pharm. Ass., Sci. Ed.* **35**, 317.

Rehbinder, P. (1954). *Disc. Faraday Soc.* **18**, 151.

Reiner, M. (1943). "Ten Lectures on Theoretical Rheology", Interscience Publishers, New York.

Reiner, M., and Riwlin, R. (1927). *Kolloidzschr.* **43**, 1.

Reynolds, O. (1885). *Phil. Mag.* **20**, 469.

Richardson, E. G. (1953). *J. Colloid Sci.* **8**, 367.

Robinson, J. V. (1949). *J. phys. Chem.* **53**, 1042.

Samyn, J. C. (1961). *J. pharm. Sci.* **50**, 517.

Samyn, J. C., and Mattocks, A. M. (1957). *J. Amer. pharm. Ass., Sci. Ed.* **46**, 310.

Schmidt, G. (1940). *Z. physik. Chem.* A**186**, 113.

Schon, S. A., and Fuerst, W. J. (1941). *Dansk. Tidsskr. Farm.* **15**, 34.

Schwarz, T. W., and Levy, G. (1957). *J. Pharm., Lond.* **9**, 672.

Schwarz, T. W., and Levy, G. (1958). *J. Amer. pharm. Ass., Sci. Ed.* **47**, 442.

Schwarz, T. W., Levy, G., and Kawagoe, H. H. (1958). *J. Amer. pharm. Ass., Sci. Ed.* **47**, 695.

Scott-Blair, G. W. (1945). *Pharm. J.* **154**, 3.

Scott-Blair, G. W. (1949). "A Survey of General and Applied Rheology", Ed. 2. Sir Isaac Pitman and Sons, London.

Scott-Blair, G. W. (1960). *J. Sci. cosmet. Chem.* **11**, 181.

Segur, J. B., Whittaker, E. L., and Miner, C. S. (1956). *Food Tech., Champaign* **10**, 625.

Seifriz, W. (1951). *Protoplasma* **40**, 313.

Seifriz, W., and Pollack, H. L. (1949). *J. Colloid Sci.* **4**, 19.

Seifriz, W., and Pollack, H. L. (1949a). *Arch. Sci. Genève* **2**, 9.

Sellers, E. S., and Wilkinson, W. L. (1959). *In* "Cosmetic Science" (A. W. Middleton, Ed.), pp. 183–199. Butterworth Scientific Publications, London.

Serrallach, J. A., Jones, G., and Owen, R. J. (1933). *Industr. Engng. Chem.* **25**, 816.

Shangraw, R., Grim, W., and Mattocks, A. M. (1961). *Trans. Soc. Rheology* **5**, 247.

Sherman, P., Ed. (1963). "Rheology of Emulsions," pp. 1, 43, 73. The Macmillan Company, New York.

Sherman, Y. (1950). *J. Soc. chem. Ind., Lond.* **69**, S-70.

Shotton, E., and White, R. F. (1960). *J. Pharm., Lond.* **12**, 108T.

Sibree, E. (1931). *Trans. Faraday Soc.* **27**, 161.

Sibree, E. (1941). *Trans. Faraday Soc.* **37**, 542.

Simon, T. H., DeKay, H. G., and Banker, G. S. (1961). *J. pharm. Sci.* **50**, 880.

Skauen, D. M., Cyr, G. N., Christian. J. E., and Lee, C. O. (1949). *J. Amer. pharm. Ass., Sci. Ed.* **38**, 618.

Sobue, H., and Ishikawa, K. (1941). *J. Soc. Text. Cellulose Ind.* (*Japan*) **5**, 369.

Storz, G., DeKay, H. G., and Banker, G. S. (1963). "The Interaction of a Macromolecular Ionic and Non-Ionic System. Rheological and Suspension Characteristics", Ph.D. Thesis, Purdue University.

Strianse, S. J. (1957). *In* "Cosmetics, Science and Technology", (E. Sagarin, Ed.) pp. 166–167. Interscience Publishers, New York.

Sumner, O. G. (1940). *Trans. Faraday Soc.* **36**, 272.

Sumner, O. G. (1954). "The Theory of Emulsions and their Technical Treatment", pp. 222–224. The Blakiston Co., New York.

Sweeney, K. H., and Geckler, R. (1956). *J. appl. Phys.* **25**, 1135.

Swindells, J. F. (1947). *J. Colloid Sci.* **2**, 177.

Swindells, J. F., Hardy, R. C., and Cottington, R. L. (1954). *J. Res. nat. Bur. Stand.* **52**, 105.

Taub, A., Meer, W. A., and Claussen, L. W. (1958). *J. Amer. pharm. Ass., Sci. Ed.* **47**, 235.

Tillman, W. J., and Kuramoto, R. (1957). *J. Amer. pharm. Ass., Sci. Ed.* **46**, 211.

Toms, B. A. (1941). *J. chem. Soc.* **54**, 542.

Vand, V. (1948). *J. phys. Chem.* **52**, 277.

Van Wazer, J. R., Lyons, J. W., Kim, K. Y., and Colwell, R. E. (1963). "Viscosity and Flow Measurement—A Laboratory Handbook of Rheology", Interscience Publishers, New York.

Ward, T. H., and Kammermeyer, K. (1940). *Industr. Engng. Chem.* **36**, 622.

Weltmann, R. N. (1943). *J. appl. Phys.* **14, 343.**

Weltmann, R. N. (1956). *J. Soc. cosmet. Chem.* **7**, 599.

Whistler, R. L. (1959). *In* "Industrial Gums, Polysaccharides and their Derivatives" (R. L. Whistler and J. N. BeMiller, Eds.), pp. 6–10. Academic Press, New York.

Whistler, R. L., and BeMiller, J. N., Eds. (1959). "Industrial Gums, Polysaccharides and their Derivatives". Academic Press, New York.

Williams, I. (1924). *Industr. Engng. Chem.* **16**, 362.

Williams, P. S. (1953). *J. appl. Chem.* (*London*), **3**, 120.

Wood, J. H., Catacalos, G., and Lieberman, S. V. (1963). *J. pharm. Sci.* **52**, 296, 375.

Zettlemoyer, A. C., and Lower, G. W. (1955). *J. Colloid Sci.* **10**, 29.

Zettlemoyer, A. C., Lower, G. W., and Walker, W. C. (1953). *J. Colloid Sci.* **8**, 116.

SOLUBILITY IN SYSTEMS CONTAINING SURFACE-ACTIVE AGENTS

B. A. MULLEY

School of Pharmacy, Chelsea College of Science and Technology, London, England[1]

[1] Present address: Pharmacy Department, Bradford Institute of Technology, Bradford 7, England.

I. Introduction

The solubility of materials in solvents is usually not markedly affected by the addition of a third component, unless it is added in high concentration or unless a chemical reaction takes place causing the solute to lose its original identity. The remarkable increase in the solubility of many materials when relatively low concentrations of surface-active agents are present, has therefore attracted a great deal of attention not only for its intrinsic scientific interest, but also because it has found many technical applications. In pharmacy it is frequently desirable to produce a solution in water or other solvents of a drug which is nearly insoluble in the medium, and for this purpose considerable use has been made of the special solvent properties of solutions containing surface-active agents. For example, aqueous solutions have been prepared of oil-soluble vitamins, hormones, steroids, antibacterial compounds and many other medicinally useful materials.

It is a matter of common experience that solutions may be divided, very broadly, into two main types, aqueous and oily. The underlying molecular interactions between molecules forming solutions are also of two types: ionic or dipolar forces predominating in the aqueous, and non-polar or London forces in the oily solutions. It is recognized that the high mutual solubility between molecules of the same class stems from the strong intermolecular interactions between them, while lack of solubility between opposite types is thought to derive from the fact that the attractive forces between like molecules are greater than those between unlike. The result of this is that in mixtures of opposite types the molecules separate into two phases.

Molecules of materials classed as surface-active agents are unusual. Not only do they possess polar and non-polar characteristics, but at least one of the two regions of the molecule is very asymmetrical and of considerable size, as shown in Fig. 1. When such molecules form solutions in water, they do so because of the strong interaction of the polar part with water molecules. However, there are powerful forces opposing solution. In particular, the strong mutual attraction between water molecules is disturbed by the interposition of the non-polar portion of the surface-active agent, and there is strong interaction between this region and the non-polar parts of other surface-active molecules. Because of the mutual attraction of like molecules, surface-active agents have only a limited solubility monomolecularly dispersed in aqueous solution. They are able to remain in solution at higher concentrations by orientating themselves in such a way that the molecular interactions of the different parts of the molecule may be satisfied. This is achieved by

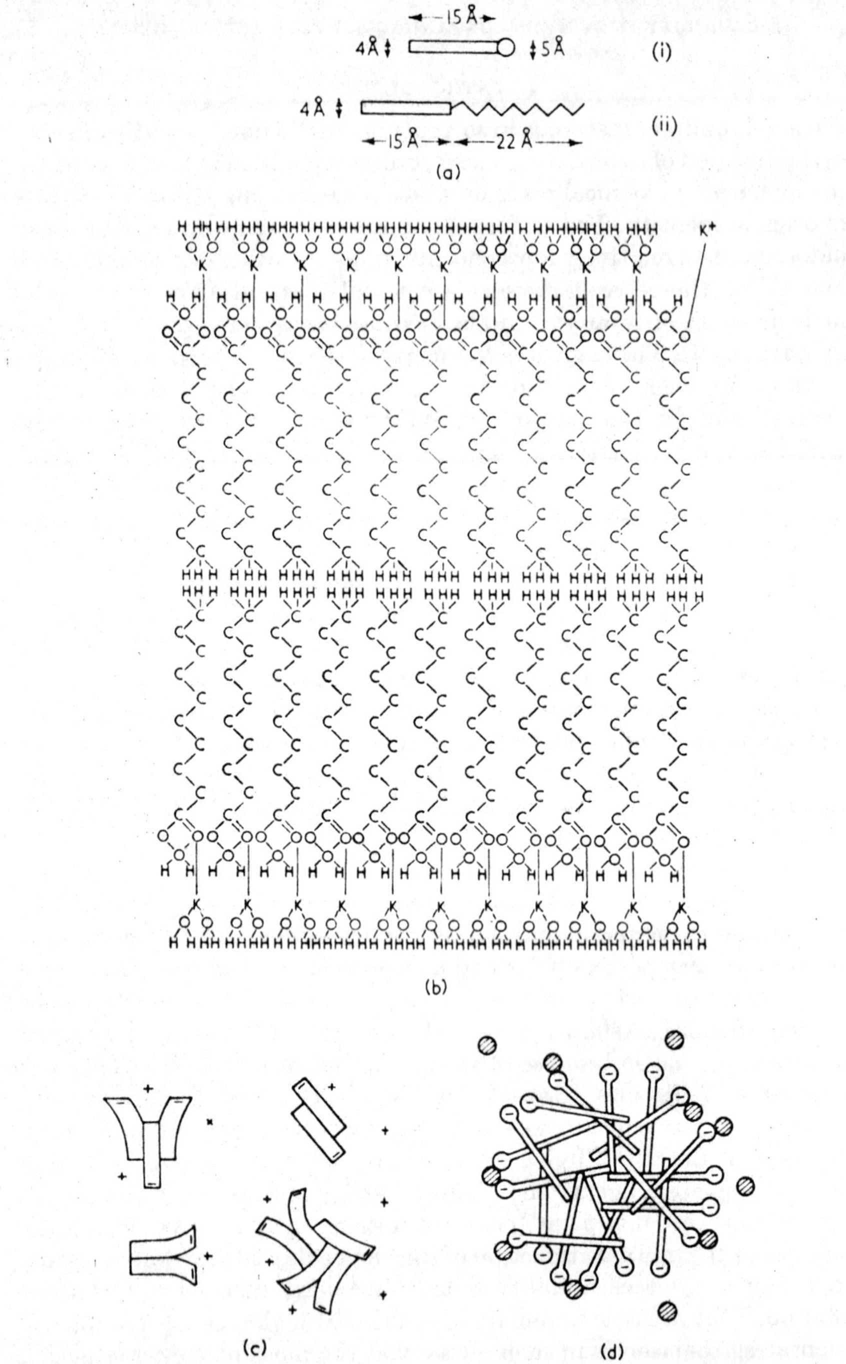

Fig. 1. (*a*) Asymmetric nature of surface-active agents. (i) The approximate dimensions of a C_{12} soap. (ii) Dimensions of a monoalkyl polyether, $C_{12}H_{25}(O.CH_2.CH_2)_6OH$, measured with the ether chain (zig-zag line) fully extended. (*b*) The McBain lamellar micelle ("neutral colloid") (McBain, 1950). (*c*) The McBain spherical ionic micelle (McBain, 1950). (*d*) Hartley spherical micelle (Hartley, 1936).

aggregation of the hydrocarbon chains and orientation of the polar part of the molecule towards the water molecules. The aggregates formed are known as micelles. A developed solution structure of this type would be impossible for less asymmetric materials of lower molecular weight. It is possible to imagine different geometrical arrangements which satisfy the molecular interactions and a number have been proposed. The best known are illustrated in Fig. 1.

The solvent properties of solutions containing surface-active agents are closely bound up with their specialized structure, since in dilute solution, when they are molecularly dispersed, materials of low water solubility do not dissolve in the solution any more than they would in pure water. Above a certain concentration, when physical measurements show the aggregation process previously described to have occurred, the solvent power of the solution is considerably increased. The concentration of surface-active agent at which this occurs is known as the critical concentration for formation of micelles (c.m.c.). It seems as if the micelles provide in the solution, a discrete region of colloidal dimensions, part of which is non-polar in character, in which materials not normally soluble in aqueous solutions can dissolve. This process has been termed solubilization by J. W. McBain.

Solution theory is not sufficiently developed to provide a precise account of solubility even in simple systems, still less so in the ones under discussion. However, there is now a considerable body of information concerning micelles; their form in solution, the critical micelle concentration for various types of surface-active agent, the solubilities of many materials in these solutions, and much useful qualitative explanation of the observed phenomena. Since the Second World War the increased availability of surface-active agents of the non-ionic type has enabled solubilized preparations for internal use to be introduced, and there is now more published information on solubilized systems from a phase equilibrium point of view which improves the descriptive basis of the phenomenon. Phase rule diagrams are particularly useful for formulation purposes, besides giving considerable insight into the nature of the systems. Several comprehensive accounts of solubilization have been given fairly recently which emphasize different aspects of the situation. This article aims to summarize the more important work discussed in these specialized monographs in a relatively simple form, and to give more information on the solubilizing properties of the non-ionic surface-active agents, which are particularly useful pharmaceutically. These compounds have been intensively studied in the last few years, especially since pure materials have been available. A section on phase equilibria in systems containing surface-active agents has been included because phase equilibrium diagrams are particularly useful when discussing the properties of the more concentrated solutions and for predicting behaviour on dilution, which is often necessary in formulation problems. Other aspects likely to be important in formulation, and a review of pharmaceutical products, are dealt with in Section VII. Finally, solubility data not previously collected together in a single source, including results for a number of materials of pharmaceutical importance, have been presented in tabular form.

II. Micelle Formation and Physical Methods of Investigation of Micellar Solutions

A. Theory of Micelle Formation

Although an analysis of micelle formation in terms of the molecular interactions which govern the formation of any solution was not given until the middle thirties (Hartley, 1936), it was recognized by McBain and others about 50 years ago that structures made up of aggregates of individual ions were present in solutions of soaps and other colloidal electrolytes. Agreement between the various workers in the field as to the form of the aggregate and whether one or more forms could co-exist in any one solution, has been much more elusive. The earlier ideas on the structure of the aggregates were mainly derived from conductivity and thermodynamic measurements on fairly concentrated soap solutions. Measurements on more dilute solutions are difficult to interpret because of the possibility of hydrolysis. Later experimental work on other types of surface-active agent, which do not suffer from this disadvantage, enabled measurements to be made on much more dilute solutions. However, two theories, which at first sight seemed to be mutually contradictory, were still propounded by Hartley and McBain. A short historical account of these theories and the experimental work on which they are based is given in the following section. More detailed accounts have been given by the originators of the two theories (Hartley, 1936; Hartley, 1955; McBain, 1950) and critical reviews have been published by other authors (Winsor, 1954; Klevens, 1950; Pethica, 1960; Moilliet *et al.*, 1961).

McBain and his co-workers made conductivity and colligative property measurements on solutions of soaps at concentrations above those now known to be the c.m.c. Some solutions were of such high concentration that a gel was formed, due most probably to the presence of a liquid crystalline phase. Generally, it is important to restrict discussion of micelle formation to the isotropic solutions formed by most surface-active agents at concentrations below those at which liquid

crystalline phases form. This is particularly so when considering micelle formation in the presence of third components since phase equilibrium studies show that a liquid crystalline phase can form at extremely low concentrations (see Section V). The conductivity at the lower concentrations measured by McBain was found to be falling to a minimum and was much less than that expected for a dissociated electrolyte of comparable strength. At higher concentrations the conductivity was found to rise again. At the same time the colligative properties of the solutions indicated that aggregates of some kind were being formed. McBain interpreted these results in terms of formation of particles of two kinds, "neutral colloid", which was thought to be predominant at the lower concentrations, and "ionic micelle" which became more important at the higher concentrations and was based mainly on the necessity of explaining the rise in conductivity in this region. In McBain's view it was not unexpected that dissociation of soap became incomplete with rise of concentration, as might be expected even with strong electrolytes of the more usual kind at high concentrations. The falling conductivity was, therefore, explained as formation of neutral colloid (Fig. 1). Neutral colloid later became identified with the McBain lamellar micelle. This particle also explained the low osmotic activity of the solution. The rise in conductivity which was found at still higher soap concentrations was, therefore, very unusual and was explained by McBain as due to the progressive formation of a homoionic aggregate (without counter ions) which would be highly conducting, more so even than completely dissociated soap in the form of single ions, because the viscous drag on such a particle in the conductivity process would be less, according to Stokes', law, for the aggregate than for the individual ions. According to McBain's later description of this particle (McBain, 1950), the McBain spherical ionic micelle, it was small, containing up to about ten ions. Possible configurations considered by McBain are shown in Fig. 1.

In the thirties, extensive measurements of conductivity over a wide concentration range were made for surface-active agents of differing chemical type. Lottermoser and Puschel (1933) made measurements on *n*-alkyl sulphates, Hartley (1936) studied cetylpyridinium salts and M. E. L. McBain and co-workers (1939) reported data for a range of sulphonic acids of varying chain length. These results were reinforced in certain cases by transport number measurements. Figure 2 shows the typical form of the conductivity curves and of thermodynamic measurements made by freezing-point determinations (M. E. L. McBain and co-workers, 1939). Some transport number measurements are shown in Fig. 3. The more extensive data available in the thirties was reinterpreted by G. S. Hartley (1936). One of his main objections to the earlier interpretation lay in explaining why the process of decreased dissociation and consequent formation of neutral colloid should become reversed at higher concentrations in favour of the ionic micelle. He also thought that

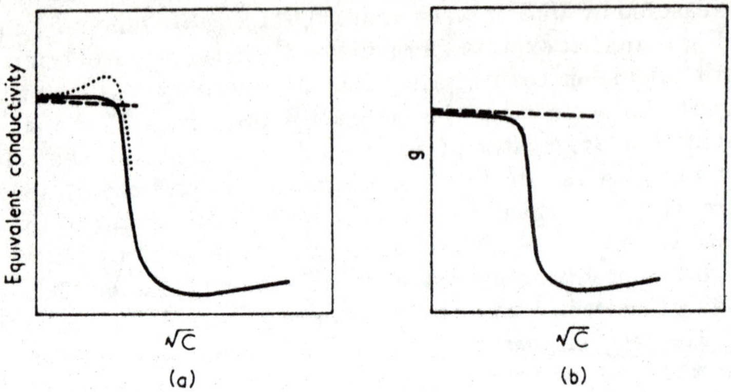

FIG. 2. (*a*) Typical curve of equivalent conductivity of a surface-active agent plotted against the square root of its concentration. The dotted line is obtained at high field strengths, with double chain salts or with other atypical surface-active agents. (*b*) Osmotic coefficient *g* against the square root of the concentration. The broken lines are the theoretical Debye-Huckel-Onsager slopes.

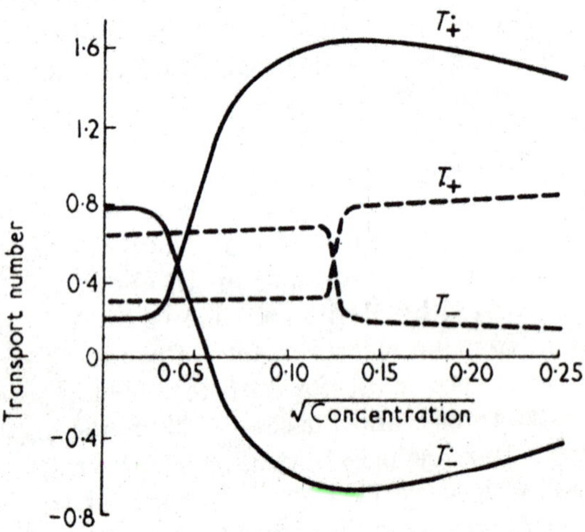

FIG. 3. Transport numbers of positive and negative radicals of ionic surface-active agents. Broken lines dodecylamine hydrochloride at 60° C. Full lines cetylpyridinium bromide at 35° C (from Moilliet *et al.*, 1961).

the lamellar micelle was unlikely to form, on the grounds that it had a pseudocrystalline structure and was highly asymmetric, whereas the solutions under discussion were isotropic and density measurements indicated the fluid nature of the solutions. At very low concentrations Hartley thought the compounds were completely dissociated, the conductivity being very close to that expected for a strong uni-univalent electrolyte. At the c.m.c. he considered the long chain ions begin to aggregate, for the reasons described in the introduction, to form particles that are spherical in shape, containing about fifty ions. Hartley visualized the micelle as having a number of counter ions attached to it (Fig. 1) by reason of the high charge that would otherwise be associated with the particle. In his view the fall in conductivity in the region of the c.m.c. was due to the low mobility of the micelle because of its associated counter ions and also because the ions attached to the micelle were no longer available to carry the current in the opposite direction. Transport number measurements especially were taken to be in agreement with these views since they showed that the conductivity of the paraffin radical rose at the c.m.c. (Stokes effect) whereas that of the other ion fell below zero, which meant that the overall fall in conductivity was due to the counter ions being carried in the other direction. According to Moilliet and his co-authors (1961), neither the negative transport number nor its rapid change with concentration is adequately explained by postulating a decrease in the degree of dissociation or the formation of almost neutral micelles. Either would account for a decrease in total conductivity but both require the mobilities of the two radicals to decrease in about the same proportion. In fact the transport number of the long chain ion increases rapidly while that of the counter ion falls (Fig. 3).

Hartley was also much influenced by a picture of micelle formation from the point of view of the law of mass action, which he had developed (Murray and Hartley, 1935) from earlier work by others (Jones and Bury, 1927; Davies and Bury, 1930). If a micelle contains m simple molecules and C is the stoichiometric concentration of surface-active agent, x the fraction aggregated and K the equilibrium constant (Alexander and Johnson, 1950) then:

$$\text{(concentrations)} \qquad \frac{m \text{ single molecules}}{C(1-x)} \rightleftharpoons \frac{\text{micelle}}{Cx/m}$$

The equilibrium constant

$$K = \frac{\text{micelles}}{[\text{single molecules}]^m} = \frac{Cx/m}{[C(1-x)]^m}$$

It may be shown if K is given any arbitrary value, how x varies with C for various values of m. It is found that when m is large (20 or more) the fraction of the surface-active agent existing as micelles, undergoes a sharp change at a particular concentration which is somewhat analogous to a phase change, and further that the concentration of single molecules above this concentration is approximately constant. These relationships are shown in Fig. 4. The form of the curves in Fig. 4 is independent of the actual value of K, only the position of the sharp change in properties being affected. The sharp breaks in conductivity, colligative property and transport number curves at the c.m.c. were thus to be expected.

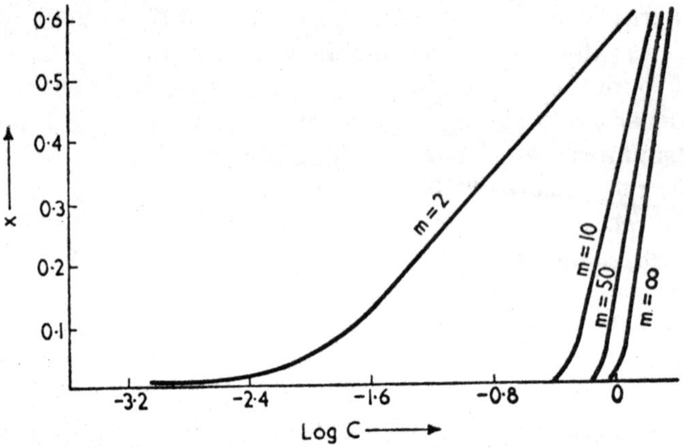

FIG. 4. Diagram illustrating that if micelle formation is a mass action process there is a critical concentration (c.m.c.) at which the fraction of solute present as aggregate changes abruptly when the aggregation number is high (from Murray and Hartley, 1935).

Hartley also considered that if an appreciable part of the surface-active agent formed particles of smaller size below the c.m.c., then the breaks in the property-concentration curves would be blurred. In his view the form of the curves made the formation of such particles unlikely. Hartley thought that the slow rise in conductivity at higher concentrations could not be due to the Stokes effect since transport number measurements show the conductivity of the long chain ions to be falling in this region. Hartley considered two possible mechanisms. The first was a loosening of the binding of the counter ions to the micelle, caused by the possibility of interaction of ionic atmospheres between micelles, which must be closer together in the more concentrated solutions. This idea seems similar to McBain's postulate of the increasing formation of a highly charged micelle. The other possible mechanism Hartley suggested was an increase in the mobility of the free ions.

McBain has maintained his interpretation of micelle formation in his more recent account (1950) and has tended to focus attention on the region near the c.m.c. The conductivity here is just above that predicted by the theoretical Onsager slope and in some cases, where the counter ion is iodate or where the lipophilic part of the molecule is a double chain, there is quite a sharp rise in conductivity at concentrations near the onset of micelle formation (Fig. 2*a*) (McDowell and Kraus, 1951). This, together with the fact that the osmotic coefficient is below that expected for an ideal electrolyte (Fig. 2*b*), was considered by McBain as being due to the formation of the small homoionic micelle. The shapes of the conductivity curves in certain of these cases are very similar to those obtained by Hartley for the compound cetylpyridinium chloride when studied at high field strengths. The influence of ionic atmospheres, which decrease conductivity, can be lessened if high field strengths are used during the measurements (Wein effect in ordinary electrolytes), and Hartley considered the rise in his case to be the Stokes effect supervening once the gegenions were removed from the micelle by the high field. The low mobility of the iodate ion has been suggested as the reason for the rise in conductivity of certain iodates, the counter ions being unable to maintain contact with the micelle (Moilliet and coauthors, 1961). In the case of the double chain compounds the rise has also been attributed to less firm binding of the counter ions, because in this case there may be a lower concentration of charges per unit area of the micelle surface (Winsor, 1954). Winsor has also suggested an alternative mechanism for the rise in conductivity in the concentrated solutions. This was by a migration of the counter ions along the micelle surface, which by Winsor's theory of micelle formation (see Section III) would tend to be nearer the lamellar type micelle in this region.

X-ray diffraction methods have been used to study solutions containing micelles in the hope of obtaining direct evidence of the structure present. Most of the interpretations have been made on the assumption that the diffraction patterns were Bragg spacings and the repeating distances were calculated by Bragg's method. The derived distances were then interpreted in relation to the forms proposed for micelles, especially those of the McBain theory. A review of the work up to 1950 has been given by Phillippoff (1950). Doubts have been expressed as to the propriety of treating the diffraction patterns as true Bragg spacings (Fournet, 1951).

Disregarding diffraction bands caused by water, three different bands have been found. (1) "S-band" or short spacing band, indicating a regularly repeating distance in the solution of 4–5 Å. This band does not vary with the solution concentration. (2) "M-band" with a spacing which varies with the chain length of the surface-active agent but is approximately independent of concentration. (3) "I-band" or long spacing band which indicates a repeating distance in the solutions greater than the first two, but decreasing with concentration of the surface-active agent. None of the bands are found in very dilute solution but the S- and M-bands have been observed at concentrations of about 5 per cent and the I-band at concentrations of about 10 per cent. These concentrations are above those on which most of the other measurements previously discussed were made. Interpretation of the S-band generally agrees that it corresponds to the thickness of the hydrocarbon chain, very similar bands being found in simple liquids containing such chains. The M-band also seems to be unequivocally associated with twice the length of a fully extended hydrocarbon chain because in solutions of any

TABLE I

Variation of M Spacings of Solutions of Surface-active Agents Compared with the Molecular Dimensions (M spacings from Matoon and co-workers, 1948).

Surface-active agent (% *w/w*)	*M Spacing* (Å) *averaged over conc. range studied*	*Twice the molecular length from "Catalin" models* (Å)
Potassium caprylate (C_8) 6–44%	29·7	30
Potassium caprate (C_{10}) 8–12%	31·7	35
Potassium laurate (C_{12}) 5–20%	35·3	40
Potassium myristate (C_{14}) 2–16%	40·3	45
Potassium palmitate (C_{16}) 1–5%	47·3	50
Sodium lauryl sulphate (C_{12}) 8–25%	37·3	40

one compound it is independent of concentration and fits all theories of micelle structure (Fig. 5) and because it increases with the alkyl chain length of the surface-active agent (Table I).

Interpretation of the I-band is more controversial. At first it was assumed that diffraction could only occur from planar spacings between micelles and strong support was thus given to the lamellar micelle. The increasing distance d_I which occurs when the proportion of water in the system is increased was also thought to be explained by this model, because this would be expected if the water was incorporated between the lamellar micelles (Fig. 5). However, Hartley (1949) pointed out that the increase in d_I was not great enough to account for all the water added on dilution and that part of it on this model must be incorporated in another way. He reinterpreted the data in terms of the spherical micelle, which he considered would be fixed in hexagonal array at the high concentrations under discussion, by the mutual repulsion between their charged atmospheres. If the long spacing corresponded to the distance between comparable regions of the micelles in this geometrical arrangement, he found that the expansion of the I-spacing was close to that expected for the degree of dilution producing the change.

In the last few years important evidence on the form of micelles in solution has been obtained by the light-scattering technique. Not only does the method give information about micellar "molecular weight",

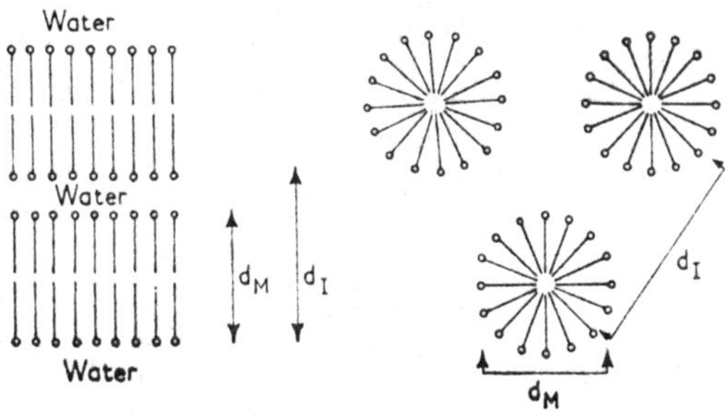

FIG. 5. The McBain lamellar micelle and the Hartley spherical micelle and the spacings supposed to give rise to the M and I diffraction haloes (gegenions not shown).

but by dissymmetry measurements it may also be used to determine the shape of the particles. The theoretical basis of light scattering was developed by Debye (for references see Table II). M. E. L. McBain and Hutchinson (1955) have given a critique of the method and a recent review in two parts has been presented by Robinson (1960). Table II shows some of the results which have been obtained. For paraffin chain salts the longer the alkyl chain length the higher the micelle molecular weight and the larger the number of molecules per micelle. Addition of salt to a solution always increases the size of the micelle. The alkyl chain length also seems to increase the micelle size in solutions of nonionic compounds, but increasing the ethylene oxide chain length has the reverse effect. The results in Table II and the dissymmetry measurements which have been made are consistent with the spherical Hartley micelle for most of the straight chain compounds. In the presence of salt or solubilized components (particularly long chain alcohols), or in the case of double chain salts, the size of the micelle increases and the molecules could not be accommodated in a sphere. Using light scattering results, Tartar (1955) calculated the micelle dimensions, assuming that

TABLE II

Micellar Molecular Weights and Aggregation Numbers for Anionic, Cationic and Non-ionic Surface-active Agents from Light Scattering Measurements

Compound	*Solvent*	*Temperature (°C)*	*Micellar M.W.*	*Aggregation No.*
$C_{10}H_{21}(CH_3)_3NBr$[a]	Water		10,200	36·4
$C_{12}H_{25}(CH_3)_3NBr$[a]	Water		15,500	50·3
$C_{14}H_{29}(CH_3)_3NBr$[a]	Water		23,500	75·2
$C_{12}H_{25}NH_3Cl$[a]	Water		12,300	55·5
$C_{12}H_{25}NH_3Cl$[a]	0·01574 M NaCl		20,500	92·4
$C_{12}H_{25}NH_3Cl$[a]	0·04598 M NaCl		31,400	141·6
$C_{10}H_{21}SO_4Na$[b]	Water	23°	13,000	50
$C_{12}H_{25}SO_4Na$[b]	Water	23°	20,500	71
$C_{14}H_{29}SO_4Na$[b]	0·01 M NaCl	23°	43,500	138
$C_{12}H_{25}SO_4Na$[c]	Water	22°	23,000	80
$C_{12}H_{25}SO_4Na$[c]	0·02 M NaCl	22°	27,000	94
$C_{12}H_{25}SO_4Na$[c]	0·4 M NaCl	22°	36,200	126
$C_8H_{17}SO_3Na$[b]	Water	23°	5500	25
$C_{10}H_{21}SO_3Na$[b]	Water	30°	9900	40
$C_{12}H_{25}SO_3Na$[b]	Water	40°	14,700	54
$C_{14}H_{29}SO_3Na$[b]	Water	60°	24,000	80
$(C_{12}H_{25}SO_3)_2Mg$[b]	Water	60°	28,600	107
$(C_8H_{17})(CH_3)_3NSO_3C_{10}H_{21}$[d]	Water		89,700	456
Octylphenol with 10 EtO units[e]	Water	23°	53,500–208,000	
$C_8H_{17}(O.CH_2.CH_2)_6OH$[f]	Water		12,450	32
$C_{12}H_{25}(O.CH_2.CH_2)_6OH$[f]	Water		84,600	188
$C_{12}H_{25}(O.CH_2.CH_2)_{23}OH$[g]	Water		37,000–48,000	
$C_{10}H_{21}(O.CH_2.CH_2)_8OCH_3$[h]	Water	30°	43,100	83
$C_{10}H_{21}(O.CH_2.CH_2)_8OCH_3$ in the presence of *n*-decane[h]	Water	30°	45,600–90,700	87–162
$C_{10}H_{21}(O.CH_2.CH_2)_8OCH_3$ in the presence of *n*-decanol[h]	Water	30°	47,800–210,300	89–351
$C_{10}H_{21}(O.CH_2.CH_2)_{11}OCH_3$[h]	Water	30°	42,900	65
$C_{10}H_{21}(O.CH_2.CH_2)_{11}OCH_3$ in the presence of *n*-decane[h]	Water	30°	44,800–54,300	67–80
$C_{10}H_{21}(O.CH_2.CH_2)_{11}OCH_3$ in the presence of *n*-decanol[h]	Water	30°	52,600–122,000	75–158
$C_{16}H_{33}(O.CH_2.CH_2)_9OH$[i]	Water		140,000	
$C_{16}H_{33}(O.CH_2.CH_2)_{12}OH$[i]	Water		1'7,000	

[a] Debye (1949); [b] Tartar and Lelong (1955), Tartar (1955); [c] Phillips and Mysels (1955); [d] Anacker (1953); [e] Kushner and Hubbard (1954), Kushner *et al.* (1957); [f] Corkill *et al.* (1961); [g] Becher and Clifton (1959); [h] Nakagawa and co-workers (1960); [i] Elworthy and MacFarlane (1962a).

the shape would be either a sphere or an oblate spheroid. He found that the number of molecules of straight chain salts per micelle was consistent with spherical or near spherical micelles, but double chain salts or inorganic salts in the solution gave numbers which were consistent with oblate spheroids of increasing eccentricity. The other results in the table, some of which are from later work and not, therefore, considered by Tartar, also agree with this view.

In conclusion it seems that in solutions of straight chain surface agents which are isotropic and below concentrations at which crystal or liquid crystal phases are formed, the evidence favours the formation of micelles of relatively small aggregation number which probably correspond closely to the Hartley spherical micelle. In the presence of salts or solubilized materials the micelles are larger and with increasing proportion of the third component at least one dimension becomes greater than twice the length of the extended hydrocarbon chain. The geometrical form of these micelles is not certain, oblate spheroids being favoured by some authors and lamellar micelles by others. It should also be realized that a solution is a dynamic system and that the micelles, though having a predominant or equilibrium form, are continually breaking down and reforming. This leads to fluctuations about the average structure (Winsor, 1954). Dervichian (1954) has stated that each solution will have a different micellar form depending on the concentration and nature of the surface-active agent and the other constituents of the solution. The average form, however, seems to be close to the spherical micelle over considerable concentration ranges but changes near the phase boundaries of the isotropic solution region, especially when salts or other solutes are present in the system.

B. METHODS OF MEASURING C.M.C.

The c.m.c. of a surface-active agent in water may be affected by the addition of a third component. However, in many cases, dilution of a solubilized preparation below the c.m.c. will result in the precipitation of the solute. A knowledge of the c.m.c., besides being useful in solubility measurements, is important because the c.m.c. corresponds to the concentration at which a radical change in the physical properties of the solution takes place, and this is a major factor in the practical use of surface-active agent solutions. For example, the antibacterial activity of phenols and other compounds in the presence of surface-active agents is very much affected by micelle formation.

Almost any physical property of a solution containing a surface-active agent changes sharply at the c.m.c. and may be used to measure it: the surface-tension, dye and conductivity methods have been particularly widely used.

1. *Surface-tension Method*

Below the c.m.c. the surface-tension of a surface-active agent solution falls rapidly with increase in concentration, usually proportionally to the logarithm of the concentration. This relationship does not hold in very dilute solution. Above the c.m.c. the surface-tension is independent of concentration. The c.m.c. is usually taken to be the point of intersection of the extrapolated straight lines of these two parts of the surface-tension

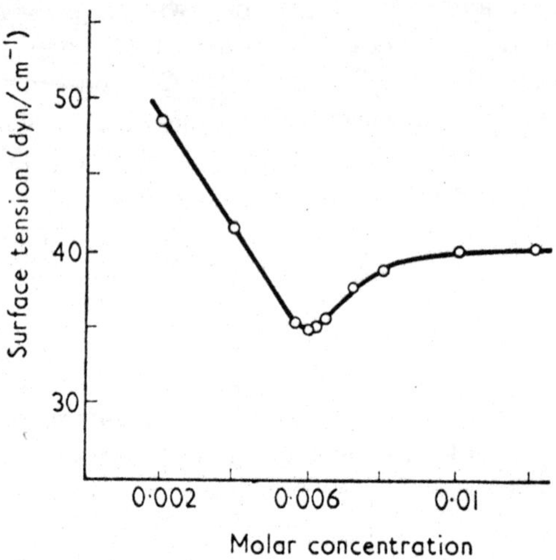

FIG. 6. Surface-tension concentration curve for sodium dodecyl sulphate at 20° C (from Powney and Addison, 1937).

curve (Williams and co-workers, 1955). Although this method of plotting implies that micelles form at one concentration this is not so, but the break in the curve does occur over a very narrow range, a convenient figure for the c.m.c. being given by this method of treating the results. The general form of the curve is satisfactorily explained by the description of micelle formation given by the law of mass action. If the surface-active species is the single molecule, then below the c.m.c. the surface-tension falls rapidly with increase in concentration since the concentration of single molecules is increasing. Above the c.m.c. the concentration of single molecules remains approximately constant and therefore the surface-tension remains constant. In practice, the surface-tension curve of many detergents is modified and frequently shows a dip near the c.m.c. (Fig. 6). This has made interpretation difficult for earlier workers since it was hard to see how negative adsorption (increase in surface-tension) could occur when the concentration of the surface-active agent was increasing. Some doubted whether Gibb's equation applied to colloidal electrolytes. Murray's suggestion (1935) that the single ions reached a maximum concentration seemed a possible explanation, but later work has shown that the dip is due to impurities in the surface-active agent and that when these are removed, no dips are found. The surface-tension curve was therefore that of a two component mixture. Below the c.m.c. the concentration of both species increase with concentration but near the c.m.c. the micelles compete with the surface for the

TABLE III

C.m.c. of Some Surface-active Agents Measured by Surface-tension

	c.m.c. (M)						
	C_8	C_{10}	C_{11}	C_{12}	C_{14}	C_{16}	C_{18}
Sodium alkyl sulphates at 50° C (Lange, 1957; Kling and Lange, 1957)	$9 \cdot 8 \times 10^{-2}$	$3 \cdot 2 \times 10^{-2}$	—	8×10^{-3}	2×10^{-3}	$6 \cdot 5 \times 10^{-4}$	$1 \cdot 9 \times 10^{-4}$
N-alkyl *NN*-dimethylglycines at 23° C (Beckett and Woodward, 1963)	$1 \cdot 7 \times 10^{-1}$	$1 \cdot 8 \times 10^{-2}$	$6 \cdot 6 \times 10^{-3}$	$1 \cdot 8 \times 10^{-3}$	$1 \cdot 8 \times 10^{-4}$	$2 \cdot 0 \times 10^{-5}$	—

fixed ratio of impurity and therefore it was possible for the concentration of single molecules to fall and the rise in surface-tension to occur (Alexander, 1942; Alexander and Johnson, 1950).

The surface-tension method has been applied to many types of surface-active agent, and some results are shown in Table III.

A difficulty occurs when the surface-tension method is applied to the longer alkyl chain compounds, because with these prolonged ageing of the surface is found. The ageing is particularly marked below the c.m.c., and can result in a gradual fall of surface-tension over a period of some hours. If the method of measuring surface-tension takes no account of ageing then there is uncertainty in the c.m.c. derived from the surface-tension curve, since different concentrations may be ageing at different rates. This is probably the explanation for differences in c.m.c. of nominally identical non-ionic surface-active agents reported recently (Table IV) of C_{16} alkyl chain length, whereas good agreement was found for shorter chain compounds prepared and measured by the same workers. For longer chain compounds it is therefore better to choose an experimental method allowing ready measure of surface ageing, for example the Wilhelmy plate, rather than the Du Nouy ring method. Whether the surface-ageing phenomena reflects non-equilibrium conditions in the bulk solution is uncertain. Carless, Challis and Mulley (1964) found good agreement between c.m.c. values measured by surface-tension and the iodine method, the latter presumably reflecting conditions in the bulk solution, whereas the c.m.c. by a surface-tension method which allows for ageing of the surface is much lower.

TABLE IV

C.m.c. (M.) for Non-ionic Surface-active Agents Measured by Surface-tension

Compound	*Carless* et al. (J. Colloid Sci., *in the press*)	*Elworthy and MacFarlane,* (1962b)	*Corkill* et al., (1961)	*Lange*, 1959; (1960)
$C_{16}E_6$	$9{\cdot}9 \times 10^{-5}$ (27°)	$1{\cdot}6 \times 10^{-6}$ (25°)	$1{\cdot}0 \times 10^{-6}$ (25°)	—
$C_{16}E_9$	$3{\cdot}6 \times 10^{-5}$ (20°)	2×10^{-6} (25°)	—	7×10^{-4} ($C_{16}E_{10}$)
$C_{12}E_6$	$8{\cdot}2 \times 10^{-5}$ (20°)	—	$8{\cdot}7 \times 10^{-5}$ (25°)	$8{\cdot}0 \times 10^{-5}$ (25°, $C_{12}E_7$)

Moilliet *et al.* (1961) have recently reviewed the literature on surface ageing.

2. *Dye and Iodine Methods*

Colour changes in indicator solutions in the presence of surface-active agents of opposite charge were first reported by Hartley, and the principle was used by Corrin and Harkins (1947) as a method of determining the c.m.c. The method is particularly useful because it may be rapidly carried out and needs only simple apparatus. The commonest dye used for anionic compounds is pinacyanol chloride. At concentrations below the c.m.c. solutions of the dye in the presence of an anionic surface-active agent are reddish in colour; above the c.m.c. the solutions become blue. A solution of the detergent and the dye above the c.m.c. are titrated with an aqueous solution of the dye (same concentration as in the detergent solution) until the first visible colour change is found. This is the c.m.c. With other dyes the fluorescent properties may change at the c.m.c. The colour changes have been investigated spectroscopically. Above the c.m.c. two bands are found at 570 mμ (α-band) and 615 mμ (β-band). The intensity of the bands increases with the concentration of the surface-active agent. Below the c.m.c. these two bands are of low intensity and a third band is found at 480 mμ (γ-band). The mechanism by which these spectral changes are brought about was generally considered to be that above the c.m.c. solubilization of the dye in the hydrocarbon interior of the micelle in monomeric form, accounts for the α- and the β-bands, because these are also found in organic solvents containing the dye. In water the absorption is at 550 mμ. Corrin and Harkins considered that the shifts could also be due to changes in aggregation of the dye because such changes are known to affect its spectrum. An investigation of other dyes failed to resolve the mechanism because in many cases no change in the spectra occurred and in others the shift did not correspond to that expected in a hydrocarbon-type environment. For example, in the case of Sky Blue FF (an anionic dye), solutions in a cationic detergent above its c.m.c. had the same colour as those in water. Below the c.m.c. the colour was different to that found in either of these environments. It seems unlikely in this case that the mechanism of the colour change is due to solution in the hydrocarbon interior of the micelle.

The dye method suffers from a number of disadvantages. Klevens (1947) found the result to be always below values determined by other methods, showing that the dye must interfere to some extent with micelle formation. Winsor (1948) used the method on a number of isomeric tetradecane sulphates and found that the colours varied with time, making the results somewhat uncertain. He noted that the c.m.c. was sometimes above and sometimes below values determined by other methods and appeared to depend on the position of the sulphate group in the alkyl chain. Although the dye method gives an approximate result it is hardly surprising that it may differ from those methods where no third component is present. For instance, Mukerjee and Mysels (1955) found with pinacyanol and sodium laurylsulphate that the colour below the c.m.c. was due to formation of a simple insoluble salt

$$C_{25}H_{25}N_2SO_4(CH_2)_{11}CH_3$$

between the large oppositely charged ions, which remained suspended in an apparently clear solution, especially if excess detergent was present. The colour could be removed if the "solution" was centrifuged. Above the c.m.c. the salt was solubilized by the detergent and the blue colour was then due to the dye being in the state found in ordinary organic solvents. The c.m.c. obtained by the dye method therefore depends on a number of factors, especially the concentration of the dye used (Fig. 7) and the c.m.c. of the detergent. The spectral changes which occur at the c.m.c. are shown in Fig. 8.

The dye method has been applied to non-ionic materials. The colour

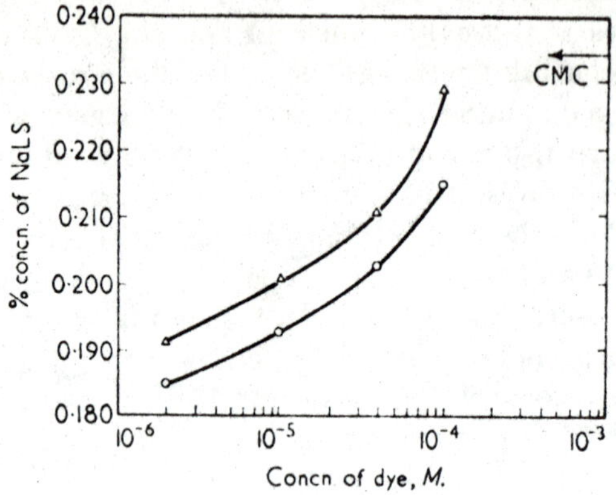

FIG. 7. Effect of concentration of pinacyanol upon the apparent c.m.c. measured by the maximum slope of spectral change (circles) and the levelling of the γ-band (triangles) (from Mukerjee and Mysels, 1955).

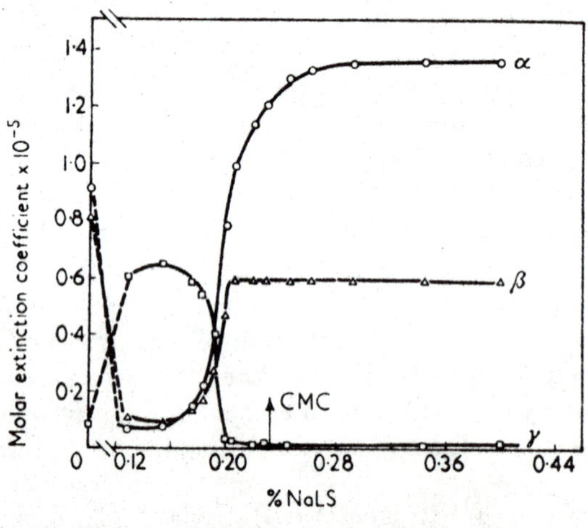

FIG. 8. Extinction coefficients at the band maxima of pinacyanol in water and in the presence of sodium dodecyl sulphate; dye conc. 1×10^{-5} M; band maxima: in water α 600 mμ, β 550 mμ; in sodium dodecyl sulphate solution, α 610 mμ, β 562 mμ, γ 485 mμ (from Mukerjee and Mysels, 1955).

changes produced are less than those found in the presence of ionic surface-active agents and can only be detected spectrophotometrically. Goto, Sugano and Koizumi (1953) measured the spectra of pinacyanol in water and in various concentrations of the non-ionic alkyl ether

$C_{12}H_{25}(O.CH_2.CH_2)_6OH$ (abbreviated to $C_{12}E_6$). Only α- and β-bands were found and both λ_{max} and E_{max} changed with concentration of the surface-active agent. These authors found the c.m.c. by plotting optical density at the absorption maxima against concentration of the surface-active agent. The break found was not sharp but occurred at about 10^{-4} M. The blurred nature of the break seems to be due to the impure character of many samples of non-ionic detergents which consist of

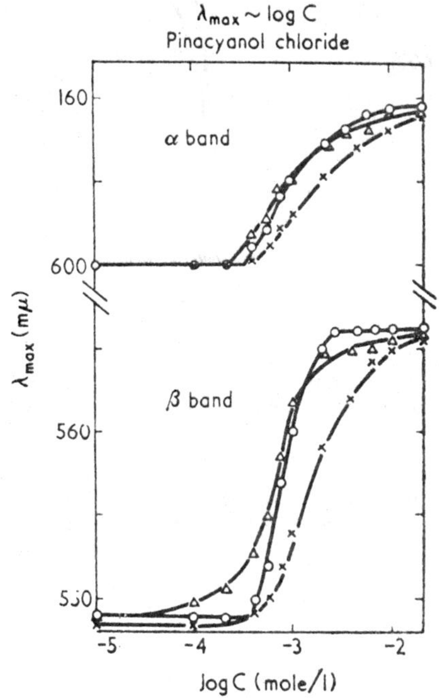

FIG. 9. The effect of molecularly distilled fractions of a dodecyl monoalkyl polyether on the α- and β-bands of pinacyanol chloride (from Nakagawa, 1958a) (see text).

mixtures of varying polyglycol chain length. This point is illustrated by more extensive measurements made on a similar compound (Nakagawa, 1958a). He used a lauryl ether which was molecularly distilled into fractions and then investigated the c.m.c.'s of three samples. The first was a fraction of average molecular weight 440 which corresponds to the formula $C_{12}E_6$. A second sample was made from three fractions of average molecular weight, 362, 440, and 472 respectively, and the third was undistilled raw material. Several dyes were used in the detection of the c.m.c. and the results were checked by other methods. All methods showed breaks in the property-concentration curve at the c.m.c. which were sharper in the order single fraction > mixed fraction > raw undistilled material. Some of Nakagawa's results are shown in Figs. 9 and 10 and in Tables V and VI. He considered that the mechanism of the

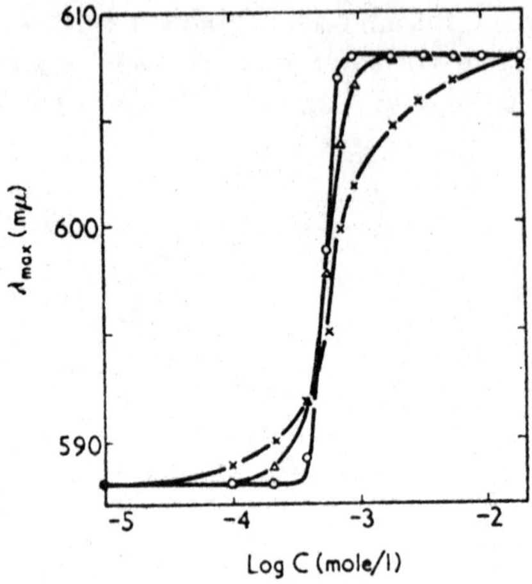

FIG. 10. The effect of molecularly distilled fractions of a dodecyl monoalkyl polyether on the spectrum of Tripan Blue (from Nakagawa, 1958a).

TABLE V

λ_{max} and ϵ of Pinacyanol Chloride in Various Solvents (from Nakagawa, 1958a)

Solvent	λ_{max} (*mμ*)	$\epsilon \times 10^{-4}$	*Dye conc.* (*mole*/*l*)
Water	ca. 525[a]	ca. 1·70	$1{\cdot}26 \times 10^{-5}$
	547	8·06	
	600	7·94	
Methanol	ca. 525[a]	ca. 2·20	$7{\cdot}32 \times 10^{-6}$
	561	8·36	
	604	18·35	
Ethanol	ca. 525[a]	ca. 1·70	$6{\cdot}25 \times 10^{-6}$
(95%)	562	7·24	
	607	16·58	
Acetone	ca. 525[a]	ca. 1·50	$4{\cdot}56 \times 10^{-6}$
	563	6·37	
	607	13·92	
Lauryl Alc.	ca. 525[a]	ca. 1·10	$3{\cdot}42 \times 10^{-6}$
	571	5·38	
	618	11·10	
PEG 400	ca. 525[a]	ca. 1·55	$1{\cdot}17 \times 10^{-5}$
	570	8·75	
	615	15·00	

[a] Shoulder.

colour change was somewhat different to that for the ionic compounds and suggested that the spectra might be explained by partitioning of the dye between the micelles and water.

C.m.c.'s for homogeneous non-ionic surface-active agents of the alkyl polyglycol type have been measured by the dye method by Lange (1960). From Nakagawa's work he judged that Eosin Yellow gave the best

TABLE VI

C.m.c. of a Monododecyl Polyglycol Ether (M.W. 440, Purified Sample) by the Dye Method at 27° C (from Nakagawa, 1958a)

Dye	*Charge of dye ion*	*C.m.c. (mole/l)*
Pinacyanol chloride	+	5×10^{-4}
Erythrocine	−	3×10^{-4}
Rhodamin 6G	+	6×10^{-4}
Eosine Yellow	−	6×10^{-4}
Trypan Blue	−	4×10^{-4}

TABLE VII

C.m.c. Values ($M \times 10^{-4}$) for some Monoalkyl Polyglycols ($C_{12}E_m$) Measured by Different Methods (from Lange, 1960)

m	*Dye solubilization*	*Surface-tension*	*Eosin method*	*Iodine method*
5	0·7	0·57	0·8	—
7	0·75	0·8	0·8	0·71
9	0·8	1·0	1·0	0·83
12	0·8	1·4	1·2	1·08

results and obtained spectra for this dye in the presence of varying concentrations of lauryl polyglycol ethers of general formula $C_{12}E_m$. Below the c.m.c. of the compound $C_{12}E_7$ the peak is at 517 mμ and it shifts to 535 mμ above the c.m.c. with concurrent changes in the density. The c.m.c. for several members of the series was measured by plotting the changes in density which occurred with concentration at 535 mμ. Below the c.m.c. this was fairly low and constant, above it increased rapidly. The results, which are shown in Table VII, indicate poor agreement with values by the surface-tension method for the compounds where $m = 5$ and 12, but where $m = 7$ and 9 the values by the two methods are very close.

A method analogous to the dye method and applicable to non-ionic compounds, was discovered by Ross and Olivier (1959). It consisted of measuring the changes in the spectrum of 30 mg/l of iodine which occur at the c.m.c. of surface-active agents of this type. According to Ross and Olivier an iodine-micelle complex formed above the c.m.c. which absorbed at 360 mμ. When the concentration of the surface-active agent

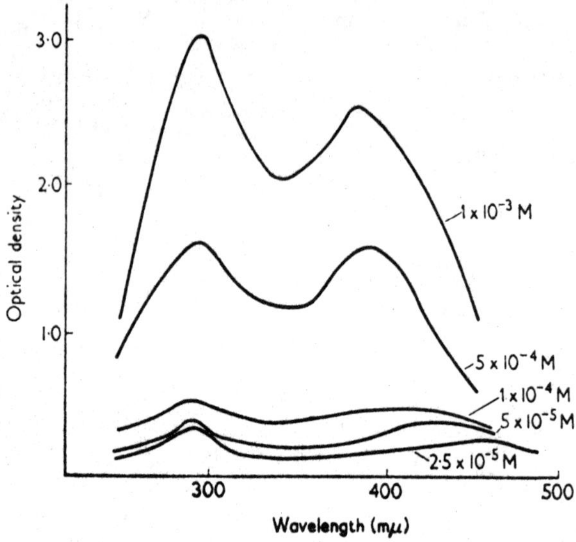

FIG. 11. Spectra of iodine in solutions of $C_{16}H_{33}(O.CH_2.CH_2)_6OH$ (from Carless, Challis and Mulley, 1964).

was further increased, progressive formation of the complex was responsible for the increased density of absorption in this region. A plot of percentage transmission against concentration of the detergent was used to show the break at the c.m.c. They found that measurements should be taken within an hour because the spectra changed with time. The method suffers from the inherent disadvantages of the dye method although precipitation of the complex does not take place. There has also been some disagreement between workers as to the position of the absorption bands and one author has found the density of absorption to decrease at the c.m.c. (Elworthy, 1960). Some of these discrepancies seem to be due to the impure nature of the compounds and once again pure compounds show much sharper breaks in the absorption density-concentration curves than commercial materials. With pure compounds the spectra of iodine in water and in the presence of non-ionic alkyl ethers below the c.m.c. showed low intensity peaks near 290, 360 and 460 mμ, while above the c.m.c. the peaks were near 290 and 390 mμ. Typical spectral results are shown in Figs. 11 and 12, and Table VII compares some results by the iodine method with two other methods. The mechanism of the spectral changes of iodine in the presence of non-ionic surface-active agents is further considered in Section VI.

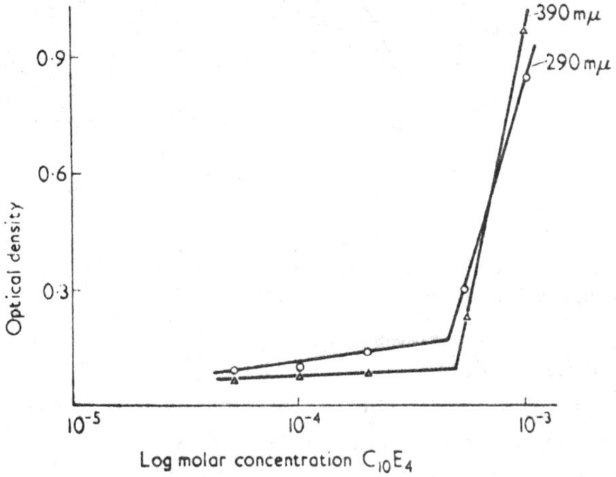

FIG. 12. Optical density of iodine at 290 and 390 mμ plotted against log molar concentration of $C_{10}H_{21}(O.CH_2.CH_2)_4OH$ (from Carless, Challis and Mulley, 1964).

3. *Conductivity Method*

More measurements of conductivity have probably been made than of any other property of colloidal electrolytes, and interpretation of the conductivity-concentration curves has played an important role in theories of micelle formation as described earlier in the chapter. The c.m.c. is given by the break in the equivalent conductivity curve where the conductivity first begins to fall. Two methods of plotting the results are commonly used. In the first the equivalent conductivity is drawn against the square root of the concentration. This method is used because strong electrolytes have a linear relation in dilute solution when plotted in this way, and the break is thus readily detected when the conductivity falls (Fig. 2). The second method plots the specific conductivity against concentration, when the c.m.c. is given by the point of intersection of the two straight lines usually found in this type of plot (Fig. 13).

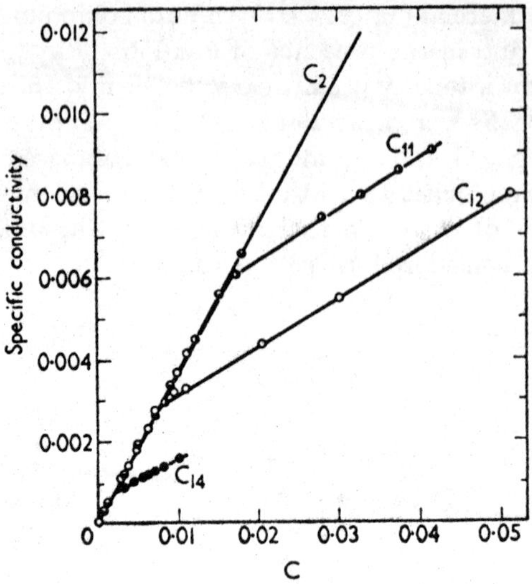

FIG. 13. Specific conductivity at 25° C of undecyl, dodecyl and tetradecyl sulphonic acids and a fully dissociated electrolyte (C_2) (from McBain, 1950).

4. *Refractive Index Method*

One of the main advantages of this method is that no interfering substance is present in the solution, a serious drawback to the dye and solubilization methods. Aggregation in many colloidal systems has been studied by the refractive index method but only a few papers have appeared in which it has been applied to micelle formation. The most comprehensive results with references to earlier work have been reported by Klevens (1948). A plot of change of refractive index against concentration usually shows two straight lines of different slopes which intersect at the c.m.c. Since the refractive index changes are small, especially where the c.m.c. is low, a sensitive method of measurement is required. Good temperature control is essential since a variation of 1° C can produce a change in refractive index of one or two in the fourth place, and the measurements often need to be accurate to the sixth or seventh place. To reduce errors a differential technique is mostly used in which the change in refractive index is measured in relation to water or a previous solution. Klevens used the method for straight chain potassium soaps from C_8 to C_{16}, for alkylamine hydrochlorides (C_{10} to C_{16}) and for a number of sodium alkyl sulphonates. Good agreement was found with measurements by other methods. Satisfactory measurements may also be made on non-ionic compounds, as is shown by the results in Fig. 14 on some monoalkyl polyethers. Comparison of the results by this method shows good agreement with c.m.c. values obtained on the same compounds by the surface-tension and iodine methods. However, the tendency for the value to be lower when a third component is present (iodine method) is apparent. Such effects have been noted by Klevens (1948), among others, when comparing values by refractive index with those obtained by the dye method.

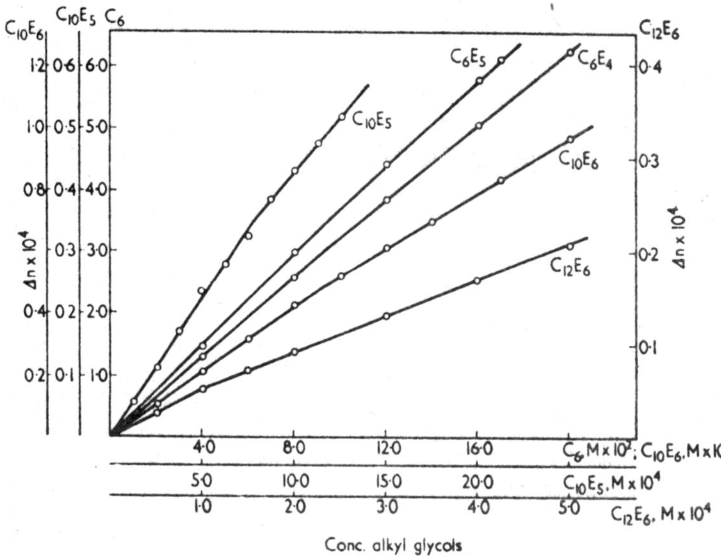

FIG. 14. C.m.c. of some non-ionic alkyl glycols (Mulley, 1958; 1960) by refractive index measurements (from Donbrow and Jan, 1963).

5. *Dye Solubilization Method*

Since the solubility of water-insoluble materials increase at the c.m.c., measurements of solubility may be used to determine it. The method is most conveniently carried out if the solute is a coloured dye, since the amount taken up may be measured colorimetrically (see Section IV). Kolthoff and Stricks (1948, 1949) have published extensive results on the c.m.c.'s of soaps by this method, using dimethylaminoazobenzene and Orange OT as the dyes. Other results, mainly for soaps, have been reviewed by Winsor (1954). More recently, Elworthy (1960) and Lange (1960), have applied the method to measurement of the c.m.c. of non-ionic compounds of the alkyl glycol type.

The values found by dye solubilization usually agree fairly well with those by other methods, but since a third component is present, in some cases the c.m.c. may be slightly affected. Usually the values are lower than those found by methods where third components are absent. Some typical solubility curves are shown in Fig. 15 and comparison of the results with those of other methods for the same compounds are shown in Table VII. The method may also be limited in some cases because it is possible that the phase separating at the solubility limit may not be the solid dye (Section IV).

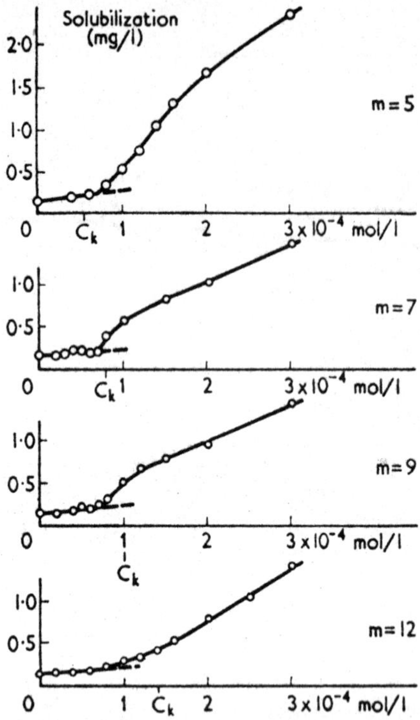

FIG. 15. The c.m.c. of some dodecyl monoalkyl ethers, $C_{12}H_{25}(O.CH_2.CH_2)_mOH$, measured by solubilization of an azo dye. C_k is the c.m.c. measured by surface-tension (from Lange, 1960).

C. EFFECT OF THE STRUCTURE OF THE SURFACE-ACTIVE AGENT ON THE C.M.C.

Since surface-active agents form micelles because they contain within the same molecule regions with differing solution tendencies, it is obvious that micelle formation will depend on the relative strength of the two interactions and that this in turn will depend on the structure of the two regions of the molecule. An expression of these interactions which was used by Winsor (1954) to describe solvent processes and which is a formal statement of the widely used concept that the properties of surface-active agents depend on their hydrophilic–lipophilic balance, may be applied to micelle formation. The resulting description is useful for qualitatively explaining the effect of the structure of surface-active agents on their c.m.c.'s. The interactions controlling micelle formation may be expressed as follows:

Forces opposing micelle formation: $A_{\bar{C}\bar{W}} = A_{L_{\bar{C}\bar{W}}} + A_{H_{\bar{C}\bar{W}}}$

Forces promoting micelle formation: $A_{\bar{C}\bar{C}} = A_{L_{\bar{C}\bar{C}}} + A_{H_{\bar{C}\bar{C}}}$

$A_{\bar{W}\bar{W}} = A_{L_{\bar{W}\bar{W}}} + A_{H_{\bar{W}\bar{W}}}$

$A_{\bar{C}\bar{W}}$ is the molecular interaction energy between the surface-active agent ($\bar{C}$) and water ($\bar{W}$) and is of two types, hydrophilic (H) and lipophilic (L). The other symbols have similar meanings. On this analysis, micelle formation occurs when the ratio of the forces promoting formation to those opposing it is unity. Thus an increase in the molecular interaction energy $A_{\bar{C}\bar{C}}$ should promote micelle formation and lower the c.m.c. This is most commonly produced by an increase in the alkyl chain length of a surface-active agent, which increases the forces promoting micelle formation mainly through the lipophilic interaction $A_{L_{\bar{C}\bar{C}}}$, because forces between molecules or parts of molecules increase in proportion to the molecular weight of the grouping. $A_{\bar{C}\bar{W}}$ is not substantially affected by an increase in alkyl chain length because both lipophilic and hydrophilic interaction between hydrocarbon and water is low (Winsor, 1954). The increase in $A_{\bar{C}\bar{C}}$ produced by extending the alkyl chain and the consequent promotion of micelle formation is indicated by the c.m.c.'s of three series of paraffin chain salts shown in Fig. 16. The figure shows that the c.m.c. decreases logarithmically as the alkyl chain length increases and therefore for chains between eight and eighteen carbon atoms the lipophilic interaction between them is directly proportional to the number of carbon atoms which they contain. Since the c.m.c. of a compound depends not only on the magnitude of the forces opposing and promoting micelle formation but also on the balance between them, it is not unexpected that for the paraffin chain salts in Fig. 16 the c.m.c.'s should be approximately equal for molecules of the same alkyl chain length, since the forces promoting micelle formation are similar in each case and the main contribution to $A_{\bar{C}\bar{W}}$ is through $A_{H_{\bar{C}\bar{W}}}$ and results from one unit charge in each series. In fact, when allowance has been made for the effect of the atoms in the head group, Klevens (1953) has shown that for potassium fatty acid salts, sodium alkane sulphonates, sodium alkyl sulphates and alkyl ammonium chlorides the c.m.c. is logarithmically related to the geometrical length of the chain and that compounds of the same chain length have the same c.m.c.

The other two series of compounds in Fig. 16 both have lower c.m.c.'s than the equivalent paraffin chain salts. It seems that this is because although $A_{\bar{C}\bar{C}}$ is similar to that of the paraffin chain salts, $A_{\bar{C}\bar{W}}$ is smaller. In the case of the betains this is because of internal neutralization of the charges in the head group (reducing interaction with water), and for the alkyl polyglycol ethers because the glycol chain is not so effective as the charge on the long chain ions. Thus in both cases the balance between the forces promoting and opposing micelle formation reach unity at concentrations below those of the paraffin chain salts. Although a unit change in

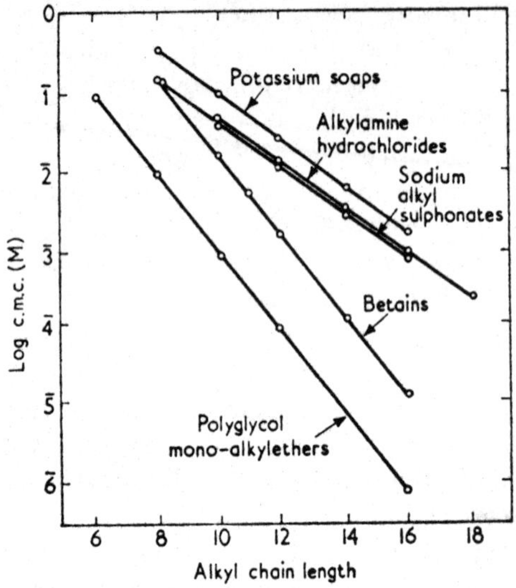

FIG. 16. The effect of the alkyl chain length on the c.m.c. of various types of straight chain surface-active agent. From values given by Klevens, 1948 (ionic compounds); Beckett and Woodward, 1963 (betains); Lange, 1960, Corkill and co-workers, 1961, Mulley and Metcalf, 1962, Elworthy and MacFarlane, 1962, and Carless, Challis and Mulley, 1964 (polyglycol monoalkyl ethers).

the alkyl chain alters $A_{L\bar{C}\bar{C}}$ by the same amount in ionic, non-ionic and betaine type compounds, the change produced in the c.m.c. in the three cases is different (different slopes for each series in Fig. 16), since this is related to the change in $A_{L\bar{C}\bar{C}}$ per CH_2 group to the total interactions opposing micelle formation, which is not the same in the three classes.

The results shown in Fig. 16 may also be expressed by equations of the form:

$$\log \text{c.m.c.} = A - Bn \qquad (1)$$

where n is the alkyl chain length of the surface-active agent, B is a constant (slope of the lines in Fig. 16), and A is a constant (intercept on the c.m.c. axis) (Klevens, 1948). Some values for these constants are given in Table VIII for a number of different classes of compound.

An increase in the polyglycol chain of non-ionic surface-active agents usually raises their c.m.c.'s. The earlier work, which reported results on commercial materials, which are mixtures of varying glycol chain lengths, has been reviewed by Schönfeldt (1959). More reliable results should be given by pure compounds produced by the Williamson synthesis and a number have recently been recorded. Lange (1960) gave results for the effect of the ethylene oxide chain on C_{12} alkyl ethers and others have been given on related C_6, C_{10}, C_{12} and C_{16} compounds by

TABLE VIII

Constants for Equations of the Form Log Molar c.m.c. = $A - Bn$ (or Bm) (Pethica, 1960) Describing the Effect of the Alkyl (n) and Ethylene Oxide Chain Length (m) on the c.m.c. of Various Classes of Surface-active Agent

	A	B
Potassium soaps, (temperature effects neglected)[a]	1·91	0·29
Alkylamine hydrochlorides (temperature effects neglected)[a]	1·38	0·27
Sodium alkyl sulphonates (temperature effects neglected)[a]	1·30	0·27
Sodium alkyl sulphates at 50° C[b]	1·46	0·27
N-alkyl *NN*-dimethylglycines at 23° C[c]	3·17	0·48
$C_nH_{2n+1}(O.CH_2.CH_2)_6OH$ at about 20° C[d]	1·03	0·51
$C_{10}H_{21}(O.CH_2.CH_2)_mOH$ at about 20° C[d]	−3·37	−0·08
$C_{12}H_{25}(O.CH_2.CH_2)_mOH$ at 23°C[e]	−4·49	−0·056

[a] Kleven's results (1948); [b] Kling and Lange (1957); [c] Beckett and Woodward (1963); [d] Carless, Challis and Mulley, (1964); [e] Lange, (1960).

Mulley and Metcalf (1962) and Carless, Challis and Mulley (*J Colloid Sci.*, in the press). Elworthy and MacFarlane (1962b) have also reported values for the C_{16} monoalkylglycols containing up to twenty-two ethylene oxide units. For C_{16} compounds some workers have found that the effect of the hydrophilic chain is the reverse of that expected (Carless and co-workers, Lange, 1959). This may be a result of the prolonged ageing of the surface found in these compounds, their c.m.c.'s having been measured mainly by the surface-tension method. The glycol chain is similar to the alkyl chain, in that its c.m.c. is related logarithmically to the glycol chain length as shown by the results in Fig. 17. Equations derived from Fig. 17 and others from the literature are given in Table VIII. The ethylene oxide chain does not affect the c.m.c. nearly as much as the alkyl chain length. For example an increase of two carbon atoms in the alkyl chain of the alkyl glycols with six ethylene oxide units per molecule, decreases the c.m.c. to a tenth of the previous value, whereas in the $C_{16}E_m$ series an increase in m from 6 to 15 only doubles the c.m.c.

Although many different chemical classes of detergent have been prepared, published data on their properties is scanty compared with that for the simple *n*-alkyl compounds. Winsor (1948) has published data for tetradecane sodium sulphates, on the effect of the position of the ionic group in the chain on the c.m.c. As the sulphate group is progressively moved to the middle of the chain the c.m.c. rises. The c.m.c.

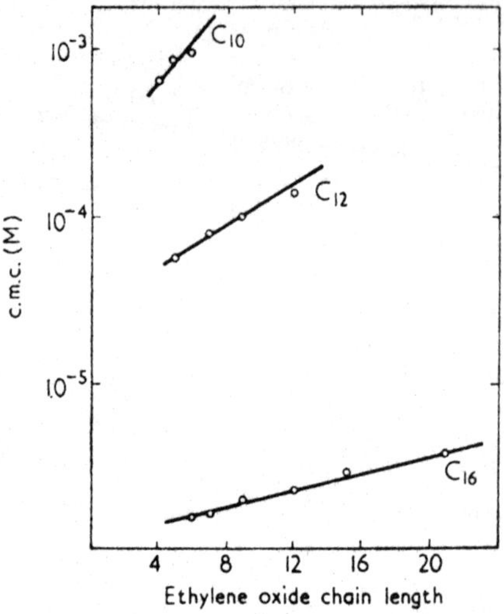

FIG. 17. The effect of the ethylene oxide chain length on the c.m.c. of C_{10} (Carless, Challis and Mulley, 1964), C_{12} (Lange, 1960) and C_{16} (Elworthy and MacFarlane, 1962b) monoalkyl polyethers.

of tetradecane-7 sodium sulphate was found to be about ten times that of the 1-sodium sulphate. This effect is analogous to that found in the double chain salts, which have higher c.m.c.'s than the corresponding straight chain compounds. Winsor (1954) quotes a c.m.c. of $8{\cdot}45 \times 10^{-3}$ M for di-*n*-hexylethyl sodium sulphate at room temperature, which is about five times that of the corresponding straight chain compound. The higher c.m.c.'s for the double chain salts and the salts with non-terminal ionic groups are thought to be due to steric factors. Not only will packing within the micelle be more difficult but the single molecules are less asymmetric than straight chain compounds and therefore may be more readily accommodated in aqueous solution because they disturb the strong cohesive forces between water molecules less (Hartley, 1941). The micelles of such compounds are also thought to be smaller than those of single chain detergents (Winsor, 1954) and they do not appear to be effective solubilizing agents (Hartley, 1941).

Compounds containing benzene rings in the alkyl part of the molecule are common commercial detergents. The ring appears to be equivalent in lipophilic character to about three-and-a-half carbon atoms of a straight hydrocarbon chain since Paquette, Lingafelter and Tartar (1943) report c.m.c. values for *n*-octyl benzene-*p*-sulphonate and the corresponding dodecyl compound as 0·011 N at 25° and 0·0012 N at 60° respectively, by a conductivity method. These values are near those for straight chain compounds of about 11 to 12 and 15 to 16 carbon atoms respectively.

D. EFFECT OF OTHER SOLUTES ON THE C.M.C.

Many solutes appear to lower the c.m.c. of surface-active agents. Salts are particularly active in this respect and affect both anionic and cationic materials. The effect is proportional to the concentration of the salt but is independent of its nature in the case of sodium and potassium chlorides, bromides, iodides, nitrates, sulphates or phosphates. The action seems to be simply one of reducing solubility of the surface-active agent by salting out. Some typical results are shown in Fig. 18. Other results have been

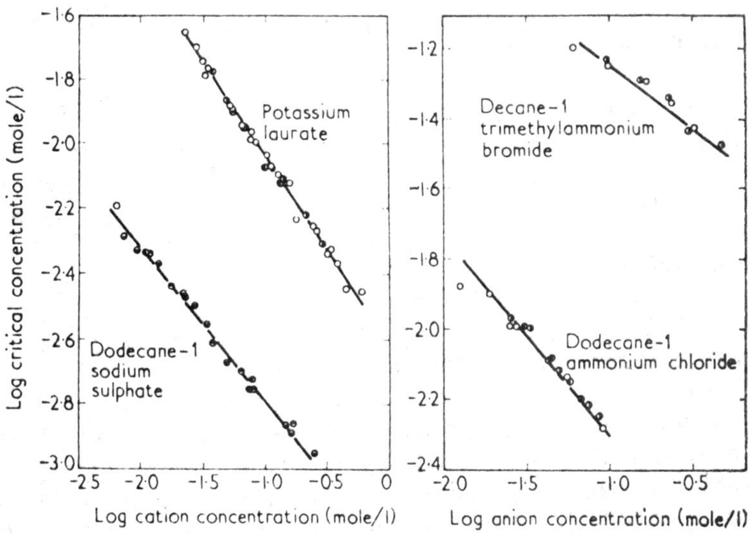

FIG. 18. Effect of salts on the c.m.c. of anionic and cationic detergents: anionic, ○ KCl, ◒ NaCl, ◑ K_2SO_4, ◓ Na_2SO_4, ◐ $Na_4P_2O_7$; cationic, ○ NaCl, ◑ $BaCl_2$, ◐ $LaCl_3$ (from Corrin and Harkins, 1947).

reviewed by Winsor (1954). Non-ionic compounds are very much less affected by salts although their c.m.c. is still depressed (Hsiao *et al.*, 1956). For a nonylphenol with 10, 15 or 20 ethylene oxide units these workers found the c.m.c. to be approximately halved by 0·86 N sodium chloride, whereas 0·5 N salt solutions depress the c.m.c. of anionic and cationic compounds to a fifth or less of the original value. The effect of various sodium salts on the c.m.c. of nonylphenol type non-ionic materials appears to be related to the lyotropic number of the anion (Fig. 19). The compounds are also affected by acids and alkalis. At low acid concentrations, the acid effect (which raises the c.m.c.) is balanced by the salt effect and the c.m.c. is about the same as in water. In strong

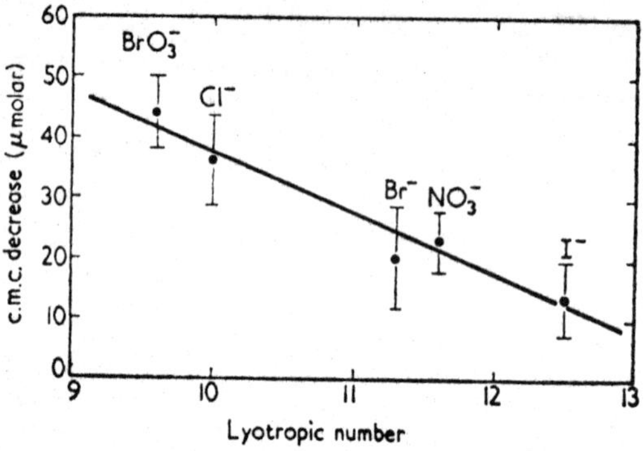

FIG. 19. Effect of 0·5 N sodium salts on the c.m.c. of a nonylphenol detergent containing fifteen ethylene oxide units per molecule (from Hsiao *et al.*, 1956).

acid the acid effect predominates and the c.m.c. is raised; e.g. the c.m.c. of a nonylphenol in 3·1 N hydrochloric acid is 150 μM (120 in water) and in 3·1 N nitric acid 290 μM. The cause of this is probably an increase in the hydrophilic nature of the ethylene oxide chain by oxonium ion formation of the ether groups. Bases decrease the c.m.c. (Hsiao and co-workers, 1956).

Many other materials also lower the c.m.c. of surface-active agents. The effects of alcohols has been studied by Herzfield, Corrin and Harkins (1950 and earlier papers), by Harva (1956) and by Lawrence and Stenson (1957). The lowering appears to be a function of the alcohol concentration at some concentration ranges and the effect is greater as the chain length of the alcohol increases. Ward and Chitale (1957) have reported the effect of α-naphthylamine, naphthalene and β-naphthol on the c.m.c. of sodium dodecyl sulphate, which was lowered from 0·006 M to 0·0036, 0·0045 and 0·005 M respectively in the presence of 5 mole per cent of these compounds. Considerable discussion on c.m.c.'s in ternary solution was made at the conference at which Ward and Chitale presented their paper and is listed under their names in the conference report. More recently the effect of certain third components on the c.m.c. of some short chain non-ionic glycols has been measured (Mulley and Metcalf, 1962) and has been found to be negligible. In this paper it was suggested that large effects were only found on the c.m.c. when ionic effects were involved. Results indicated that it was possible for some of the supposed

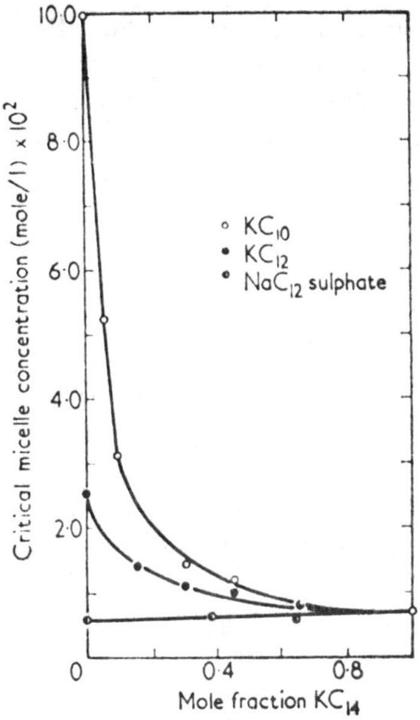

FIG. 20. C.m.c. of mixtures of potassium myristate and other soaps at 25° C (from Klevens, 1948).

shifts in c.m.c., usually judged by a break in some property/concentration curve, might in fact be due to phase changes occurring when third components are present in the solution.

The c.m.c. of mixtures of surface-active agents has received some attention because commercial materials are usually mixtures of various chain lengths and because mixtures have desirable properties in some respects. Some results obtained by Klevens (1948) are shown in Fig. 20. These show that the c.m.c. of a mixture is not proportionate to that expected from the c.m.c.'s of the individual components and the fraction of each present, but that micelle formation is induced at concentrations near that of the compound with the lowest c.m.c. even when it is present in a mixture in a relatively small proportion.

E. EFFECT OF TEMPERATURE ON THE C.M.C.

A rise in the c.m.c. of paraffin chain salts is normally found when the temperature of their solutions is increased, but the effect is quite small. Presumably the rise results from the increased thermal motion of the molecules which occurs with rise in temperature in any solution and which would be expected to militate against aggregation processes such as micelle formation. When the c.m.c. is measured by the dye method anomolous results have been found for the effect of temperature, an apparent decrease being found (Klevens, 1947). This is probably bound up with the mechanism of the dye method and does not indicate a true effect on micelle formation. Non-ionic compounds show a decrease in

TABLE IX

Effect of Temperature on the c.m.c. of Some Ionic Compounds and a Non-ionic Glycol (Wright *et al.*, 1939; Corkill *et al.*, 1961)

Compound	*Temperature and c.m.c. (molar)*		
	40°C	60°C	80°C
C_{10} *n*-alkyl sulphonate	0·040	0·043	0·058
C_{12} *n*-alkyl sulphonate	0·011	0·012	0·014
C_{14} *n*-alkyl sulphonate	0·0025	0·0033	0·0046
	35°	48°	80°
Sodium myristate	0·0068	0·0072	0·0092
	15°	25°	35°
$C_{12}H_{25}(CH_2.CH_2.O)_6OH$	$10{\cdot}8 \times 10^{-5}$	$8{\cdot}7 \times 10^{-5}$	$7{\cdot}2 \times 10^{-5}$

c.m.c. when the temperature is raised. In this case the effect is probably related to the reduced solubility of these compounds at higher temperatures. Decreased solubility and reduced c.m.c. for these compounds probably reflects the effect of temperature on the hydration of the hydrophilic chain. Table IX shows the effect of temperature on the c.m.c. of some ionic and non-ionic surface-active agents. Other values have been given by Klevens (1948).

III. THEORY AND MECHANISM OF SOLUBILIZATION

In the introduction it was pointed out that increased solubility in the presence of a surface-active agent was coincident with the formation of micelles. It is obvious that the increased solubility must in some way result from an association of the solute with the micelle. The simplest view which has been put forward is that the water-insoluble material dissolves in the hydrocarbon interior, almost as if the latter formed a separate phase finely dispersed in the solution. This view implies that the absolute amount of material which can be dissolved in a surface-active agent solution should be near the amount that would dissolve in a volume of hydrocarbon equivalent to the volume of paraffin chains present in the micelles. Thus the solubility should increase in proportion to the concentration of the surface-active agent and should be greater when the alkyl chain length increases. Although this view is probably an over simplification quite a lot of the solubility data in the literature fits in qualitatively and even quantitatively with such an explanation (M. E. L. McBain and Hutchinson, 1955). For example, Hartley (1938) calculated that the solubility of *trans*-azobenzene in the hydrocarbon interior of cetyl pyridinium chloride micelles was quite close to its solubility in *n*-hexadecane. Many solubility curves indicate that once micelles are fully formed, the solubility of the material is directly proportional to the concentration of the surface-active agent over a wide range (Table X). The effect of increased volume of micelle interior on the solubilization of a dye by some potassium soaps is shown in Table XI. This data has been analysed by M. E. L. McBain and Hutchinson (1955, p. 59) as follows. At 0·33 N soap concentration the ratio of Orange OT dissolved for the C_{10}, C_{12} and C_{14} soaps is about 1 : 3 : 5·8, whereas the relative volumes of the micelle (assuming the micelles are spheres of radius equal to the length of an extended hydrocarbon chain) would be in ratio 1 : 1·7 : 2·7. Allowing for the modifications which might be necessary because this is a very idealized picture of the micelle "then the relative volumes of the micelles may well be in a ratio close to that of the amounts of dye solubilized". Furthermore, if solubility is controlled by the volume of hydrocarbon available in the micelle interior then a change in nature of the ionic head group of the surface-active agent should have little effect on the amount dissolving. Table XII shows this to be approximately true, at least for cetylpyridinium salts where the solute is azobenzene.

Although this picture accounts approximately in several systems for the absolute amount of material dissolving, M. E. L. McBain and Hutchinson suggested that a truer view is given if solubilization is seen as a partition between the micelle and water, i.e. treating the micelle as a separate phase. Making the assumption that the presence of surface-active molecules has no effect on the solubility of a solute in the aqueous phase, they thought that solubilizing power should be measured by the ratio of moles of solute dissolved per mole of surface-active agent to moles of solute per mole of water. Some selected values calculated by these authors are shown in Table XIII. It can be seen that the solubilizing power of the surface-active agent for materials of increasing molecular

TABLE X

The Effect of Concentration (Volume of Hydrocarbon in the Micelle Interior) on the Number of Milligrams of the Dye Dimethylaminoazobenzene (DMAB) Solubilized by Different Concentrations of a Homologous Series of Soaps at 30°C (from M. E. L. McBain and Hutchinson, 1955, p. 53).

Soap	*Soap concentration, mole/l*			
	0·05	0·10	0·15	0·20
K caprate	1	1·5	30	64
K laurate	40	110	180	255
K myristate	125	255	380	510

TABLE XI

The Effect of the Alkyl Chain Length (Volume of Hydrocarbon in the Micelle Interior) on the Number of Grams of Orange OT Solubilized per Mole of Soap at 25°C at Different Soap Concentrations (from McBain and Johnson, 1944 and McBain and Green, 1946)

Soap	0·08 N	0·16 N	0·33 N	0·84 N
K caprate	0·20	0·22	0·32	0·35
K laurate	0·87	0·97	0·96	1·01
K myristate	1·90	1·84	1·85	1·87

TABLE XII

Solubilization of Azobenzene by Cetyl Pyridinium Salts at 25°C (from Hartley's results, 1938)

	Chloride	*Sulphate*	*Acetate*
Concentration of detergent, molarity × 10^4	41·8	39·6	40
Concentration of solute, molarity × 10^4	6·42	6·06	5·81

size rises, although the absolute solubility decreases as is usually found in any series of compounds when the molecular weight is increased. Thus the water solubility of octane is only about one-tenth that of hexane whereas its solubility in the micelle is nearly one-half that of hexane. The solubility of octane in a micellar solution does not decrease nearly as much as its solubility in water. Materials of low water solubility are thus partitioned in favour of the micelle much more than those of higher

TABLE XIII

Distribution Constants for Dodecylamine Hydrochloride, Potassium Laurate and Potassium Myristate Solutions (from M. E. L. McBain and Hutchinson, 1955)

Solute	*Molality of soap*	*Solubility in water, mole:mole*	*Solubility in micelle, mole:mole*	*K [Micelles] [Water]*
			Dodecylamine Hydrochloride	
Hexane		$2·8 \times 10^{-5}$	0·75	$2·7 \times 10^{4}$
Heptane		9×10^{-6}	0·54	6×10^{4}
Octane		$3·2 \times 10^{-6}$	0·29	9×10^{4}
Benzene		$1·6 \times 10^{-4}$	0·65	4×10^{3}
Octylamine		$2·8 \times 10^{-5}$	0·13	$4·6 \times 10^{3}$
n-Octanol		$8·2 \times 10^{-5}$	0·18	$2·2 \times 10^{3}$
			Potassium Laurate	
Benzene	0·085	$1·6 \times 10^{-4}$	0·43	$2·5 \times 10^{3}$
	0·213	$1·6 \times 10^{-4}$	0·59	$3·7 \times 10^{3}$
n-Heptane	0·088	9×10^{-6}	0·087	9×10^{3}
n-Octanol	0·1	$8·2 \times 10^{-5}$	0·4	5×10^{3}
			Potassium Myristate	
Benzene	0·076	$1·6 \times 10^{-4}$	0·244	$1·5 \times 10^{3}$
	0·114	$1·6 \times 10^{-4}$	0·246	$1·5 \times 10^{3}$
n-Heptane	0·114	9×10^{-6}	0·246	$2·7 \times 10^{4}$

water solubility. Polar compounds which usually show increased solubility when compared with similar non-polar molecules are on this view of solubilization much less strongly dissolved by micelles, as is shown by the lower K values of such compounds in Table XIII.

The foregoing seems a reasonably satisfactory explanation of solubilization if only restricted ranges of data are considered. But, as M. E. L. McBain and Hutchinson have pointed out, such a simple view would not be expected to apply to materials which have a fairly high solubility in surface-active agent solutions, because the additive might modify the micelle and therefore introduce a new factor into the situation. A similar complication would be expected where the solutes themselves have a polar-nonpolar character because these materials are thought to be solubilized by orientating themselves in the micelle, or by adsorption on the micelle (Lawrence, 1937; Ward, 1940; Harkins and Oppenheimer, 1949). In many cases it seems more suitable to think of the additive and the surface-active agent interacting to form a new micelle, possibly considerably increased in size or modified in form (Section II). In such cases the explanation of solubilization as solution in the interior of a basically unmodified micelle would not be applicable. McBain in particular thought that solution in the interior of the micelle did not explain much of the solubility data and quoted results for dimethyl phthalate (McBain and Huff, 1948) which is insoluble in hydrocarbon type solvents and therefore could not be dissolved by the simple mechanism. It is not suggested in such cases that solubilization is not a solution process, but rather that the effect of the additive on the micelles, and possibly its special orientation within the micelle, make the solubility dependent on the new environment formed by mutual solution of all the components, which may have special characteristics not found in any single component or pair of components on their own. At present there seems little likelihood of being able to quantitatively account for solubilities in these special cases.

It is usually assumed that solubilization in solutions containing non-ionic surface-active agents is analogous to that found for the paraffin chain salts and in many respects this appears to be true. Solubilization is associated with micelle formation because it begins at the c.m.c. (Mulley and Metcalf, 1962) as in the case of other surface-active agents. There are other similarities. For example, the amount of material solubilized is proportional to the concentration of the surface-active agent over a considerable range (Sjöblom, 1956; Mulley and Metcalf, 1956; Guttman and co-workers, 1961; Carless and Mitchell, 1962). The view that solubilization by non-ionic surface-active agents is a solution process within the micells is further considered in some detail in Section VI. Other mechanisms have been proposed, e.g. that solubilization is a binding phonomonon botwoen the surface-active agent and the solute (Patel and Kostenbauder, 1958). The properties of the solubilized systems sometimes suggest different mechanisms for ionic and non-ionic micelles. For example, Riegelman (1960) found different degrees of protection afforded benzocaine against base hydrolysis in these two classes. But in general, solution within the micelle explains most of the published data.

P. A. Winsor (1954) has proposed a theory to explain changes in solubility when such factors as the alkyl chain length of the surface-active agent are altered. He thought that the solubility was affected by changes in the micelle form present in the solution. Solubility increases when there is any change tending to make the average form nearer the lamellar type micelle; and decreases when changes occur which have the reverse effect. According to Winsor the interactions conditioning the miscibility of an organic liquid O and water W are of two types, hydrophilic and lipophilic, and may be represented as:

1. Opposing miscibility: promoting separation

$$A_{OO} = A_{L_{OO}} + A_{H_{OO}}$$
$$A_{WW} = A_{L_{WW}} + A_{H_{WW}}$$

2. Promoting miscibility: opposing separation

$$A_{OW} = A_{L_{OW}} + A_{H_{OW}}$$

where A_{OO} is the molecular interaction between the "Oil" (O) molecules and is lipophilic ($A_{L_{OO}}$) (London forces) and hydrophilic ($A_{H_{OO}}$) (polar forces). The other symbols have analogous meanings. From this viewpoint, water and hydrocarbons are immiscible because the combined interactions between like molecules are greater than those between unlike, and the interactions are therefore best satisfied by the formation of two separate phases. The co-solvent action of a third molecular species $\bar{C}$, depends, according to Winsor, on the strength and balance of the molecular interactions between $\bar{C}$ and the normally immiscible molecules ($\bar{O}$ and $\bar{W}$):

Interactions:

$$A_{CO} = A_{L_{\bar{C}\bar{O}}} + A_{H_{\bar{C}\bar{O}}}$$
$$A_{CW} = A_{H_{\bar{C}\bar{W}}} + A_{L_{\bar{C}\bar{W}}}$$

Balance: R

$$\frac{A_{CO}}{A_{CW}} \qquad \frac{A_{L_{\bar{C}\bar{O}}} + A_{H_{\bar{C}\bar{O}}}}{A_{L_{\bar{C}\bar{W}}} + A_{H_{\bar{C}\bar{W}}}}$$

Surface-active agents are thus very effective co-solvents because they have strong interactions with both water and oil molecules. The action is mediated by the $\bar{C}$ molecules forming bridges between $\bar{O}$ and $\bar{W}$ regions in a solution in which considerable intermolecular organization occurs. The process of organization is micelle formation. Since such solutions are fluid, the organized regions may have a variable form depending on the "dispersing tendencies" (i.e. tendencies to become convex) on the $\bar{O}$ and $\bar{W}$ faces of the $\bar{C}$ region bridge. The ratio of the dispersing tendencies is denoted by R and is given by the above expression. A diagrammatic expression of Winsor's ideas is given in Fig. 21. In his view, there is in any solution a dynamic equilibrium giving micelles of predominately one type depending on whether R is greater or less than unity. The probability of one form or the other will increase as the mean value of R recedes from unity. He further states, "The intermicellar equilibrium shown in Fig. 21 does not mean that perfect S_1, S_2 and G micellar forms are present in equilibrium, but rather that a fluctuating micellar form may be regarded as resolved into S_1 and S_2 forms in equilibrium with G micelles." In Winsor's view solubilization or co-solvent action is at a maximum when R is near 1. Using these concepts, Winsor has described a number of general methods of influencing solubilization which are shown in Table XIV.

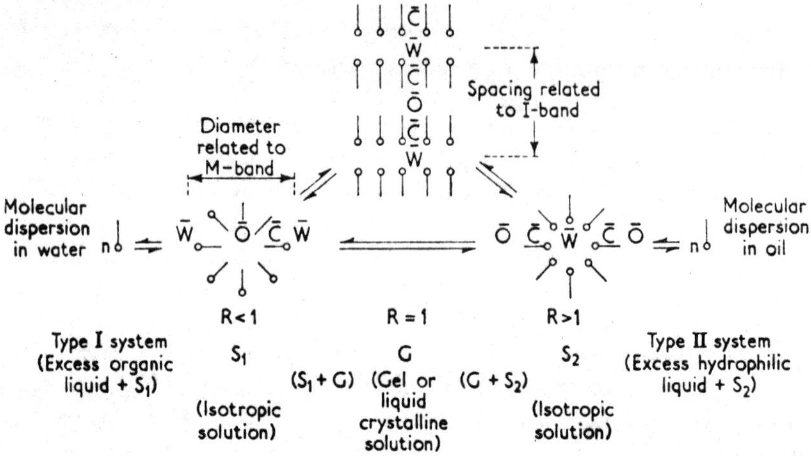

FIG. 21. Intermicellar equilibrium and associated phase changes shown by certain series of amphiphilic solutions (from Winsor, 1954).

It should be noted that Winsor's description was in general derived from experiments in systems considerably more complex than those discussed up to now. The concentration of the surface-active agent was usually high (20 per cent) and was achieved by using compounds with non-terminal ionic groups, which have a much lower crystallizing tendency than most detergents. Also inorganic salt and mixtures of oil solutes were usually present. The dramatic changes in solubility brought about by small changes in composition are not commonly observed in lower concentration systems. The effects Winsor describes are related to those regions of the phase equilibrium diagrams discussed in Section V where, in simpler three-component systems, changes from aqueous to oily type solutions occur with small composition changes, whereas lower down on the diagrams much greater composition changes are necessary for the same sequence of events to be seen. However, the same general principles seem to apply even in the more dilute regions.

Attempts have been made to obtain evidence for the mechanism of

TABLE XIV

General Methods Influencing Solubilization by Displacement of the Intermicellar Equilibrium in the Amphiphilic Phase of a System containing initially an Organic Liquid O_1, an Amphiphilic Salt C_1 and Water or an Aqueous Solution of an Inorganic Salt W_1 (from Winsor, 1954)

Method		Effect on solubilization in initial system of		Effect on R, $R \propto A_{\bar{C}O}/A_{\bar{C}W}$ i.e. as $\frac{A_{H\bar{C}O}+A_{L\bar{C}O}}{A_{H\bar{C}W}+A_{L\bar{C}W}}$	Probable mechanism of influence on R
Number	*Details of method*	*Type I*	*Type II*		
$I(a)$	Reduction in relative proportion of W_1	Increased solubilization of O_1	Removal of excess W_1	Increased	$A_{\bar{C}W}$ diminished by mass action
$I(b)$	Addition to O_1 of an oil-soluble compound of more polar (hydrophilic) character than O_1. Alternatively this may be regarded as the addition to C of an amphiphilic compound more lipophilic than C_1	Increased solubilization of O_1	Increased precipitation of aqueous layer	Increased	Reduction of $A_{H\bar{C}W}$ by incorporation of amphiphilic additive in C layer and/or increase of $A_{H\bar{C}O}$
$I(c)$	Increase in relative lipophilic character of C_1, e.g. by increase of molecular weight, substitution of an organic for an inorganic gegenion or by certain changes in constitution	Increased solubilization of O_1	Increased precipitation of aqueous layer	Increased	$A_{L\bar{C}O}$ increased and/or $A_{H\bar{C}W}$ diminished
$I(d)$	Addition to W_1 of an inorganic salt	Increased solubilization of O_1	Increased precipitation of aqueous layer	Increased	$A_{H\bar{C}W}$ diminished
$II(a)$	Reduction in relative proportion of O_1	Removal of excess O_1	Increased solubilization of W_1	Decreased	$A_{\bar{C}O}$ diminished by mass action
$II(b)$	Addition to W_1 of a water-soluble organic liquid of more lipophilic character	Increased precipitation of organic liquid	Increased solubilization of W_1	Decreased	$A_{L\bar{C}W}$ increased
$II(c)$	Increase in relative hydrophilic character of C_1, i.e. method $I(c)$ in reverse	Increased precipitation of organic liquid	Increased solubilization of W_1	Decreased	$A_{L\bar{C}W}$ increased and/or $A_{L\bar{C}O}$ diminished
$II(d)$	Addition to O_1 of a less hydrophilic oil-soluble component, e.g. medicinal oil, i.e. method $I(b)$ in reverse	Increased precipitation of organic liquid	Increased solubilization of W_1	Decreased	Reverse of mechanism of method $I(b)$

solubilization by X-ray diffraction measurements but interpretation of the results is even more controversial in these systems than in the simple binary solutions containing surface-active agent and water alone. M. E. L. McBain and Hutchinson claim (1955) that neither of the two main competing theories of micelle formation fit the diffraction patterns very well. The main changes in the patterns of some of the simpler solubilized systems that have been studied seem to be: (1) with non-polar solutes both the M- and the I-bands increase in length of spacing; (2) with polar solutes either there is no effect on the M- or the I-band, or small decreases are found. These results have been interpreted in terms of the different mode of incorporation of the two types of solute within the micelle (Harkins and Oppenheimer, 1949) (see Fig. 22). Although

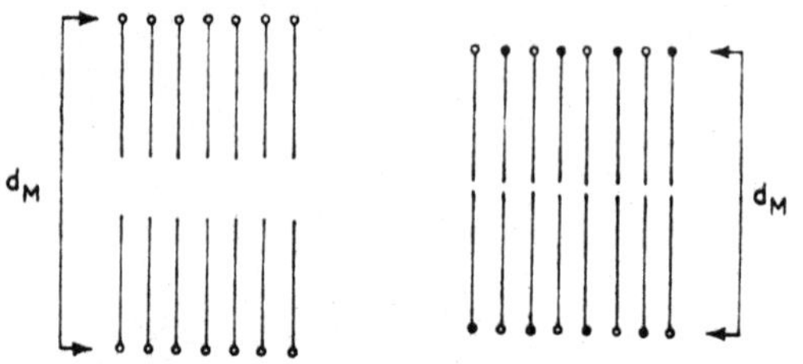

FIG. 22. Effect of solubilized materials on X-ray diffraction band d_M. Hydrocarbon solute d_M increased; polar solute (molecules with solid heads) d_M unaffected (see text).

expansion of d_I (see Fig. 5) would be expected on this model for hydrocarbons, quantitative agreement between the expansion and the amount added is not found on the lamellar micelle model (Hartley, 1955). Hartley has claimed that the spherical model fits the expansion reasonably well. The X-ray evidence does indeed seem to indicate that there is a difference between solubilization of polar and non-polar solutes. This is consistent with the light scattering data mentioned earlier which also showed that polar solutes had a greater effect on micelle size than the non-polar materials.

Further evidence on the mechanism of solubilization has been sought by spectroscopic measurements on solubilized materials, because it is well known that the solvent environment affects the spectra of many compounds. Although the evidence is not unequivocal, non-polar solutes give similar spectra when solubilized, to those given in hydrocarbon solvents, whereas polar solutes do not (Mulley and Metcalf, 1956; Riegelman and co-workers, 1958; Guttman and co-workers, 1961; references to other work, particularly that from Ekwall's School, are given in the last paper).

In conclusion, it may be said that the evidence points to the theory of simple solution in the micelle interior for slightly soluble materials as being reasonably satisfactory. At higher surface-active agent concentrations, where the structure of the solutions may change drastically, treatment as a pseudo two-phase system is less convincing.

IV. Measurement of Solubility and Methods of Representing Solubility Data

A. SYNTHETIC AND ANALYTICAL METHODS

Basically, methods of determining solubilities in surface-active agent solutions are the same as those used in any system (Weisberger, 1959). The actual technique chosen depends on the particular system being studied and in the form in which the results are required. The synthetic method is especially useful if simple methods of analysis are not available. In this method the solute is added in gradually increasing amounts to a solution of the surface-active agent at the temperature at which the solubility value is required. The solubility will lie between two values; at the lower the solute will be just below and at the other just above its solubility. The mean between these is usually taken. When the solute is such that equilibration is rapid, a single solution may be used and the solute added in increasing proportion until the solubility limit is reached.

Detection of the end-point is not difficult if the phase separating has a refractive index considerably different from that of the solution. A milkiness is seen in the mixture when the solute is in excess of its solubility. Simple visual determination of the concentration at which this occurs usually suffices. If the turbidity is difficult to detect, instrumental methods may be used (Klevens, 1950, p. 5). For materials which give coloured solutions, particularly the solid dyes, a convenient extension of the method has been used (Klevens, 1950, p. 7). It consists of adding excess dye to solutions of the surface-active agent of varying concentration, equilibrating, taking an aliquot of the solution and determining the amount of dye solubilized using a reference curve. This method may give a misleading result if no check is made of the phase or phases separating at the solubility limit because a three-component system is not invarient at any one temperature when three phases are in equilibrium (vapour is one phase) unless one of them is solid. The point is illustrated by reference to Fig. 42 on page 145. At low concentrations of the alkyl glycol the phase separating at the solubility limit is pure chloroxylenol and therefore addition of excess chloroxylenol does not affect the composition of the aqueous phase. At higher concentrations the phase separating is a liquid and when excess phenol is added the composition of the aqueous phase is given by the composition of the dilute phase at the end of the tie line drawn through the total composition of the mixture and cutting the binodal BCD. The point is important because there is good reason to believe that the phase separating at the solubility limit in many solubilized systems is liquid or liquid crystal even when the solute is a solid (see Section V).

The synthetic method may also be used when a complete phase diagram is required. The results are most accurate and the end-point readily detected if the mixtures are arranged so that phase boundaries are crossed at approximately 90°. Phase changes involving separation of a liquid crystal phase may be detected by viewing the sample in plane polarized light. Isotropic solutions may be readily distinguished from liquid crystal because liquid crystal phases are birefringent and much more viscous. Mixtures of liquid crystal and liquid phases usually have a high viscosity and appear cloudy. Single liquid crystalline phases are clear and boundaries between such regions can often be detected visually (Lumb, 1951). The "triangularly staggered walk" technique described by Boffey *et al.* (1959) is particularly useful in the preliminary stages of working out a phase diagram. Regions in which equilibria between solid and liquid crystal phases occur are often difficult to investigate, and microscopic observation in an apparatus such as the Kofler Micro Cold Stage (C. Reichert Optische Werke A.G., Wein) is helpful. Thermal analysis and dilatometric measurements are also useful in these regions (Vold, 1941).

The analytical method of determining solubility is used when it is possible to assay the components of a system (Dervichian, 1957). Very high speed centrifugation may be necessary to separate the phases when liquid crystal is present (Dervichian, 1957; Ekwall *et al.*, 1960). For three-component mixtures determination of two is sufficient to fix the composition of any phase, and determination of even one component may enable the diagram to be drawn in appropriate regions by applications of phase rule principles.

High molecular weight solids of low solubility may give rise to equilibration difficulties. Equilibration times of 24 to 60 h have been reported when hydrocarbons such as *n*-heptane, benzene and ethylbenzene are solubilized (Heller and Klevens, 1946), and up to 60 days for benzanthracene and dibenzanthracene (Klevens, 1950). Similar difficulties were earlier reported by McBain (1942). Supersaturation at solubility limits where solid phases are involved may be troublesome, particularly as surface-active agents are known to inhibit crystallization. There have even been reports of supersaturation of liquid phases (Lester-Smith, 1932) and of solubilities differing when the order of mixing the components is changed (Carless and Nixon, 1960). In the majority of cases solutions produced by surface-active agents appear to be in true equilibrium and it is this assumption that underlies treatment of solubilization as a true solution process (McBain and McBain, 1936).

B. REPRESENTATION OF SOLUBILITY DATA

1. *Solubility Curves*

Solubility results are usually plotted on two types of solubility curve which are shown in Fig. 23. The first is best if the concentration at which solubilization begins is required and it readily enables the weight of the

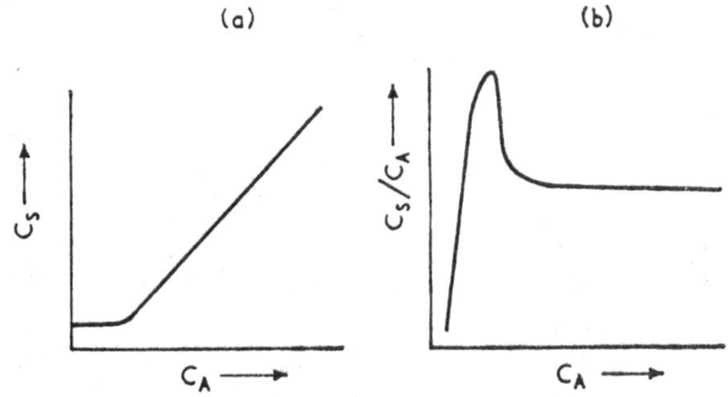

FIG. 23. Solubility curves for solubilized systems. (*a*) Ordinary solubility curve. (*b*) Differential solubility curve. C_s/C_a is the molar ratio of the solute and surface-active agent concentrations (from Hartley, 1938; Moilliet and co-authors, 1961).

solute, which would dissolve in any concentration of the surface-active agent solution, to be calculated. Differential curves are more suitable for interpretation of the mechanism of solubilization and for information about micelle formation (Klevens, 1950, pp. 16–17). The marked changes in solubility (both negative and positive) often found in this type of plot near the c.m.c. indicate not only the onset of micelle formation but also the possible occurrence of phase changes.

2. *Phase Diagrams*

The simplest solubilized systems are of three components, surface-active agent, solute and solvent. They may be completely described by means of a three-component phase rule diagram and this method has been increasingly used in the study of these systems in recent years. Such diagrams have a number of properties (Campbell and Smith, 1951) which are particularly useful in formulation (O'Malley *et al.*, 1958; Mulley, 1959; Martin, 1960; Boon *et al.*, 1961). For example, in Fig. 24 point *a* represents a composition containing a certain ratio of surface-active agent to solute and all points along the line joining *a* to the water corner (*a*A) represent compositions containing an increasing proportion of water but a constant proportion of surface-active agent to solute. Similarly any composition within the triangle diluted with water, for example *b*, traverses compositions represented by points along the line joining it to the water corner (*b*A). Any point along the water surface-active agent axis joined to the solute corner C shows the effect of increasing concentrations of solute on a solution of the detergent of concentration shown by the original point (e.g. *c*′C). Knowledge of the phase diagram

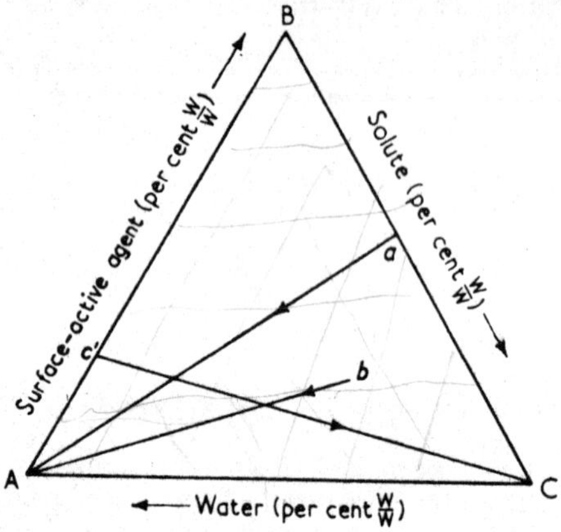

FIG. 24. Properties of ternary phase equilibrium diagrams useful in the formulation of solubilized products (see text).

for the system therefore makes it possible to predict the effect of dilution on a product (*b*A) and shows the proportion of surface-active agent necessary to dissolve the solute (*a*A). It also gives the concentration of surface-active agent necessary to produce a solution of the required strength.

Representation of systems of more than three components is more complicated. It may be done on a triangular diagram by keeping the concentration of one of the components constant when the effects of varying the other three may be shown (Boon *et al.*, 1961), or by construction of a solid model (Campbell and Smith, 1951).

V. PHASE EQUILIBRIA IN SYSTEMS CONTAINING SURFACE-ACTIVE AGENTS

A general classification on a phase rule basis of the complex phenomena found in solubilized systems is very useful for comparison between systems. In the last few years a considerable number of diagrams have been worked out extending the early work by McBain, which was mainly on soaps, to many other types of surface-active agent. Broadly speaking there seems to be a general pattern in the nature of the phases found and the regions in which they occur, for both binary solutions of surface-active agents and ternary systems where a third solute is present. The particular concentrations and temperatures at which analogous regions are found varies with the chemical nature and the molecular weight of the surface-active agent and in the three-component systems with the nature of the third component, but, in general, appropriate choice of temperature and proportion of each component will show the general phase behaviour in any system. The use of such diagrams in formulation has already been pointed out and also, as Winsor has stated (1954, p. 92), solubility limits and mechanistic interpretations of them by comparison between different systems should only be made if the phase change which occurs is of similar type.

A. BINARY SYSTEMS

Binary phase diagrams for a number of non-ionic surface-active agents of different types have been published (Weston, 1953; Chakovskoy, 1956; Mulley, 1961; Balmbra Clunie *et al.*, 1962; Mulley and Metcalf, 1961) and a number of these diagrams are shown in Figs. 25 to 29. Diagrams for anionic detergents and soaps have been given by McBain and his co-workers (McBain *et al.*, 1938; Gonick and McBain, 1946 and other papers) (e.g. Fig. 30) and by Vold (1941), Bergeron (1954) and Luzzatti *et al.* (1957, 1958). Cationic materials have not had the same attention and no phase diagrams appear to have been published for these surface-active agents. Dealing with the ionic type first, these mostly form clear isotropic solutions in water, providing the lipophilic group is not too large and the concentration is not too high. This is the region which has been investigated most thoroughly by the methods described in Section II and is the region which probably contains the Hartley spherical micelles. The solubility is markedly dependent on the temperature and the alkyl chain length. For example, Fig. 31 shows, in the case of the sodium alkyl sulphonates, that only the C_{10} compound is soluble to any extent in water at room temperature (about 0·8 and 12 per cent at 20° and 30° respectively; the solubility of the C_{12} compound is only about 0·26 per cent at 30°). The compounds used in these measurements were pure and illustrate the tremendous difference between them and technical materials of nominally similar structure. The curves in Fig. 31 also show the remarkable effect of temperature on the solubility for many surface-active agents. On the lower temperature part of each curve solubility increases slowly with temperature until at a critical point the curve shows a break and the solubility a dramatic increase. This temperature is known as the Krafft point and the solubility of the surface-active agent at this point is usually near the c.m.c. The reason for the

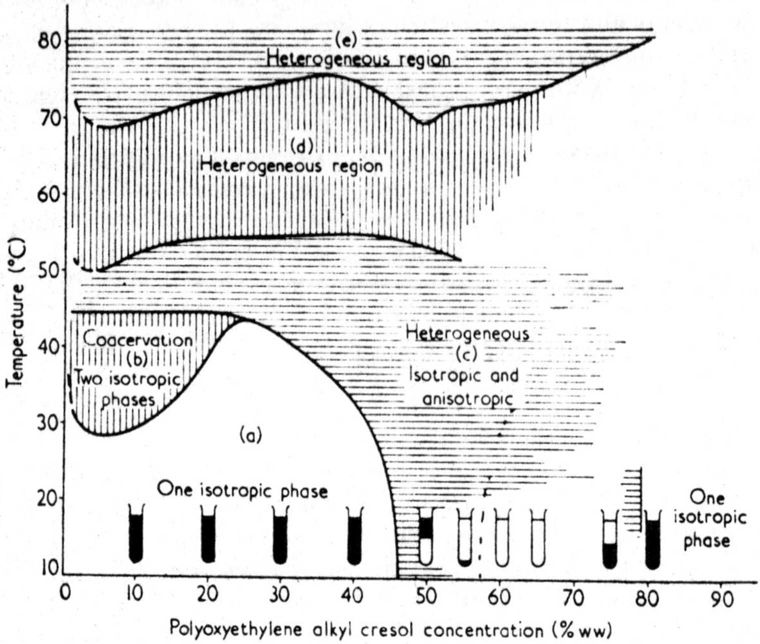

FIG. 25. Solubility diagram for a polyoxyethylene alkyl cresol in water (from Weston, 1953).

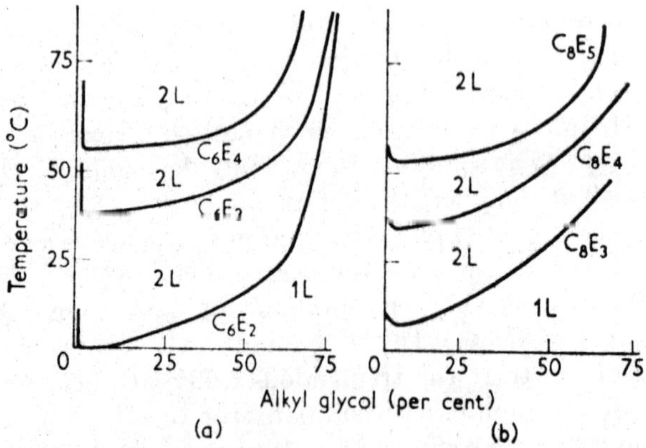

FIG. 26. Phase equilibrium diagrams for (*a*) monohexyl, and (*b*) mono-octyl polyoxyethylene glycols. (Redrawn from diagrams published by Chakovskoy, 1956).

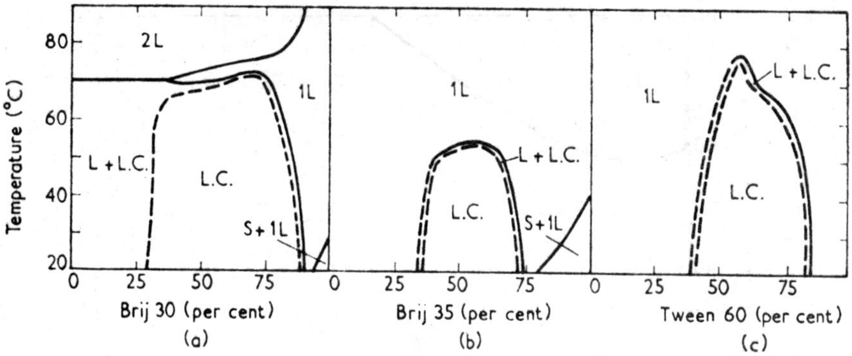

FIG. 27. Phase diagrams of some commercial surface-active agents. (*a*) Brij 30 (lauryl ether with about 3·5 ethylene oxide units per molecule). (*b*) Brij 35 (lauryl ether with about 21 ethylene oxide units per molecule). (*c*) Tween 60 (polyoxyethylene sorbitan monostearate (from Mulley, 1961 and unpublished results).

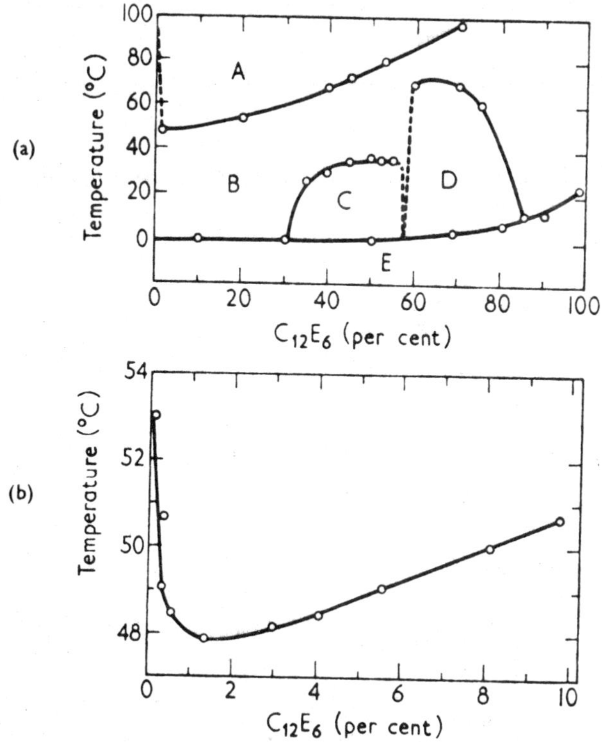

FIG. 28. Phase diagram for $C_{12}H_{25}(O.CH_2.CH_2)_6OH$ + water (from Balmbra and co-workers, 1962). (*a*) A, two isotropic liquids; B, one isotropic liquid; C, middle phase; D, neat phase; E, solid + ice. (*b*) The two liquid phase region.

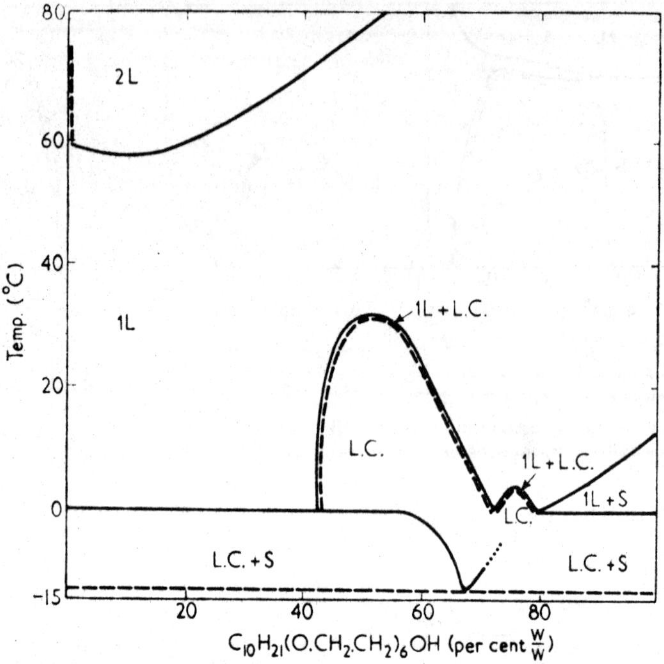

FIG. 29. Phase diagram for the system $C_{10}H_{25}(O.CH_2.CH_2)_6OH$ + water (from Mulley and Metcalf, *J. Colloid Sci.*, in the press).

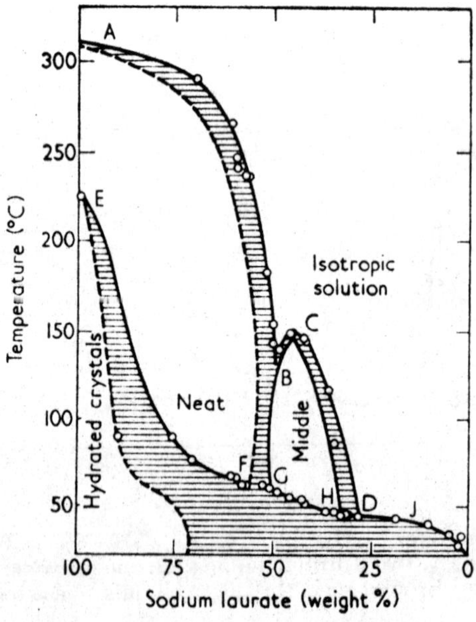

FIG. 30. The system sodium laurate + water (from McBain and co-workers, 1938).

break is bound up with the aggregation which occurs at the c.m.c. and has been discussed by Murray and Hartley (1935) and by Winsor (1954, p. 31). A solubility curve indicates the maximum solubility of a material at a temperature and shows that the chemical potential of the solid and liquid phases is equal at this point. Below the c.m.c. the chemical potential of the solid and liquid phases increases regularly with rise in temperature and therefore the solubility curve shows a regular increase.

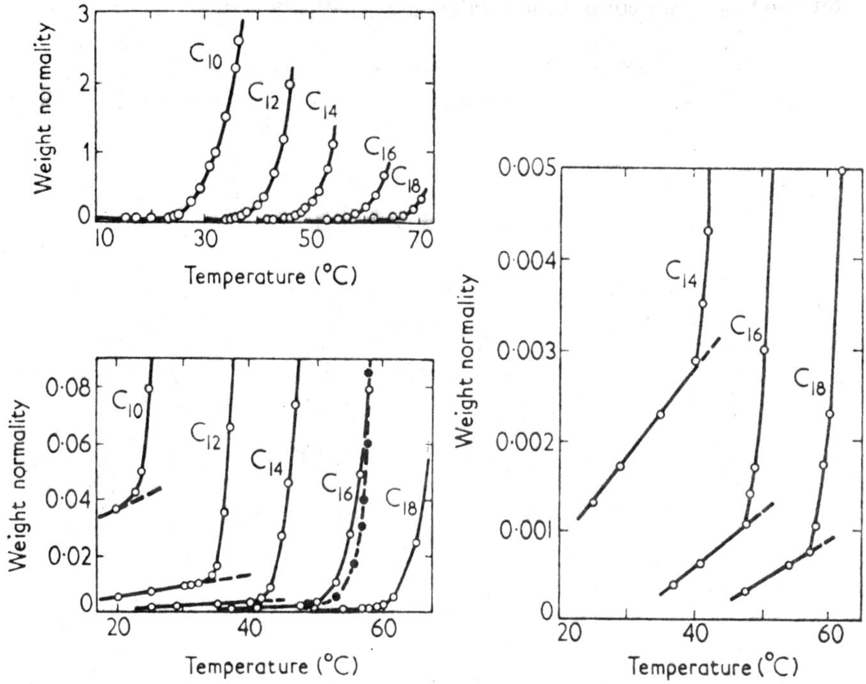

FIG. 31. Solubilities of the sodium salts of the higher alkyl sulphonates (from Tartar and Wright, 1939).

Above the c.m.c. the regular increase in chemical potential of the solid phase which increases solubility continues, but the rate in the liquid phase is much reduced, as is shown by the colligative properties of the solution. A much greater rate of change of concentration in the liquid phase is therefore necessary in order to produce equality of chemical potential in the phases in equilibrium at the solubility limit. This, beginning at the Krafft point gives a rapid increase of solubility with rise of temperature. Surface-active agents having a low crystallizing tendency (shown by low melting points) are thus more soluble than others in regions where solution is limited by separation of solid, which probably explains the high solubility of materials such as the non-terminal chain tetradecane sodium sulphates and hexanolamine oleate (Fig. 32).

The solubility of the ionic surface-active agents is limited at higher temperatures by the separation of a liquid crystalline phase. The concentration at which this occurs may be as high as 20 to 30 per cent for the lower alkyl chain materials but shifts rapidly to much lower concentrations for the higher chain materials (probably 1 to 2 per cent for the C_{18} chain compounds) (Tartar and Wright, 1939).

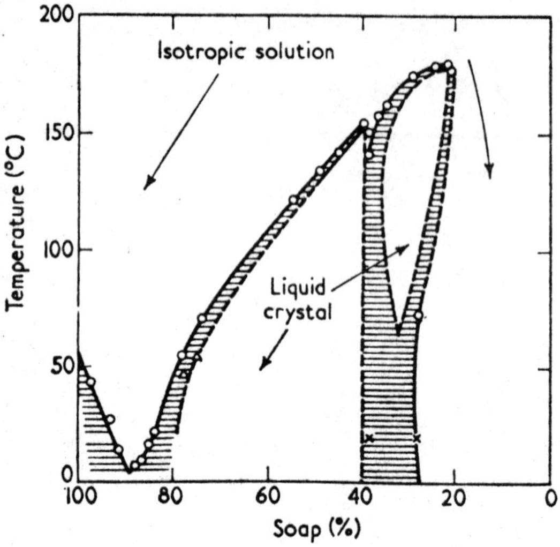

FIG. 32. Phase diagram for the system hexanolamine oleate + water (from Gonick and McBain, 1946).

Non-ionic materials form isotropic water solutions at room temperature in concentrations up to 30 to 50 per cent if sufficient hydrophilic groups are present in the molecule to produce much water solubility at all. Those with alkyl chains of C_8 and below are completely miscible with water (Fig. 26). The alkyl chain length does not exert so marked an effect on solubility at room temperature for these compounds since even those up to C_{18} are soluble in concentrations up to 20 to 30 per cent (Mulley and Metcalf, 1956). The number of ethylene oxide groups necessary to produce solubility in compounds of the polyglycol monoalkyl ether type is shown in Table XV. Most of the non-ionic type compounds do not show the Krafft phenomena because solubility is not limited by separation of a solid phase but by formation of liquid crystal (Figs. 25, 27, 28 and 29). This statement might find exception in certain higher members which have higher melting points, because there are indications that the compound $C_{16}E_6$ shows solubility changes with temperature analogous in some respects to the ionic compounds (Mulley, 1960). At room temperature the solubility is low and the phases in equilibrium above the solubility limit are solid and liquid. Solubility rises quite rapidly with temperature but then decreases at about 30° when solubility is limited by separation of a second liquid phase. Except for the separation of liquid at the higher temperature the phase diagram may be quite similar to those found for the ionic surface-active agents.

A major difference for the non-ionic compounds is the decrease in solubility found at higher temperatures (Figs. 25 to 29). When temperature increases sufficiently a second liquid phase separates which is the cause of the well-known clouding phenomenon. The temperature at which this occurs changes with alkyl and ethylene oxide chain length, as might be expected (Schönfeldt, 1959; Mulley, 1960). Organic compounds with a lower consolute point are usually considered to form hydrogen bonds with water, precipitation with rise of temperature being due to the temperature sensitivity of such bonds (Copp and Everett, 1953). The most likely structure for the second liquid phase, according to Hartley (1955), is the inverse spherical micelle. He thought that the reason for its formation in relatively dilute solution compared with other types of surface-active agent was the great length of the polyglycol chain which could cause micellar interaction at quite low concentrations, and therefore he considered that the inverse oleophilic micelle was favoured in quite dilute solutions of non-ionic surface-active agents.

TABLE XV

Solubility and cloud point (° C) of some Polyethylene Glycol Monoalkyl Ethers $C_nH_{2n+1}(CH_2.CH_2.O)_mOH$ (from Mulley, 1960)

Alkyl group	*m*				
	2	3	4	5	6
Hexyl (3% w/v)	+	37	67·5	75	80·5
Decyl (0·1% w/v)	+	+	18	36	60
Dodecyl (0·1% w/v)	—	+	—	25	48
Hexadecyl (0·1% w/v)	+	+	+	+	32

+ = insoluble.

Returning to the ionic materials, the liquid crystal phases found seem to be of two main types, usually called neat and middle in accordance with McBain's original nomenclature for soaps. Middle soap phases separate at the lower concentration. It is generally considered that the liquid crystal phases found in surface-active agent systems are of the smectic type (Boffey *et al.*, 1959). The separation into two definite regions may be related to the phenomena found in the solid phase where different crystal modifications are due to changes in the orientation of the alkyl chains with respect to the layer lattice planes (Hartley, 1955). Each liquid crystal phase is surrounded by a two-phase region in which an isotropic liquid is in equilibrium with neat or middle soap. Sometimes an intermediate region between the liquid crystal phases, which is apparently isotropic, has been reported by McBain's school. This region has also been reported and studied by Luzzati *et al.* (1957, 1958) for compounds with alkyl chains longer than C_{12}. They point out that it would be possible for a phase with an ordered structure of cubic symmetry to be isotropic in polarized light and that this corresponds to one of the ways of close packing uniform spheres, a structure suggested by Hartley for solutions of surface-active agents at high concentrations. The liquid crystalline phases are also found in non-ionic systems although they are not so stable to temperature. The two-phase regions surrounding the liquid crystal phases are usually extremely narrow and difficult to detect in these systems (Mulley and Metcalf, *J. Colloid Sci.*, in the press).

Ionic surface-active agents where the smaller ion is inorganic usually have high melting points and form liquid crystal phases on melting, with possibly a number of crystal and other liquid crystal modifications also appearing (Fig. 30). Non-ionic materials in the pure state usually melt to form isotropic liquids with no liquid crystal phase. This difference seems to be bound up with the different hydrophilic groups present in the two types and with the more intense nature of the ensuing transition between the two regions of the surface-active molecule in ionic compounds. The structure of the high concentration liquid region found in the non-ionic systems is uncertain but is probably unorganized with the molecules randomly dispersed.

B. TERNARY SYSTEMS

A number of workers have published phase diagrams for ternary systems in which water and a surface-active agent are two components and the third is an organic material which may be regarded as the solubilized component; although this is by convention and it is better to think of the systems as mutual solutions, no single component fulfilling one function. References to this work are given with Figs. 33–46 which show a number of the published results. The main classes of surface-active agent have been studied although the alkyl chain length has usually been short. This is because very high viscosity and consequent difficulty in separation of the phases is found with the longer chain compounds. Only a restricted range of solutes have been used in any one type of surface-active agent and on the whole more results have been reported for compounds which may be regarded as polar solutes.

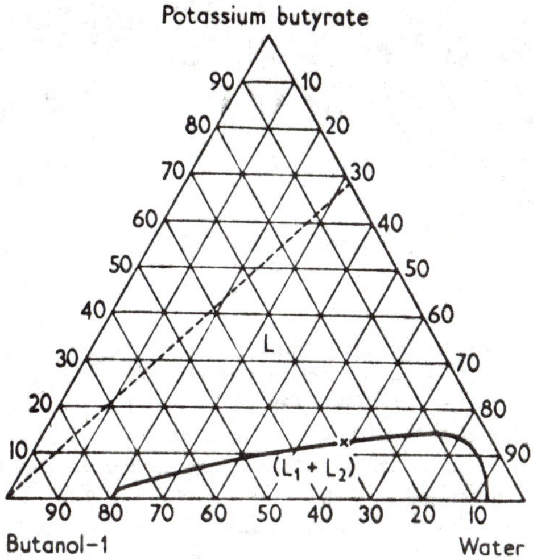

FIG. 33. The system potassium *n*-butyrate + butanol-1 + water at 25° C (from Lumb, 1951).

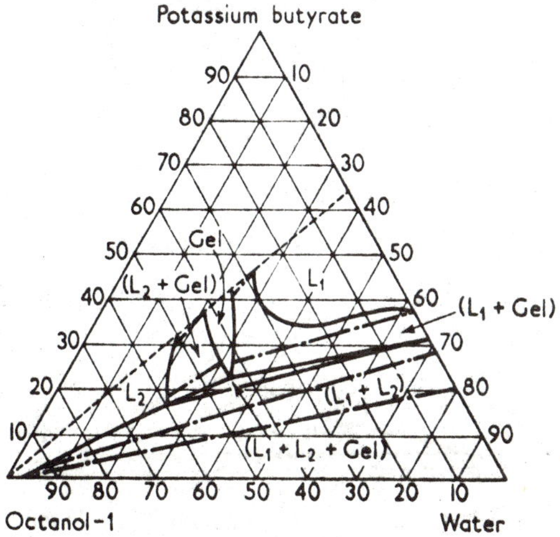

FIG. 34. The system potassium *n*-butyrate + octanol-1 + water at 25°C (from Lumb, 1951).

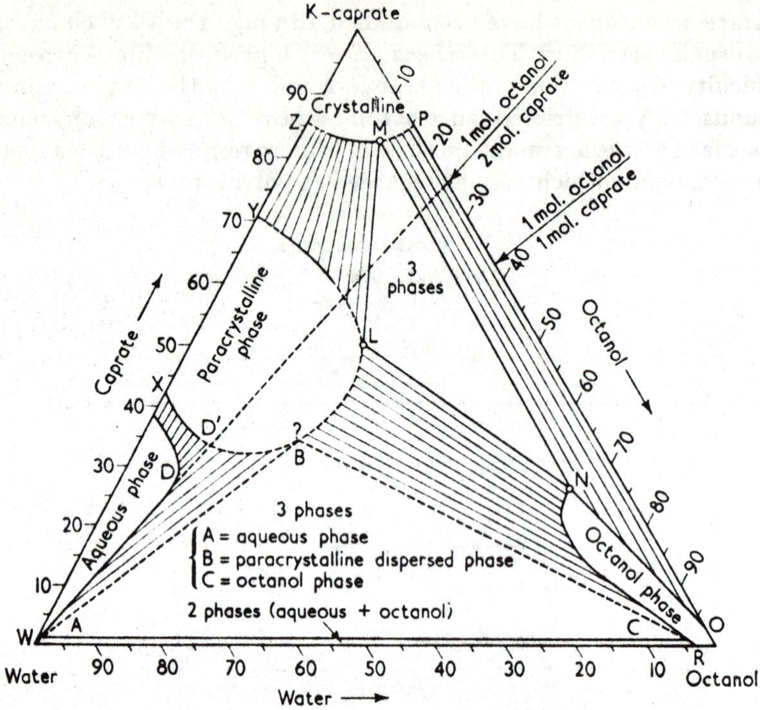

FIG. 35. Phase diagram of the system potassium caprate + n-octanol + water at 21–22° C (from Dervichian, 1957).

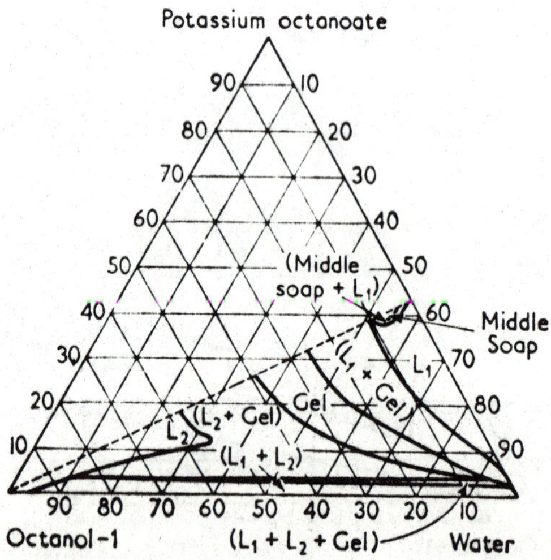

FIG. 36. The system potassium n-octanoate + octanol-1 + water at 25° C (from Lumb, 1951).

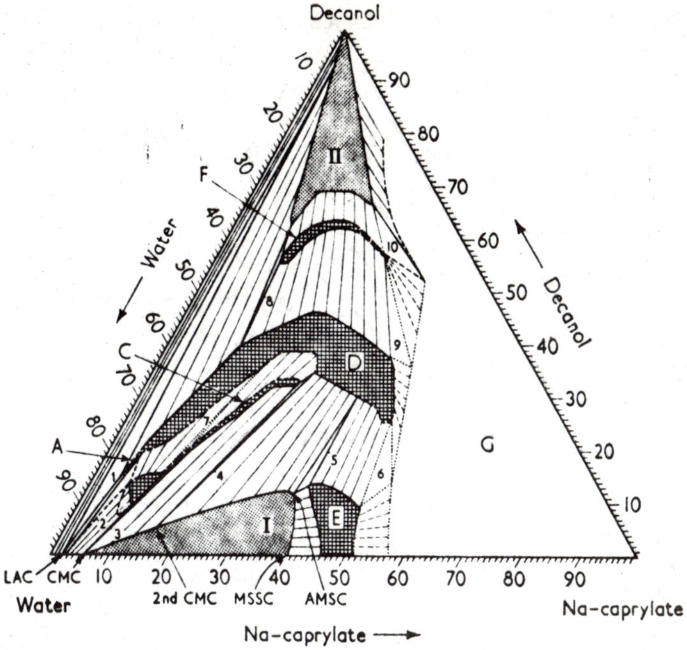

FIG. 37. Phase diagram for the system sodium caprylate + decanol + water at 20° C. I, homogeneous, isotropic aqueous solutions; II, homogeneous isotropic decanol solutions; A, B, C, D, E, F, homogeneous mesomorphous phases; 1–10 three phase triangles (from Ekwall and co-workers, 1960).

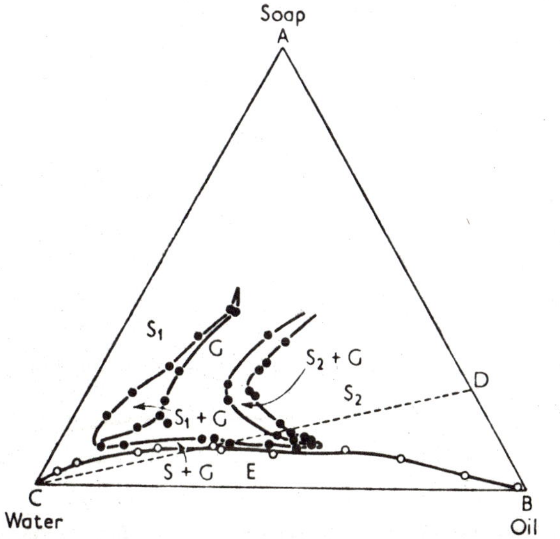

FIG. 38. Phase diagram of the system lauryldimethylbutyl ammonium bromide + C_6H_5Cl + water at 30° C (from Palit *et al.*, 1959).

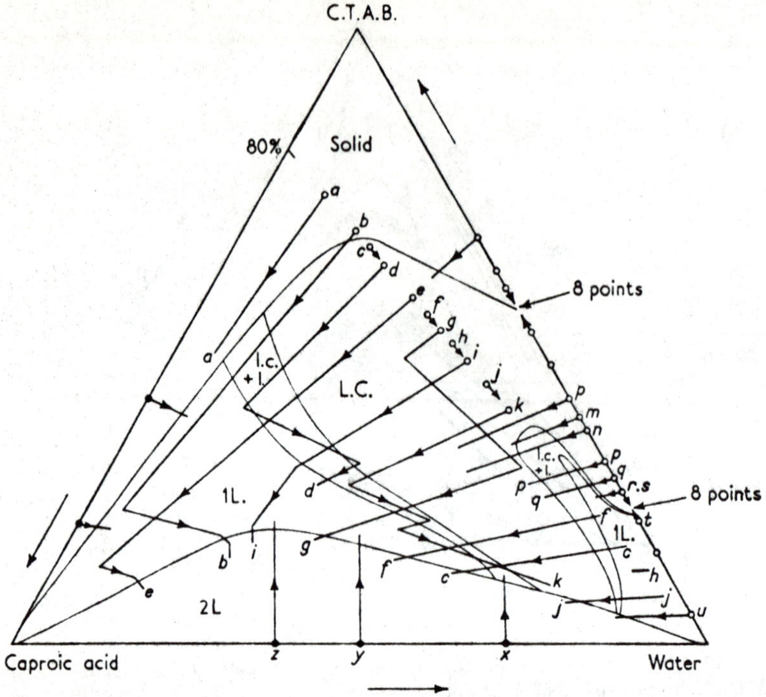

FIG. 39. The cetyltrimethylammonium bromide + caproic acid + water system at 27·5° C, showing phase boundaries and "triangularly staggered walk" technique (from Boffey and co-workers, 1959).

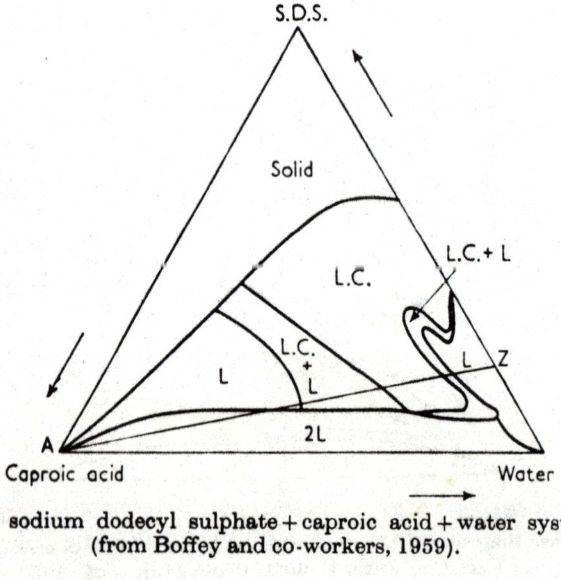

FIG. 40. The sodium dodecyl sulphate + caproic acid + water system at 25° C (from Boffey and co-workers, 1959).

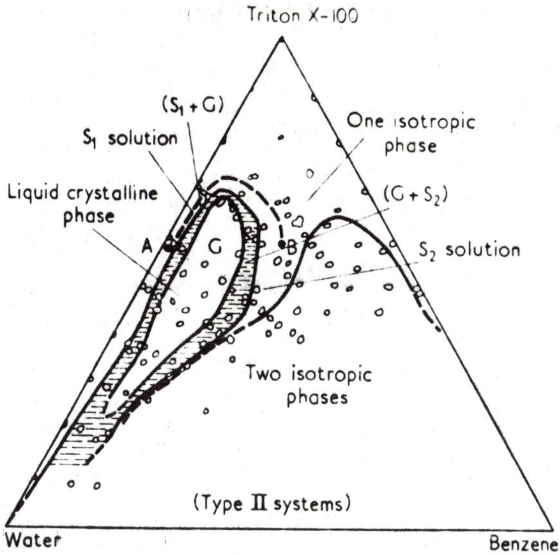

FIG. 41. Phase diagram for the system Triton X-100 (di-isobutylphenol derivative with 9 to 10 ethylene oxide units per molecule) + benzene + water (from Marsden and McBain, 1948 with phase nomenclature added by Winsor, 1954).

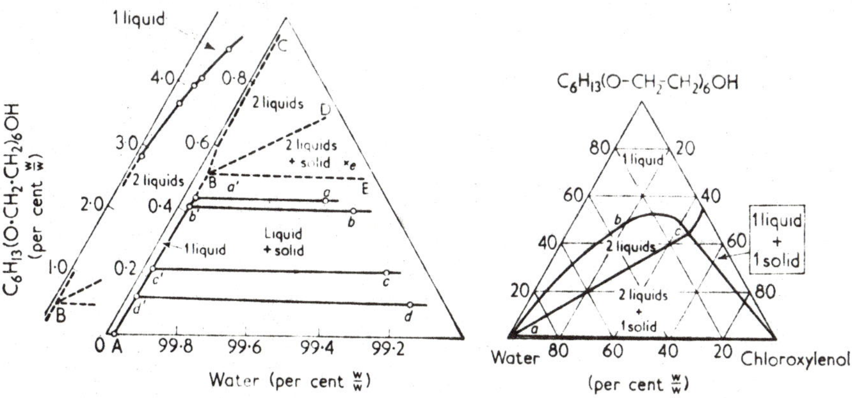

FIG. 42. The system $C_6H_{13}(O.CH_2.CH_2)_6OH$ + 4-chloro-3,5-xylenol + water at 20° C (from Mulley and Metcalf, 1961; Mulley and Metcalf, 1962).

In the lower left-hand corner in most of the systems an isotropic liquid phase forms, analogous to that containing hydrophilic micelles in the binary surface-active agent-water systems. In this region the water-insoluble material may be regarded as brought into solution by the special nature of the micellar solution. Another isotropic phase is found at high concentrations of the water-insoluble material. These solutions

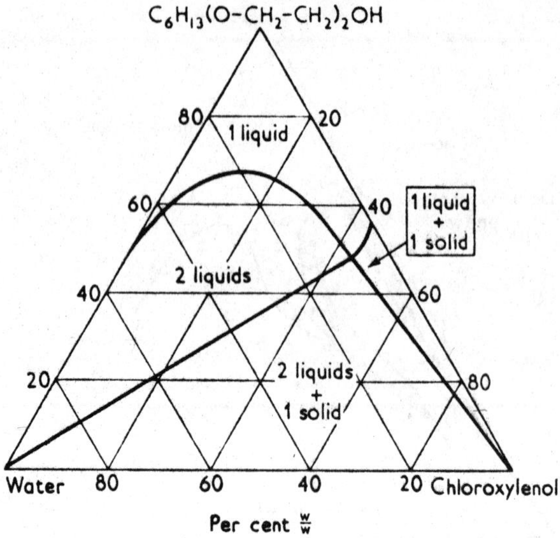

FIG. 43. The system $C_6H_{13}(O.CH_2.CH_2)_2OH$ + 4-chloro-3,5-xylenol + water at 20° C (from Mulley and Metcalf, 1961; Mulley and Metcalf, *J. Colloid Sci.*, in the press).

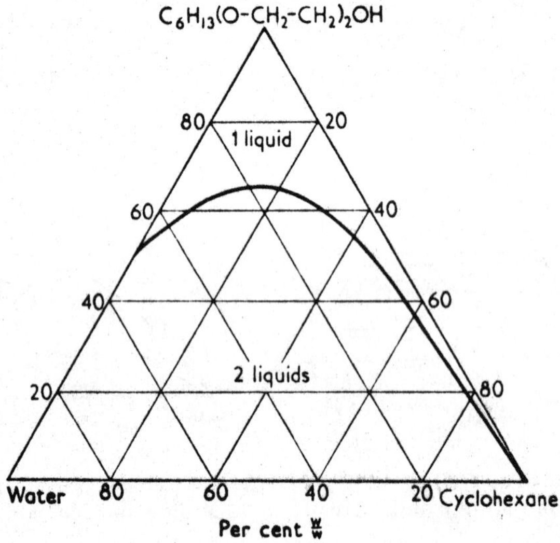

FIG. 44. The system $C_6H_{13}(O.CH_2.CH_2)_2OH$ + *cyclo*hexane + water at 20° C (from Mulley and Metcalf, 1961; Mulley and Metcalf, *J. Colloid Sci.*, in the press).

have not been studied in nearly so much detail but are usually considered to contain micelles of the inverse kind, water being solubilized in an organic environment. At low concentrations of the surface-active agent a two-liquid phase region occurs in most systems; in this region insuffi-

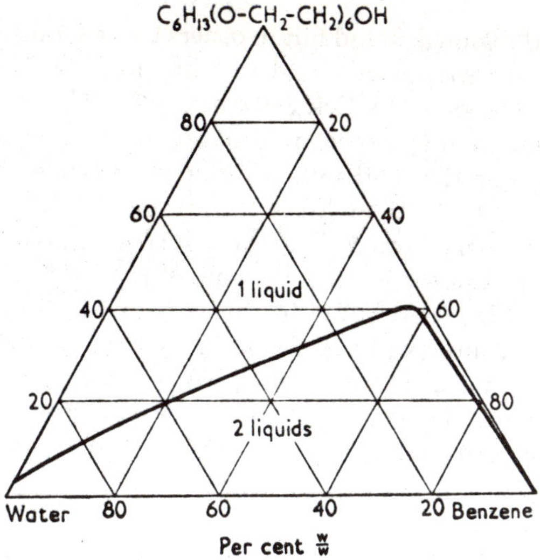

FIG. 45. The system $C_6H_{13}(O.CH_2.CH_2)_6OH$ + benzene + water at 20° C (from Mulley and Metcalf, 1961; Mulley and Metcalf, *J. Colloid Sci.*, in the press).

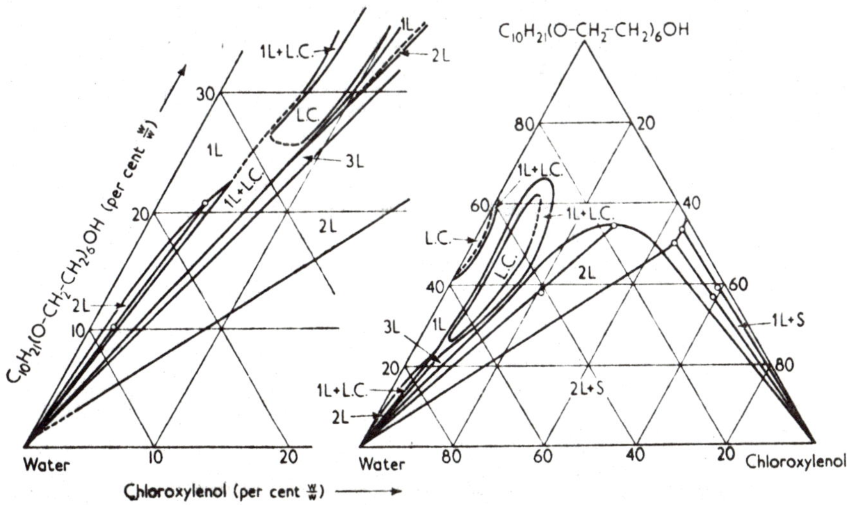

FIG. 46. The system $C_{10}H_{21}(O.CH_2.CH_2)_6OH$ + 4-chloro-3,5-xylenol + water at 20° C (from Mulley and Metcalf, 1961; Mulley and Metcalf, *J. Colloid Sci.*, in the press).

cient surface-active agent is present to produce complete miscibility and the two conjugate phases are of the hydrophilic and lipophilic micelle types. In many cases the liquid crystalline region in the binary system is considerably extended in the ternary. For shorter chain compounds only one liquid crystal region is found but in others two regions corresponding to middle and neat soap occur, and in long chain systems a complex situation has been reported by Eckwall *et al.* (1960). The six homogeneous liquid crystal regions they report were recognized by separation under high-speed centrifugation and by the different microscopic appearance of the phases (Fig. 47), although the "textures" seem to be analogous to those reported by Hyde *et al.* (1954) (Fig. 48) in different regions of the single liquid crystal phase in their system. Whether these are separate phases is doubtful but they could be the ternary liquid crystal solution derivatives of the complex phases found in pure soaps as they appear on the ternary diagram in a sequence which suggests that this is so. In many of the figures the liquid crystal phases curve in from the top of the diagram, appearing from left to right in the order found in the binary system.

The liquid crystal phases are probably to be regarded as the liquid crystal analogue of a solid solution. It is smectic in type (Boffey and co-authors, 1959) (Fig. 49) and is the region in which the McBain lamellar micelle may be regarded as fully formed. It forms at low concentrations in ternary solutions containing solutes of the long chain alcohol type because of the closer packing allowed when repulsion between the ionized head groups of the surface-active agent is reduced by interposition of the alcohol (Fig. 49), by the strong interaction of the alkyl chains and by the necessity of separating the water away from these chains (Lawrence, 1958; Boffey and co-workers, 1959). In certain systems Boffey *et al.* (1959) has calculated from the composition range over which liquid crystal forms, that the water layer in the smectic liquid crystal phase can be up to 110 Å thick and must be held by solution forces to the ionic head and the polar hydroxyl group of the solute. Its remarkable stability to temperature is evidence of its quasi crystal structure. The systems containing non-ionic materials show similar liquid crystal regions. The composition which has maximum stability to temperature corresponds in some systems to two molecules of water per ethylene oxide unit. The temperature stability in these systems where no ionic forces exist is remarkable, being even greater in relation to the melting point of the crystal than in the ionic compounds. This may be due to the possibility of the long hydrophilic chain penetrating to all parts of the water layer in the smectic sandwich, which reduces the tendency for the water to form a separate phase.

The other regions of the diagrams correspond to equilibria between the phases already described. In the base of the figures a two liquid phase region is found, one being aqueous and the other organic in type. On each side of the liquid crystal phase are regions containing both isotropic

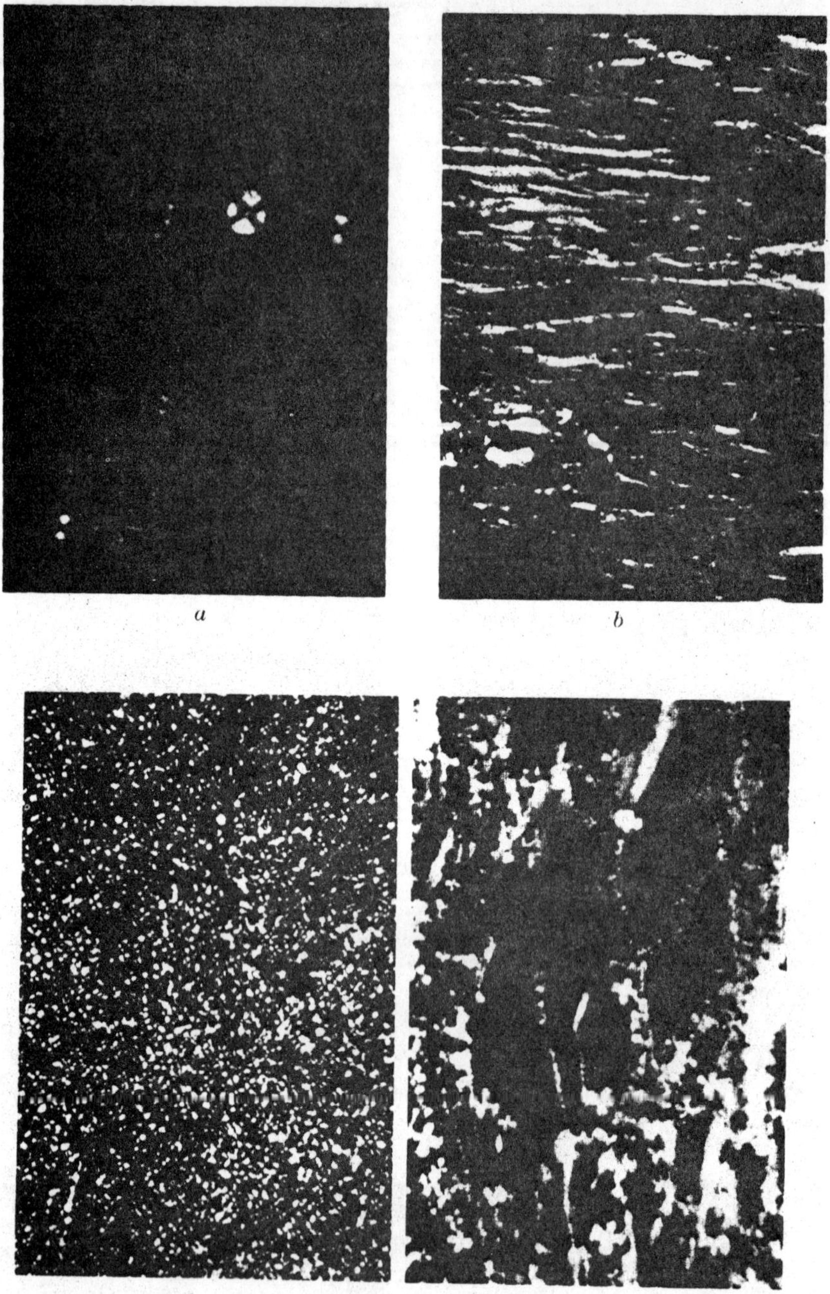

a *b* *c* *d*

Fig. 47.

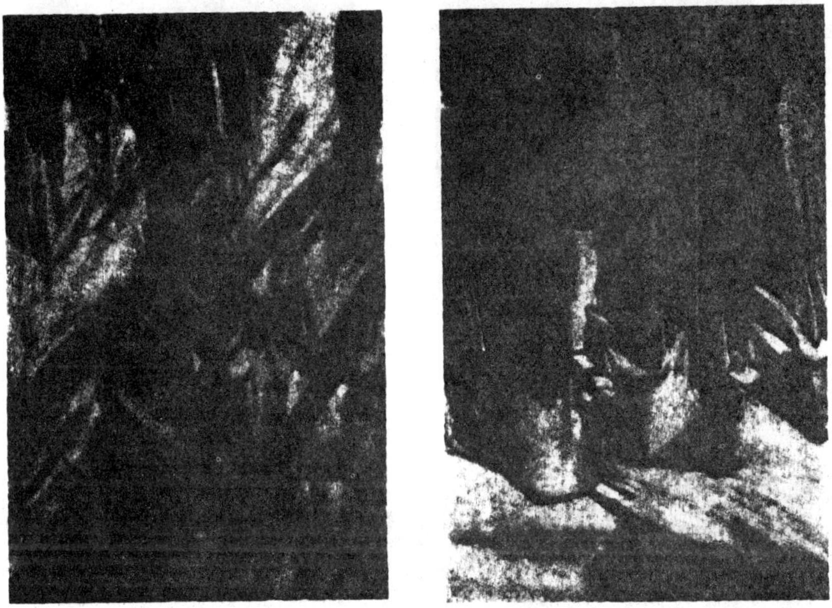

e *f*

FIG. 47.

FIG. 47. Microscopic appearance in polarized light of the liquid crystal phases in the system sodium caprylate + decanol + water at 20° C (× 300) (from Ekwall and co-workers, 1960, see Fig. 37). Composition of the system shown in each photograph (per cent w/w) is given in the order sodium caprylate, decanol, water. (*a*) Phase B; 8·5, 9·5, 82·0. (*b*) Phase C; 25·5, 31·9, 42·6. (*c*) Phase D; 28·0, 42·1, 29·9. (*d*) Phase D; 11·9, 41·1, 47·0. (*e*) Phase E; 44·0, 6·0, 50·0. (*f*) Phase F; 12·8, 60·1, 27·1.

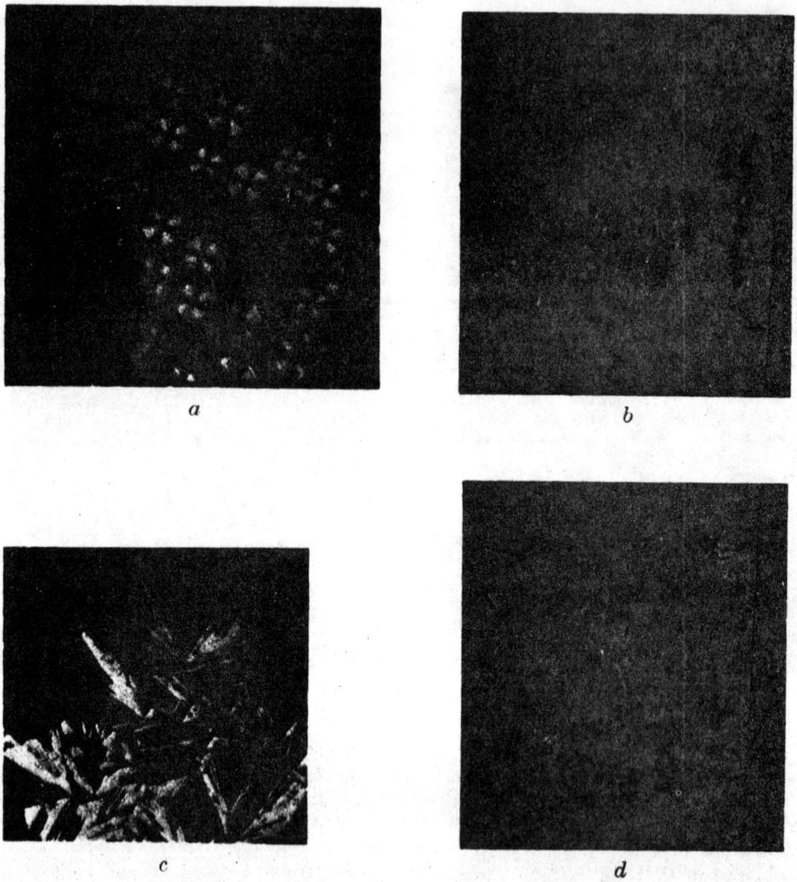

FIG. 48. Forms of liquid crystalline phase. (*a*) Anisotropic spherulites. (*b*) Striated texture found in the high viscosity region of the system. (*c*) Focal conics. (*d*) Batonnets (from Hyde *et al.*, 1954).

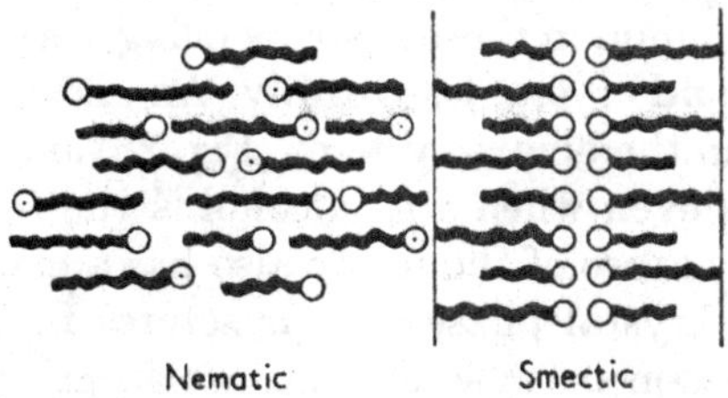

FIG. 49. Possible molecular arrangements in the liquid crystalline phase found in systems containing surface-active agents. The smectic form is most likely (from Boffey and co-workers, 1959).

liquid and liquid crystal phases, and of these one of the isotropic phases is aqueous and the other organic in nature. Between this region and the base of the figure is an invarient three phase region with two liquid and one liquid crystal phase in equilibrium. Where the organic component is a solid and if the surface-active agent itself is a solid then equilibria involving solid phases are superimposed on this pattern (Mulley and Metcalf, 1962).

Equilibria at low concentrations of the surface-active agent are of interest for the light they throw on the c.m.c. and its changes in the presence of third components, especially regarding detection of the c.m.c. by the dye and solubilization methods. Figure 42 shows phase equilibria for one system near the c.m.c. It is apparent that plots of solubility in this case would give changes in direction of the curve which, in the absence of checks on the phases found, might give a false value to the derived c.m.c. With longer chain compounds (Ekwall *et al.*, 1960; Mulley and Metcalf, *J. Colloid Sci.*, in the press), it seems likely that even more complicated phase changes can occur near the c.m.c., probably involving liquid crystal phases. Although changes resulting in the separation of bulk phases are probably paralleled by changes in the micelle form in the solutions, it does not seem correct to regard them as points at which micelles of a new type are formed (i.e. c.m.c.'s) because changes in the micelle form may have been taking place in such solutions before separation of a bulk phase. The phase change possibly represents the culmination of the process.

The effect of the surface-active agent on these equilibrium diagrams is mainly controlled by the chain length and chemical type. Those with shorter chains do not form the liquid crystal phases so readily, a solute of C_8 chain being necessary to produce extensive regions with C_4 soaps. With longer chain materials the regions of liquid crystal expand rapidly. It is noteworthy that Lumb's diagrams show the poor solubilizing power of the short chain compounds at low concentrations, the regions of aqueous isotropic liquid in these systems being very small. Non-ionic compounds form liquid crystal less readily. An alkyl chain longer than C_8 seems necessary in the binary systems (Fig. 26) and longer than C_6 in the ternary systems even when a C_8 alcohol is the solute (Mulley and Metcalf, 1962). The nature of the solute also has a marked effect on the formation of liquid crystal phases. Polar solutes favour separation of liquid crystal while non-polar solutes do not form liquid crystal until higher concentrations of surface-active agent and solute are present (Nakagawa and co-workers, 1960). The areas of miscibility in the systems are increased by rise of temperature, as might be expected (McBain and Field, 1933; Lumb, 1951; Winsor, 1954; Lawrence, 1958), but the picture is complicated in non-ionic systems by the lack of solubility of the agent itself when the temperature is raised. This was discussed in the binary systems. However, it seems to depend on the region of the diagram considered, solubility being increased in regions where liquid crystal and solid phases form (Mulley, 1961).

Although the general pattern of the diagrams for most systems is that described above, some show additional features and phases. Winsor has described regions in which three apparently isotropic phases are in equilibrium. Although two main types of micelle structure are normally considered possible, the three phases found do not all appear to have a specialized structure because in a non-ionic system (Mulley and Metcalf, *J. Colloid Sci.*, in the press) at least one of them seems to be of very low concentration, in fact below the c.m.c., and therefore unorganized with the components molecularly dispersed.

The pattern of phases found in so many systems strongly supports the general concepts of micelle formation advanced especially by Winsor (1954). Addition of a water-insoluble material to a solution of surface-active agent containing Hartley micelles gradually modifies the micelle form by the mechanism previously mentioned, until precipitation of liquid crystal occurs. Continuing addition of the organic additive first progressively reduces the volume of the aqueous phase until a single smectic phase is found, and then causes the smectic phase to disappear, leaving a single organic phase, with the water solubilized by inverted oleophilic micelles. Polar and non-polar solubilization may be distinguished by the different effect they have on liquid crystal formation. The non-polar solute cannot assist orientation of the surface-active molecules to the same extent and therefore liquid crystal is formed only at very high surface-active agent concentrations. The general effects of chain length of surface-active agent and chain length and nature of solute on the phase equilibrium pattern is closely allied to the changes expected in the micelle form by the general analysis of solution processes given by Hartley (1955) and by Winsor (1954).

VI. Some Factors in the Formulation of Pharmaceutical Products Containing Solubilized Materials

It is obviously difficult to give an account of all the possible factors involved in the formulation of solubilized preparations, many problems being specific to the particular system under consideration. For instance, the nature and proportion of the surface-active agent is important in cases where an active product is required while in other cases the only concern may be getting the drug into solution, its use not being affected by the nature or proportion of the solubilizing agent. Incompatibilities between certain solutes and solubilizing agents may also be a controlling feature. Examples of this are the inactivation of phenols by non-ionic surface-active agents and the interaction between anionic agents and cationic materials which may lead to precipitation of a complex. Despite the difficulties, a number of possible factors are considered below which may be some guide to the complex situations met with in formulation.

A. CHOICE OF SURFACE-ACTIVE AGENT

The general properties of the main classes of surface-active agent may be a controlling factor in the choice of an agent for its solubilizing action. In the anionic group the soaps are precipitated by divalent ions and are only suitable for use at alkaline pH. The potassium salts are often used because they are more soluble than the corresponding sodium compounds. Soaps with an organic cation may have advantages in respect of solubility. Paraffin chain salts of the strong acids are not so readily precipitated by divalent ions and are stable over a wider pH range. Cationic surface-active agents are not widely used as solubilizing agents because of their antibacterial activity, which is undesirable in most cases, and because they are more toxic than the other classes. The non-ionic compounds have many advantages. They are not sensitive to salts or pH, are almost non-toxic and have, in most cases, a very high solubility. They are the only class sufficiently non-toxic to have been widely used in internal preparations. The main incompatibilities of the three classes have already been mentioned.

A major difficulty in choosing a surface-active agent is that published information on their properties has been obtained with highly purified materials or with commercial products of unknown purity. It may be difficult to transfer these results to those for any particular commercial sample of a compound. Solubility of the surface-active agent itself is a property which very much depends on purity. Carefully purified materials unmixed with compounds of different chain length often have low solubility, particularly the longer chain compounds (Section V), whereas commercial materials have much higher solubility mainly because the lipophilic part of the molecule is a mixture of varying chain length. Even when results have been related to a particular commercial product, control may prove a problem owing to batch variation. There is no simple test to measure solubilizing power and it is preferable to have a test based on the formulation itself.

An important factor in choosing a surface-active agent is the comparative solubilizing efficiency of the wide range of surface-active agents available, which is controlled by such changes in structure as the alkyl chain length, the length of the ethylene oxide chain in non-ionic compounds, the nature of the ionizing group and its point of attachment to the molecule, and the branching of the chain. These factors have been extensively discussed by Klevens (1950), Winsor (1954) and by M. E. L. McBain and Hutchinson (1955). In the following discussion the data have been reconsidered together with more recent measurements, and emphasis placed on the view that solubilization depends on solution within the micelle and that therefore an appropriate measure of solubilizing efficiency is the weight of solute dissolved per unit volume of micellar material (approximately proportional to weight).

The effect of alkyl chain length on solubilizing efficiency for the straight chain potassium soaps with solutes of polar and non-polar nature has been considered by Klevens (1950, p. 20). The solutes were dimethylaminoazobenzene, *n*-heptane, 1-octanol, ethylbenzene, 1-heptanol and the soaps were from C_8 to C_{14}. Solubilizing efficiency was measured as moles of solute solubilized per thousand grams of soap solution at a soap concentration of 0·3 M. The results show increased solubilizing power for all solutes with increase in alkyl chain length. The effect is particularly marked at all chain lengths when considering the solubility of hydrocarbons. For the alcohols the effect of chain length of the soap is marked below C_{11} but above this the solubility is almost independent of chain length. Interpretation of the results may be complicated for the shorter chain soaps because of their high c.m.c., and comparison with the higher members should take account of this. If solubilization depends on solution within the micelle, better comparison between soaps is given on the basis of moles of material solubilized per gram of hydrocarbon in the micelle interior since it is obvious that each mole of the higher soaps contains a greater volume within which a solute may dissolve and would therefore be expected to be more effective solubilizers. Comparison on a weight basis allows for the effect of molecular weight. Table XVI shows the effect of this factor in the solubilization of hydrocarbons. The longer chain compounds are still more effective than the shorter and therefore simple solution in the volume of hydrocarbon in the micelle interior is not the only factor. Micelles composed of longer chains, and therefore larger, are more effective, volume for volume, than the smaller micelles of the short chain compounds, possibly for the simple geometrical reason that solutes are more easily accommodated in the large micelles. Factors other than simple solution within the micelle appear to be operating in the solubilization of long chain alcohols. The results above, in conjunction with others where the effect of the chain length of the solute alcohol has been considered (Klevens, 1950, p. 36) show that in some cases the solubility of alcohols *decreases* when the chain length of the soap increases and also

TABLE XVI

Solubility of Ethylbenzene in 0·5 M Soap Solutions at 25° (from Klevens, 1950)

Soap	*Moles of micellar soap per 1000 g of solution*	*Moles ethylbenzene dissolved*	*Weight of soap, g*	*Weight of hydrocarbon interior, g*	*Moles of oil per mole of micellar soap*	*Moles of oil per g of micelle interior* $\times 10^3$
KC_{10}	0·0405	0·087	85	56·4	0·214	1·54
KC_{12}	0·475	0·212	113	79·3	0·446	2·67
KC_{14}	0·494	0·427	132·4	96·3	0·866	4·43

that they need a solubilizing agent of approximately equal or greater chain length to give good solvent action. In these cases more specific factors are affecting solubility which are probably associated with packing of the alcohols into the micelle in fairly definite molecular ratio (Dervichian, 1957). The material separating at the solubility limit is not excess alcohol but a liquid crystalline phase rich in the surface-active agent and the alcohol. This liquid crystal formation is induced by increase in chain length of the solute and the solubilizing agent, and this is responsible for lower solubility with the increase in chain length of the soap.

In Section III it was pointed out that if solubilizing action was a solution process within the micelle it would be independent of the nature of the inorganic part of the surface-active molecule. Results for cetyl pyridinium salts (Table XII) showed this to be largely true. It should also be independent of the nature of the ionic head group. This appears to be approximately so in certain other cases. For example, the solubility of Orange OT is the same in the sodium and the potassium C_{12} soaps (Kolthoff and Stricks, 1948). These authors also found dimethylaminoazobenzene to have the same solubility in each pair of the C_{10}, C_{12} and C_{14} sodium and potassium soaps of equal chain length. However, in certain cases cationic compounds have been reported to be superior. Klevens (1950, p. 24) has collected solubility data for *n*-heptane, dimethylaminoazobenzene and C_7 to C_{10} straight chain alcohols in soaps, sulphonates, sulphates and a cationic surface-active agent of similar alkyl chain length which shows that solubility is quite near that to be expected for the volume of hydrocarbon in the micelle interior in each case, excepting the case of *n*-heptane in the C_{12} amine hydrochloride which is about four times as effective as the other compounds of the same chain length. According to Winsor (1954) this is because the hydrophilic interaction of the cationic head group with water is less than that of the anionic compounds, moving the intermicellar equilibrium to the right and thus in his view giving increased solubility. It may be noted that there is less difference between the solvent power of the compounds when dimethylaminoazobenzene is the solute.

Branching in the chain of the surface-active agent, or attachment of the ionic group to a non-terminal position in the chain, usually decreases solubilizing efficiency. This was found by Hartley (1941) for sulphonated dialkyl esters of dihydric phenols. The solubilizing power of Aerosol AY (diamyl sulphosuccinate) for dimethylaminoazobenzene is below that of a C_{14} soap (similar number of carbon atoms) although above that of a C_{10} soap (Kolthoff and Stricks, 1948). Complex systems of four or more components have been considered by Winsor (1954). He measured the amount of *cyclo*-hexanol required to produce S_1, G and S_2 solutions in mixtures of *cyclo*-hexane, water and non-terminal chain salts such as tetradecane sodium sulphates, octane sodium sulphates and undecane ammonium chlorides. Although the amount of the alcohol necessary to produce a clear solution was less for the non-terminal salts than for the 1-salts, the total amount of water-insoluble material that could be held in S_1 solution is usually greater for the salts with terminal ionic groups. In certain cases this was not so because of the greater tendency for the systems with the straight chain compounds to precipitate liquid crystal especially when long chain alcohols were the solutes. Another characteristic of these systems was the narrow range of compositions included between Type I and Type II systems for the non-terminal salts. The 1-salts were not so sensitive to change in composition. It should be noted that these statements apply to one concentration range only and may not be true of other concentrations. The situation may be analogous to the simpler ternary systems, phase diagrams of which are shown in Section V. With increased concentration of the surface-active agent the range of compositions between aqueous type solutions and oily solutions becomes narrower. The comparisons made by Winsor may simply be a consideration of different stages in the phase equilibrium pattern in the systems.

Little information on the solubilizing power of non-ionic surface-active agents compared with that on ionic agents has appeared in the earlier literature. McBain and his co-workers (McBain *et al.*, 1948) reported that hexanolamine oleate and two non-ionic materials were more effective solubilizers on a mole per mole basis than potassium laurate. The effect of the polyglycol chain length has been considered by Cohen (1952) and by Moore and Bell (1959). Cohen used dodecyl polyglycols with 7, 12, 27 and 45 ethylene oxide units per molecule, and measured the solubility of hexane, toluene, benzene and heptanol-1 in 0·1 N solutions of the compounds. The ethylene oxide chain affected solubility considerably on a mole per mole basis, as plotted by Cohen, but not in the same direction or to the same extent for each solute. Moore and Bell measured the solubilities of diphenylmethane and phenylethyl alcohol. Some of these results are presented in Table XVII with others showing the effect of the alkyl chain on solubilizing power. They show that the dominating factor in the solubilizing power of a non-ionic surface-active agent is the weight (directly related to volume) of the hydrocarbon interior of the micelles. On a weight basis the longer ethylene oxide chain compounds are not very effective. Further comparative results for non-ionic, anionic, cationic and betaine type compounds are shown in Table XVII. The comparisons have not always been made at equivalent concentrations, but since the published results show that once micelles are fully formed solubility is proportional to concentration, no significant difference would be found no matter what concentrations were considered. Since the c.m.c. of some of the compounds is high, surface-active agent which is non-micellar has been allowed for as well as the amount of solute which might be expected to dissolve in the water present where this is a significant part of the total amount dissolving. Owing to the wide differences between the head groups and in the molecular weight of the inorganic ion, which is difficult to equate between compounds, comparison has been made on the basis that the whole of the molecule takes part on solubilization. This partly explains the relatively low efficiency of Cetrimide (high atomic weight of bromine) and the rather high efficiency of Cetomacrogol ($C_{16}E_{22}$), where the calculation includes the hydrocarbon chain only, there being no head group or inorganic ion. It is also possible that the high efficiency of the non-ionic

TABLE XVII

The Effect of Ethylene Oxide Chain Length on the Solubilizing Power of Non-ionic Surface-active Agents (C_nE_m) and Comparison of their Solvent Power with that of Other Materials

Solute — *Solubility (g solute per g of hydrocarbon in the non-ionic surface-active agent; values for ionic materials and those in brackets for the non-ionic compounds are in g solute per g of total surface-active agent)*

Solute	$C_{16}E_m$, 10%						
m	10	14	18	24	30	45	60
Diphenylmethane[a]	0·94 (0·31)	0·75 (0·20)	0·77 (0·17)	0·80 (0·14)	0·48 (0·07)	0·69 (0·07)	0·40 (0·03)

Solute	$C_{12}E_m$, 0·1 M	
m	27·6	40
Hexane[b]	0·31 (0·04)	0·26 (0·02)
Toluene[b]	0·93 (0·11)	0·70 (0·06)
Benzene[b]	1·43 (0·17)	1·43 (0·12)
Heptanol[b]	3·78 (0·45)	3·57 (0·33)

Solute	$C_{16}E_{22}$, 0·1 M[c]	C_6E_6, 13%[d]	$C_{10}E_6$, 19·5%[d]	Pot. laurate 0·134 M[e]
Chloroxylenol	1·39 (0·24)	1·15 (0·26)	0·58 (0·19)	0·60

Solute	$C_{16}E_{22}$ (0·03 M)	Pot. laurate (0·25 M)	Cetrimide (0·03 M)
n-Hexaldehyde	1·42 (0·28)	1·27	1·10
n-Heptaldehyde	1·23 (0·24)	1·11	0·655
n-Nonaldehyde	0·74 (0·14)	0·57	0·48
n-Decaldehyde	0·69 (0·13)	0·38	0·36
n-Undecaldehyde	0·53 (0·10)	0·32	0·26
Methylinoleate	0·20 (0·04)	0·11	0·07
	(0·1 M)	(0·5 M)	(0·14 M)
cyclo-Hexane	0·41 (0·08)	0·21	0·17
	(0·1 M)	(0·225 M)	(0·14 M)
Benzaldehyde	0·85 (0·17)	0·70	0·44
	(0·1 M)	(0·225 M)	(0·11 M)

Solute	*N*-alkyl *NN*-dimethylglycines					
	C_8(8·5%)	C_{10}(8·5%)	C_{11}(8·5%)	C_{12}(7·7%)	C_{14}(8·8%)	C_{16}(11·4%)
Benzaldehyde	0·91	1·20	1·5	0·72	0·48	0·42

[a] Moore and Bell (1959); [b] Cohen (1952); [c] Mulley and Metcalf (1956); [d] Mulley and Metcalf (1961); [e] Berry and Bean (1953). Solubilities in the lower part of the table are taken from Carless and Nixon (1960), Nixon (1958), Carless and Mitchell (1962), Swarbrick and Carless (1963).

compound could be partly due to the glycol chain playing some part in solubilization. From Table XVII it appears that, notwithstanding the very different nature of the surface-active agents, solubility of quite a wide range of compounds is surprisingly closely related to the weight of micellar material and does not particularly depend on its nature. This would be expected if the theory of solution within the micelle is correct. For non-ionic compounds the glycol portion does not appear to be a controlling factor, except for the solubilizing action of compounds containing only a few ethylene oxide units above the number necessary to produce a soluble surface-active agent, good comparison with other surface-active agents being obtained by considering only the hydrocarbon chain. Further data which would probably show a similar picture has been recently published by Goodhart and Martin (1962). Suggestions that solubilization is controlled by more specific factors such as complex formation or absorption on the surface of the micelle are not supported by the data. Polar solutes are often considered to be solubilized by orientation of their molecules in the micelle and therefore the mechanism by which they dissolve to be different from non-polar solutes. The results, however, show that their solubility is proportionate to the volume of hydrocarbon micellar material and independent of the nature of the head group. This indicates that solubilization even of polar materials is probably a solution process within the micelle. Differences between the solubilizing agents, which chemically speaking are considerable, would be expected to be much wider if solubilization were not a simple solution process. However, factors other than solution in the micelle obviously play a part, particularly with the long chain polar solutes, because solubility can decrease even when a longer chain surface-active agent (and therefore increased weight of micellar material) is used. In such cases association between the long chains of solute and solubilizing agent reduces solubility because liquid crystal is precipitated. However, even here a solution process probably still predominates otherwise one would expect more dramatic changes in solubility.

In conclusion, all straight alkyl chain surface-active agents appear to be approximately equivalent when the volume of micelle interior is the basis of comparison. Since this is so it should be possible to calculate from a single measurement the approximate solubility of a solute in any of the straight chain compounds over a wide range of concentration. There are, however, a number of exceptions. Thus, for long chain polar solutes liquid crystal formation with the longer chain surface-active agents may limit solubility. In such cases more solute may be dissolved by using a shorter chain or branched chain surface-active agent. Another important conclusion is that non-ionic compounds having long glycol chains are relatively ineffective solubilizing agents on a total weight basis because the length of the glycol chain does not greatly increase solubilizing power.

B. EFFECT OF THE NATURE OF THE SOLUTE ON SOLUBILITY

No adequate quantitative explanation of the effect of the chemical or physical nature of solutes on their solubility in solutions of surface-active agents has been advanced. However, as in solubility phenomena generally, qualitative comparison of the effect of a number of properties such as polarity, charge, molar volume (molecular weight), chain length, branching and substitution in a molecule, and its melting point on solubility, have been made. In general the solubility is less for materials of high molecular weight, high melting point and low polarity.

TABLE XVIII

Effect of Chain Length, Presence of Polar Groups, Cyclization and Polynuclear Ring Formation on Solubility (selected from values collected by Klevens, 1950)

Amount solubilized in 0·1 N *potassium laurate, sodium octadecenoate and dodecylamine hydrochloride (moles per litre) and in* 0·5 N *potassium laurate (g per litre) at* 25°C.

	KC_{12}		NaC_{18}	$C_{12}HCl$
n-Hexane	0·18		0·46	0·75
n-Heptane	0·12		0·34	0·54
n-Octane	0·08		0·18	0·29
n-Dodecane	0·005		0·009	0·063
n-Octylamine	0·07		0·07	0·13
n-Octanol	0·29		0·59	0·18
n-Dodecanol	0·03		0·13	0·052
Benzene	0·29		0·76	0·65
Toluene	0·13		0·51	0·49
Ethylbenzene	0·20		0·40	0·38
			0·5 N KC_{12}	
Benzene	30·6	Phenanthrene		1·21
Ethylbenzene	22·0	Anthracene		0·155
n-Butylbenzene	14·9	1,2-Benzanthracene		0·145
Naphthalene	4·26	1,2,5,6-Dibenzanthracene		0·024

Solubilizing solids is more difficult than solubilizing liquids of approximately corresponding molecular weight because the latent heat of fusion opposes the change of state (Winsor, 1954; Hartley, 1955). For the same reason solids with higher melting points are less soluble at a given temperature than those of lower melting point, provided the heat of fusion of the lower melting substance is not notably greater (Winsor,

1954, p. 135). Although solubilization is frequently only slightly affected by temperature it seems possible that this is not the case at temperatures near the melting point of solids. In fact, Lawrence has spoken of a "Krafft Point" in solubilization.

Increase in the chain length of a normal paraffin or the addition of an alkyl group to a benzene nucleus decreases solubility. Cyclization enhances solubility when relatively short chain compounds are compared with their single ring analogues (Klevens, 1950, p. 30). Klevens has also collected data to show that double ring compounds are usually less soluble than the corresponding straight chain materials. Presumably this is because such molecules are less readily organized into the micellar regions of the solution than non-cyclic compounds which have a less rigid configuration. Unsaturated materials are more soluble than the corresponding saturated compounds but branched chain compounds have approximately the same solubility as their normal isomers.

Much of the solubility data in this article supports these very general statements and more is collected together in Table XVIII.

C. EFFECT OF OTHER COMPONENTS ON THE SOLUBILIZING ACTION OF SURFACE-ACTIVE AGENTS (CO-SOLUBILIZING AGENTS)

For many purposes the solubilizing action of the surface-active agent itself may suffice but where the activity of a preparation is affected by the proportion of the agent used, or where it is difficult to get sufficient solute into solution by the action of the colloid alone, addition of other components to a solubilized system may have the desired effect. Many complex solvent systems which are difficult to correlate with the more scientific work on solubilization have been developed in specific instances on an empirical basis. Some examples are analysed in Section VII.

Electrolytes have been found to have a considerable effect on solubility; a two- or three-fold increase is found in a number of cases although in some systems solubility decreases in the presence of salt (Winsor, 1954, p. 95; M. E. L. McBain and Hutchinson, 1955, p. 85). Example of increased solubility is shown in Figs. 50 and 51. The increase seems to occur particularly when the solute is a hydrocarbon; in the case of polar materials it is often reduced. The nature of the phase or phases separating at the solubility limit in the latter case are almost certainly not equivalent to that in the hydrocarbon systems and have not been determined in much of the published work. It seems quite likely that the decreased solubility is due to the precipitation of a liquid crystalline phase, possibly because of the general depressant effect of salts on the solubility of surface-active agents. The effect of salts may be partly explained by the increase in the proportion of micellar soap which they are known to bring about by a lowering of the c.m.c. However, this cannot be the whole explanation since solubility is affected by the nature of the salt (Fig. 51) whereas the change in c.m.c. is not; also the increases in many

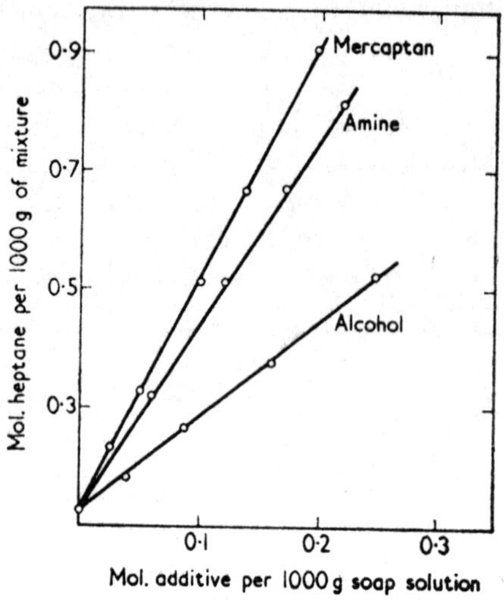

FIG. 50. The effect of added octyl alcohol, octylamine and octylmercaptan on the solubility of *n*-heptane in 0·35 M potassium myristate solution (from McBain, M. E. L., and Hutchinson, 1955).

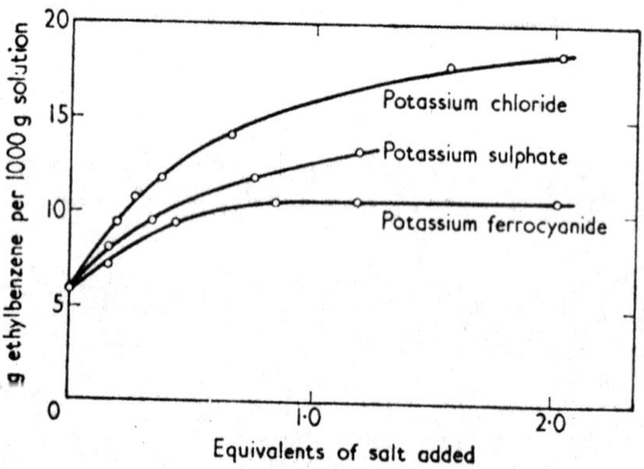

FIG. 51. The effect of salts on the solubilization of ethylbenzene by 0·1 M potassium myristate solution (from Stearns and co-workers, 1947).

cases are much greater than could be accounted for even if the whole of the soap formed micells. The solvent power of the micellar material must be affected in some way by the salt. It seems most likely that the effect is linked with the increase in micellar size which is known to take place in the presence of salts. The increased solvent power per unit weight of micellar material when the micelle increases in size was referred to in a previous section, when longer chain compounds were found to have a greater solvent power than the shorter chain materials. This statement is equivalent to Winsor's view that the micellar equilibrium shifts to the right in the presence of inorganic salt.

The addition of other, non-electrolyte, additives to a solubilized system (usually materials which are relatively insoluble in water but more readily solubilized than the solute under consideration), often enables more of the less soluble solute to be dissolved. This process has been called co-solubilization (Kolthoff and Graydon, 1951). The use of

TABLE XIX

Effect of Added Hydrocarbons on the Solubility of Orange OT in Soap Solutions (from Green and McBain, 1947)

	0·1 N *Potassium oleate*		
Soap hydrocarbon	*Benzene*	*Toluene*	*None*
ml hydrocarbon/25 ml solution	0·167	0·0112	—
mg dye/100 ml solution	47·5	41·75	27·0
g dye/mole soap	4·750	4·175	2·7
moles dye/mole soap	0·0181	0·0159	0·01
moles hydrocarbon/mole soap	0·752	0·421	—

benzene and toluene as co-solubilizing agents for Orange OT in potassium oleate solutions has been studied by Green and McBain (1947). Some of their results are shown in Table XIX. Seventy-five per cent of the amount of hydrocarbon known to dissolve in the soap solution was added and the solubility of Orange OT in the soap and co-solubilizer measured in the usual way. The authors calculated that the solvent power of the surface-active agent and co-solubilizer was not strictly additive although not too far removed from the amount expected from the known solvent power of the soap and the bulk solvent power of the hydrocarbon additive. In other cases the co-solubilizing action of additives has been found to be greater than can be explained on the bulk solvent power of the co-solubilizer (M. E. L. McBain and Hutchinson, 1955, p. 108). Examples are found in the action of polar materials, such as long chain alcohols, on the solubility of hydrocarbons in soap solutions (Fig. 50). It has been suggested that the mechanism of the action of hydrocarbons as co-solubilizers is due simply to the increase in micelle volume which they give. In the case of the polar solutes the large increases in solubility found could be due to a considerable modification in the micelles themselves, possibly again an increase in size.

D. EFFECT OF TEMPERATURE ON SOLUBILIZATION

The effect of temperature on solubilization does not appear to have been widely measured. Winsor (1954, p. 82) has indicated that the mechanism by which change of temperature affects solubility is complex because not only is the micelle structure involved but also the solubility characteristics of the solute itself, which may change though not always in the same direction as the change effected by the micelles. Micelle formation of ionic compounds in relatively dilute solutions does not seem to be markedly affected by temperature. For example the c.m.c. is almost unchanged. Since variation in temperature does not greatly affect the miscibility of hydrocarbon and water, one would expect this to be the case when hydrocarbons are solubilized. In the case of solids, however, there is a marked increase in solubility with rise of temperature. This is probably associated with the lower stability of the crystal lattice of solids at higher temperatures (Winsor, 1954, p. 135). Results obtained with solid dyes of high melting point also show this effect (Kolthoff and Stricks, 1948). Increase of solubility with rise of temperature is also likely to occur for an analogous reason, where the phase separating at the solubility limit is liquid crystal. The solubilizing power at different temperatures of non-ionic compounds of the glycol type is complicated by the effect of temperature on the solubility of the glycols themselves. Solubilizing power may be reduced almost to zero beyond a critical temperature, particularly for the shorter chain compounds. Solubility is, however, likely to be increased when the temperature is raised at concentrations where liquid crystal phases occur (Section V).

E. TOXICITY OF SURFACE-ACTIVE AGENTS AND OTHER MATERIALS IN THE PRESENCE OF SURFACE-ACTIVE AGENTS

Possible toxic effects of surface-active agents both externally and internally are of considerable importance because the compounds are extensively used as domestic and industrial detergents and leave traces of material undecomposed by sewage disposal in many supplies of drinking water. Studies which have been made of the toxic effects of detergents from these sources show that for many pharmaceutical applications toxicity is not likely to be a problem. But more caution is necessary in using products, such as vitamin solutions, where prolonged dosage is given internally or where the solute itself may be considerably more toxic in the presence of a surface-active agent.

The harmful effect of dilute aqueous solutions of soaps and synthetic detergents on the skin of the hands is well known. Such solutions produce reddening of the skin and have a defatting action which may lead to mild dermatitis or more serious conditions in sensitive individuals. In comparative tests of detergents in domestic conditions, synthetic detergents usually appear to be more irritant than the soaps but the severity of the action is considerably modified for all products by external factors such as the use of hand creams and the weather conditions at the time of the tests. Laboratory work on the comparative irritancy of compounds and formulated products are usually done by means of patch tests in which a patch of material soaked with the solution is applied to the skin under standardized conditions. An extensive review of skin irritancy has been published by Stüpel (1955) and a number of other references to test procedures and results are given by Schwartz and his co-authors (1958). The reaction produced depends on the concentration used, the frequency of application and the duration of the test. Under severe test conditions most agents can act as primary irritants and cause severe skin damage. For most people allergic or sensitized reactions are not a problem but there are a few who are sensitive to surface-active agents. As an example of the effects produced on normal skins the following will serve. 0·2 ml of a 4 per cent solution of built detergent and soap products applied to the backs of male human subjects at 48-h intervals show a gradual increase in erythema and oedema, classed as from mild to definite erythema or even slight papule formation, in from five to thirteen applications. Most subjects show no breakdown of the normal defensive mechanism of the skin and recovery of the area with no trace of the patch is shown within a few days of stopping the test. Challenge patches applied after a few weeks usually show no sensitization (Hedley, 1955). Correlation between laboratory tests and "in use" tests is poor and often little difference between soaps and other detergents is noted in the laboratory. Short chain soaps, especially when excess alkali is present, are more irritant than the longer chain compounds. The mechanism by which these effects are produced is uncertain. The defatting action has already been referred to. Ekwall (1954) has observed the effect of painting pure Tween 80 on skin. Two applications increased the bulk of the subcutaneous adipose tissue and caused a considerable enlargement of its cells with a decrease in the number and a change in the morphology of the mast cells. After a further two paintings a day for 4 days the connective tissue fibrils were much thicker than normal. Apparently Tween 80 had become concentrated in the fat cells and changed the properties of the lipoid contents in a hydrophilic direction so that the amount of water in the cells was markedly increased. It is possible that modification of the tissues in this way could result in internal transport changes possibly including an internal defatting action.

Orally, surface-active agents differ widely in toxicity between the main classes. LD_{50} values for typical groups are 50 to 500 mg/kg for the quaternary ammonium compounds; 2 to 8 g/kg for anionic materials such as the sulphates and sulphonates; 5 to 50 g/kg of body weight for non-ionic compounds (Schwartz *et al.*, 1958). Within each range, compounds having aromatic nuclei in their lipophilic chains have the higher toxicities. Chronic oral toxicities of anionic, cationic and non-ionic materials have been studied by Fitshugh and Nelson (1948) and by Barail (1954). Polyethylene glycols have been studied by Smyth and his co-workers (1955), who fed dogs and rats with diets containing up to 8 per cent of these materials with little apparent ill-effect. Six grams of Span 60 or Tween 60 have also been fed to humans for 28 days with no observable effect (Waldstein and Schoolman, 1952) and other oral studies have been made by Chow and co-workers (1953), Jones and co-workers (1948) and by Krehl *et al.* (1955), who found that polyethylene glycol esters produced no reaction in rats or cats. Non-ionic compounds may therefore be considered to have a low oral toxicity.

Little use appears to have been made of solubilized materials administered by injection mainly because of the toxic effects of surface-active agents, often including a strong haemolytic action on blood cells (see, for example, Ross and Silverstein, 1954; Pethica and Schulman, 1953). Soehring and co-workers (1951) quote toxicity of 0·4 to 1·5 g/kg body weight for non-ionic material injected intravenously into rodents.

Solubilized steroid preparations for application to the eyes have been successfully marketed, using Triton WR-1339 or Tween 80 as solubilizing agents (Triton WR-1339, Rohm and Haas Co., Philadelphia, U.S.A.) (Guttman and his co-authors, 1961), despite the strong irritant action of most other surface-active agents to the eye (Shelanski, 1952; Schwartz *et al.*, 1958).

Although surface-active agents would be safe for most applications, cases have been reported where the action of solubilized carcinogenic hydrocarbons is much enhanced by the presence of surface-active material, so much so in some cases that the solutions have been used to increase tumour incidence so that the carcinogenesis is more readily studied. Non-ionic compounds appear to affect the activity of the hydrocarbons more than others (Saxen and Ekwall, 1950). The mechanism is not simple, however, and under some conditions the studies show that hydrocarbon deposited at a site (prolonged contact increasing activity) may disperse more rapidly in solubilized preparations than in other solvents (Ekwall, 1954). In surface application at high concentration of a carcinogenic hydrocarbon, the influence of the nature of the solvent is not great, but when low concentrations of the hydrocarbon are used the action of the solvent becomes more important, increasing the activity of the hydrocarbon at higher concentrations of the surface-active material. Ekwall thinks that the use of surface-active agents in food, cosmetics, toothpaste, etc., may all help to promote the action of carcinogens in the body. There seems to be good reason for caution (Van Abbe, 1955), and the prolonged use of preparations known to contain cancer producing agents in the presence of surface-active agents of the non-ionic type (e.g. Coal Tar Solution U.S.P.) seems unwise, although the practice is not thought to be objectionable by all authors (Harris, 1956).

There are a number of examples in which the properties of solubilized materials are desirably modified. Among others the lower toxicity under certain conditions of phenols in soaps may be noted. Solubilized iodine preparations are also less toxic than other iodine solutions (Allawala and Riegelman, 1953a).

VII. Review of Pharmaceutical Products

A. PHENOLIC DISINFECTANTS

One of the first and most important uses of the solubilizing action of soaps was the production of water miscible solutions of higher phenols. These were developed at the end of the nineteenth century to replace aqueous solutions of phenol itself which were expensive for general disinfection purposes, had their activity rapidly diminished by dilution, and were very toxic. The earlier preparations were usually solutions of coal tar fractions containing complex mixtures of phenols, but in the nineteen-thirties solutions of synthetic higher chlorinated phenols were developed and more recently still the "germicidal soaps" (Finch, 1958; Sykes, 1958).

The character of the solutions based on coal tar phenols depends on the nature of the coal tar fraction used in their preparation and on the proportion of soap used to solubilize them. Those preparations containing the lower phenols are usually formulated with sufficient soap to retain them in solution at all dilutions with water (Lysol and "black fluids"), whereas the high boiling phenols are formulated so that on dilution an emulsion is formed ("white fluids"). The latter often contain a "carrier" which is a hydrocarbon or other suitable organic liquid which assists in the formation of a stable emulsion in the diluted preparation. Table XX lists some of the more important characters of the various types of preparation.

Lysol-type solutions, which contain mainly cresols, are very widely used. Their activity is affected by the type and proportion of soap used in their preparation. High proportion of soap usually makes a product that dilutes satisfactorily but the activity is often lowered (Table XXI).

TABLE XX

Phenolic Disinfectants Based on Solubilized Coal Tar Fractions

B.p. Coal Tar fraction	*Phenolic constituents*	*Rideal Walker coefficient*	*Chick Martin coefficient*	*Examples*
195–205°	Mainly cresols	Low range (2 or 3)	About 2	Lysol B.P.
216–221°	Xylenols and *m*- and *p*-ethyl-phenols	Medium range (6)	About 3	Sudol (Finch, 1953)
230° and above (high boiling tar acids)	Complex mixtures of homologues above the xylenols	High range (20)	About 4	"White fluids"

TABLE XXI

Effect of the Nature and Proportion of Soap on the Activity of Lysol-type Preparations (from Berry and Stenlake, 1942)

Oil or fatty acid (f.a.) used to prepare potassium soaps	*Amount of soap used (% w/v)*	*Phenol coefficient at* 17·5°C *Typhoid*	*Staph.*	*Strep.*
Arachis oil (f.a.)	15·7	1·6	2·0	3·9
Linseed oil B.P.	35	1·5	1·4	5·0
Linseed oil B.P.	18	2·2	1·8	5·6
Linseed oil B.P.	13	2·4	2·0	5·6
Coconut oil (f.a.)	16	2·9	2·4	6·0
Oleic acid	17·5	1·6	1·3	3·2

Figure 52 represents possible preparations of this type and illustrates the wide variation possible within official specifications. In general, unsatisfactory dilution would result if the proportion of soap were too low or if it came from a source containing longer chain-type soaps, since the latter increase the regions of the diagram over which liquid crystal phases form. Coal tar fractions containing hydrocarbon impurities or too great a proportion of higher boiling phenols would not

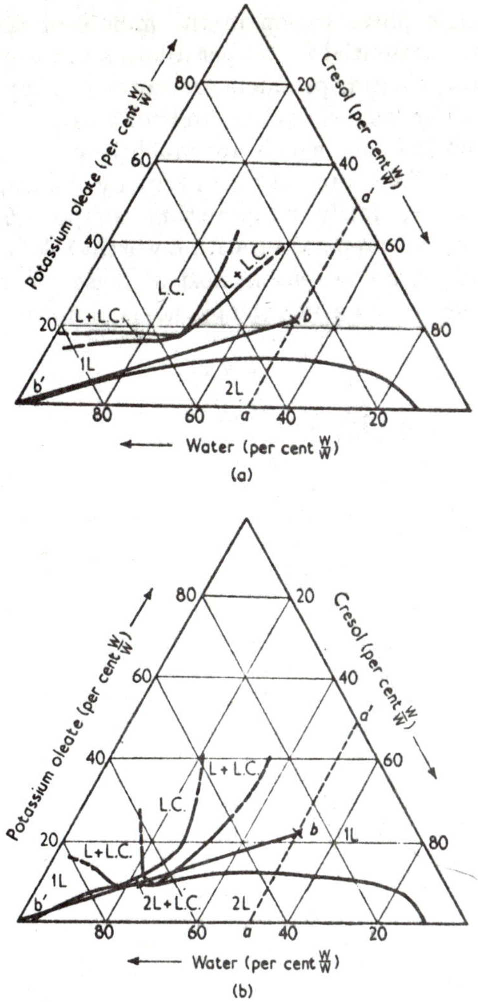

FIG. 52. Phase equilibrium diagram of the system potassium oleate + cresol + water at 20° C. (*a*) and (*b*) show the effect of different samples of potassium oleate. 2L, two isotropic liquid phases; LC, single liquid crystal phase; L + LC, liquid + liquid crystal phases; 2L + LC, three phase region. *aa'*, Compositions with approximately 50 per cent v/v of cresol (possible Lysol preparations). *b* Is Lysol B.P. *bb'*, Compositions traversed on diluting Lysol B.P. with water.

dilute properly because of an expansion in the two liquid phase region in the lower part of the diagram. This region is also affected by the proportion of the various cresol isomers present in coal tar fractions within this boiling range (Bailey, 1923). The presence of glycerin formed during the preparation of the soap, and the use of soap blends, would probably help to widen the single phase region in the middle of the diagram, the presence of which is essential for proper dilution of the product.

Few of the crude coal tar products are suitable for application to the skin because of their necrotic action and for this purpose solutions of higher chlorinated phenols, which are much less toxic, have been developed. Such solutions are official in many Pharmacopœias. The synthetic phenols are fairly high-melting compounds and a major difficulty is to obtain a preparation with a worthwhile proportion of the phenol in solution. For this reason most of these preparations have a complex solvent system in which the phenol is in mutual solution in the concentrated form with alcohol, soap and an organic solvent which is usually a terpene derivative. At the concentration used, an emulsion is formed, after dilution with water, in which most of the phenol is in solution in the oily phase, only a part of it being solubilized in the soap micelles. The activity of the product is markedly affected by the nature and proportion of soap used in the preparation. High proportion of organic solvents usually reduce the activity as shown in Table XXII. The selective action of the preparations on the two organisms used in this study seems to be due to the activity of the pine oil solvent itself on one of the organisms but not on the other. With such a complicated solvent system a wide variation in properties can be produced and many different formulae have been suggested in which the solvent system and the phenols incorporated are changed. The principles

TABLE XXII

The Effect of the Proportion of Organic Solvent on the Activity of Chloroxylenol Preparations Containing 2·5% Chloroxylenol, 30% Potash-Castor oil soap, 12·5% Alcohol and 0 to 10% of Pine Oil as organic solvent (from Moore and Walker, 1939)

	Phenol coefficient		*Calculated phenol coefficient per unit of phenol and Pine Oil*	
% of Pine Oil	B. Typh.	S. aureus	B. Typh.	S. aureus
0	2·0	0·6	80	24
2·5	2·1	0·75	42	15
5·0	2·4	0·45	32	6
7·5	3·0	0·1	30	1·0
10·0	3·6	0·03	28·8	0·2
10·0 (no phenol)	1·5	0·01	15	0·14

on which such formulations appear to be based are that the solvent system should be one in which the phenol is not precipitated as solid on dilution and that the proportion of organic solvent should be as low as possible, although sufficient to form a stable emulsion so that the whole system is saturated as much as possible by the phenol. Assuming that the phase relationships for these multicomponent systems are similar to those found in three component systems containing non-ionic glycols,

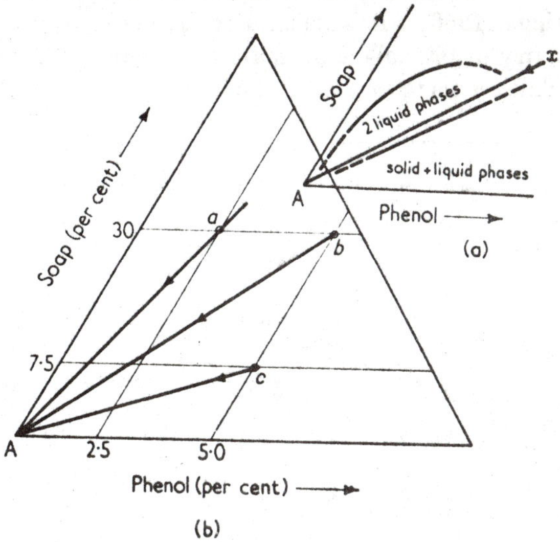

FIG. 53. Diagrammatic representation of chloroxylenol formulations, (alcohol and organic solvent components omitted). (a) Probable form of the phase diagram. *x*A shows compositions traversed on dilution. (b) Composition diagram for three preparations. *a*. 2·5 per cent phenol, 30 per cent soap, 0 per cent pine oil; *b*, 5 per cent phenol, 30 per cent soap, 5 per cent pine oil, 12·5 per cent alcohol (from Moore and Walker, 1939); *c*. Chloroxylenol Solution B.P. (See text).

Fig. 53 expresses these principles. The position of the phase boundaries within the figure will change with the nature and proportion of the components. A high proportion of soap and organic solvent will cause the region containing solid phase to diminish. The two liquid phase region will expand if the proportion of organic solvent is high. Maximum activity for any given preparation should be found if the composition at the dilution used is close to the boundary between these regions, i.e. in Fig. 53 the lines *a*A, *b*A and *c*A should be the boundary between the two liquid phase region and the region containing solid phases.

In simple solution the antibacterial activity of the phenol is logarithmically related to its concentration but in solutions containing surface-active agents at concentrations high enough to form micelles the activity is not related to the overall concentration in solution because the micelles compete with the free water for the phenol so that only part of it is available for interaction with bacteria. The effect may be regarded as a partition phenomenon so that the concentration of the phenol in the aqueous phase depends on the "partition coefficient" of the phenol (Section III) and the ratio of the volume of the micellar "phase" to the aqueous "phase" (Alexander and Trim, 1946; Berry and Bean, 1948; Berry and Briggs, 1956; Allawala and Riegelman, 1953a). Below the c.m.c. the activity of phenols is dramatically increased by the surface-active agent. This seems to be due to the increased uptake of the phenol

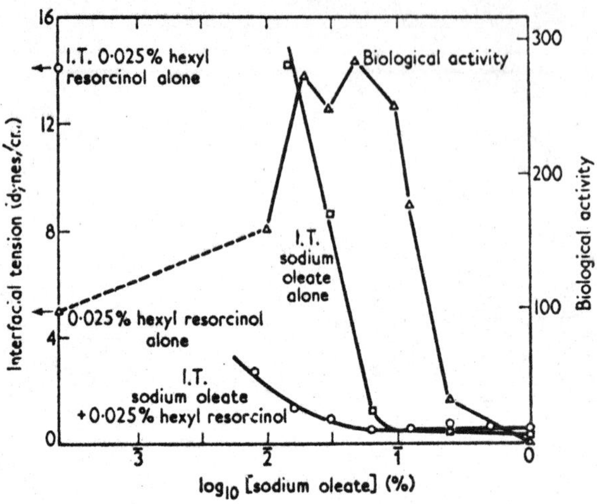

FIG. 54. Properties of sodium oleate—0·025 per cent hexyl resorcinol mixtures. Interfacial tension against nujol and biological activity measured by the rate of penetration of hexyl resorcinol as a percentage of control (0·025 per cent hexyl resorcinol alone) (from Alexander and Trim, 1946).

on the biological surface by the high surface activity of a loose complex between the phenol and the surface-active agent (Alexander and Trim, 1946). The permeability of the bacterial surface may also be increased in the presence of a surface-active agent. The principles are shown in Figs. 54–57. In Fig. 54 the activity of a fixed concentration of the phenol increases rapidly below the c.m.c. of sodium oleate because of increased uptake and/or increased permeability of the biological surface, but above this concentration the activity falls because micelles are being formed in increasing numbers and compete with the biological surface for the phenol. Figure 55 shows a similar picture although here the phenol and the soap are kept in the same ratio. Below the c.m.c. the activity increases because the phenol concentration is increasing and is being potentiated by the action of the soap. At the c.m.c. micelles compete for the phenol and the activity decreases. At still higher soap concentrations the activity again increases. The reason for this is

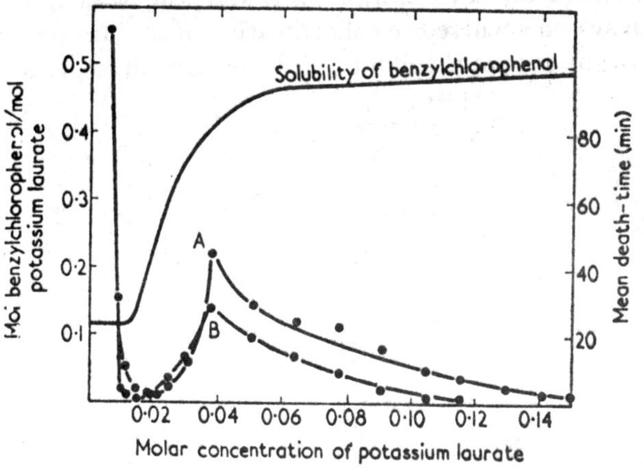

FIG. 55. The bactericidal activity against *Bact. coli* of solutions with constant benzylchlorophenol/potassium laurate ratio and increasing potassium laurate concentration, and the relation of the activity to the solubility of benzylchlorophenol. A, 0·066M benzylchlorophenol/M potassium laurate. B, 0·078M benzylchlorophenol/M potassium laurate (from Berry and Bean, 1951).

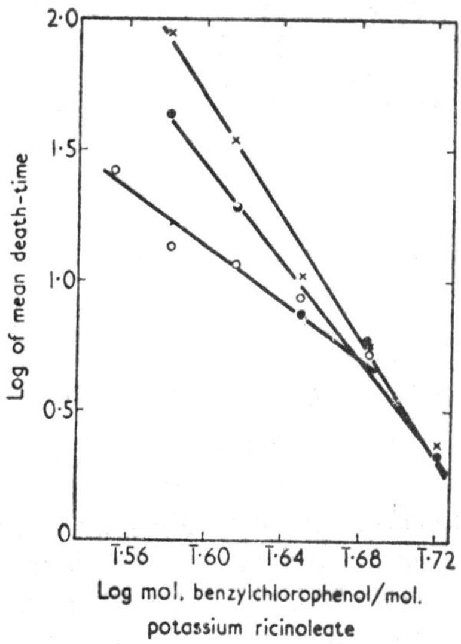

FIG. 56. The effect on the death time of *E. coli* of varying the benzylchlorophenol–potassium ricinoleate molar ratio in solutions with constant potassium ricinoleate concentration. Crosses, 0·25M; solid circles, 0·04M; open circles, 0·075M (from Berry and Briggs, 1956).

uncertain, since if the activity is controlled simply by the concentration of the free phenol one would expect it to decrease. In the quoted case the increase may be due to the activity of the soap itself, but similar effects have been found for several systems where the soap has only a low activity. In systems where the concentration of the surface-active agent is kept constant (above the c.m.c.) and the concentration of the phenol

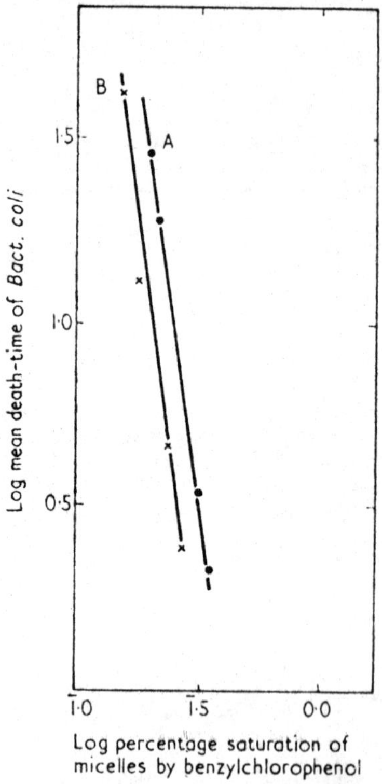

FIG. 57. Relation between the percentage saturation of micelles by benzylchlorophenol and the log mean death time of *Bact. coli* (from Berry and Bean, 1951).

is increased (capacity of the system fixed, Allawala and Riegelman, 1953a) one would expect activity to increase regularly since both micelles and aqueous "phase" are being progressively saturated with the phenol. This is shown in Fig. 56 (Berry and Briggs, 1956). The results in Fig. 57 illustrate the same principles since all the phases in the system will be in equilibrium and the concentration of the phenol "free" in the aqueous phase will increase in the same proportion as that in the micelles.

These factors are obviously vital in the formulation of solubilized antibacterial solutions. The aim should be to use as low a proportion of soap to phenol as possible while still keeping the required physical properties of the preparation. This is fulfilled by keeping as low down on the phase diagram as is consistent with the formation of a solution or with white fluid type products by using as low a concentration of surface-active agent as will give a satisfactory emulsion. The situation is closely analogous to that of materials in two-phase systems, where it has been shown that activity is mainly dependent on the concentration of the material in the aqueous phase (Bean *et al.* 1961).

B. IODOPHORS

Iodine preparations have been widely used as skin antiseptics, usually in alcoholic solutions containing alkali iodides which increase the low solubility of the element in water alone (Sykes, 1958). The solutions have a number of disadvantages, including an irritant action on skin, a rapid loss of iodine from a painted surface, due to the high vapour pressure of iodine, and the staining properties of the solution. The use of iodides to increase the solubility by forming ionized iodine also decreases the activity of the product because only unionized iodine is a strong germicide. Iodine dissolved in solutions of surface-active agents have a number of advantages over the traditional preparations, and the solutions have been used as general disinfecting agents, particularly in the dairy industry. Their properties have been reviewed by Davis (1962) and Woodward (1962), and references to many papers are given in the bibliography published by the Chilean Iodine Educational Bureau. Because no iodide is present the solutions have good activity and the vapour pressure of the iodine in the solution is low. Therefore they are relatively odourless and the iodine is not so readily lost from surfaces. They are also much less irritant and have low toxicity (Cantor and Shelanski, 1956). The detergent action of the solvent system is an advantage in many applications and the solutions have much less tendency to stain cloth and apparatus.

Although it has been suggested that surface-active agents of any of the three main classes may be used as the solubilizing agent, the non-ionic type is generally used, presumably because many of the others precipitate in the presence of iodine. For many purposes solutions containing 1 to 2 per cent of iodine are used solubilized by a suitable proportion of the surface-active agent. Little information has been published on the solubility of iodine in such solutions but the results of Allawala and Riegelman on the solubility of iodine in solutions of a nonyl phenol polyglycol ether (Antarox A-400) (Fig. 58) which contains about 10 ethylene oxide units per molecule show that the proportion of iodine solubilized changes proportionately with the concentration of the surface-active agent. Most of the proprietary preparations are made strongly acid, usually by the addition of phosphoric acid to the solution. Not only is iodine more effective bacteriologically at acid pH but also

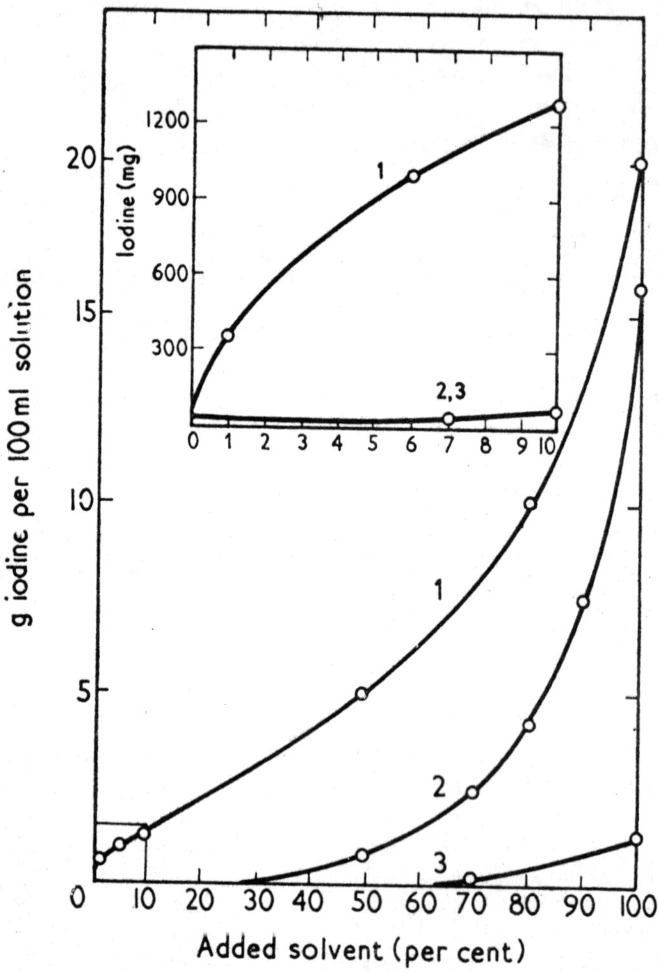

FIG. 58. Solubility of iodine in aqueous solutions containing: 1, Antarox A-400 (nonyl phenol polyoxyethylene glycol derivative) at 25° C; 2, ethyl alcohol at 15° C; glycerin at 25° C (from Allawala and Riegelman, 1953a).

the liberation of free iodine from the solubilized form is better in acid conditions. Figure 59 shows how the addition of phosphoric acid to an iodophor affects the proportion of iodine titratable with thiosulphate. Acid solutions also appear to be more stable (Allawala and Riegelman,

1953b) because a proportion of the iodine added cannot be titrated with thiosulphate, and this proportion increases with storage time (Woodward, 1962). This interaction is reduced in acid solution.

The mechanism by which the iodine is solubilized by the surface-active agents has received considerable attention (Allawala and Riegelman, 1953b; Rossetti, 1959; Woodward, 1962). Most of the iodine added may be tritrated with thiosulphate and therefore the "complex" formation to which the increased solubility has been attributed is readily reversible to unionized iodine. There does not seem to be any reason for attributing

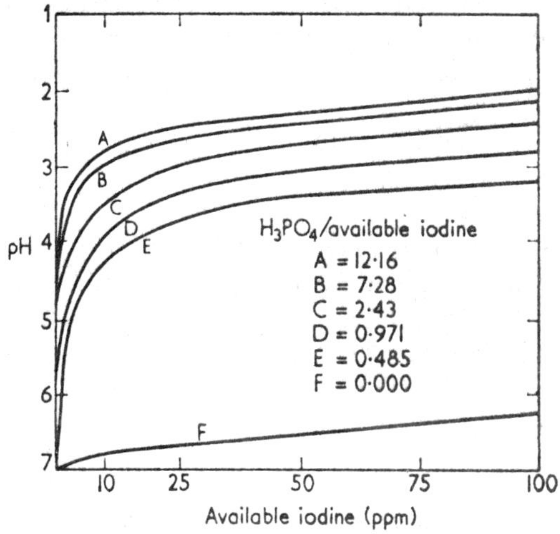

FIG. 59. pH of iodophor solution plotted against concentration of available iodine for various ratios of phosphoric acid to available iodine (from Brost and Krupin, 1957).

the increased solubility to anything other than a solvent effect of the micelles though simple solution in the interior of the micelle may not predominate since it is probably the solvent action of the polyglycol region of the micelle which is involved in this case. However, part of the iodine is not titratable with thiosulphate and is irreversibly bound to the surface-active agent or to decomposition products from it. Part of the iodine also seems to be converted to ionic species. According to Allawala and Riegelman (1953b), who investigated the interaction with polyethylene glycols of various chain length, the amount of iodine lost was increased by the longer chain compounds and did not proceed further after 24 h. Part of the lost iodine was found to be organically bound. For the alkyl phenol polyglycol Antarox-A 400 about 23 per cent of the iodine was lost from the solution. They proposed the following reaction to explain the results:

$$\mathrm{RO.CH_2.CH_2.(O.CH_2.CH_2)_n.O.CH_2CH_2.OH}$$
$$\Big\downarrow \mathrm{I_2+H_2O}$$
$$\mathrm{RO.CH_2CH_2.(O.CH_2.CH_2)_{n-1}.O.CH_2.CH_2.OH+ICH_2.CH_2.OH+HOI}$$

Rossetti (1959) studied the interaction of iodine with polyethylene glycols by spectroscopy. The effect of time on the interaction and the changes in pH of the systems were also recorded. She found a continuous decrease in free iodine, an initial increase in the formation of polyiodide (I_3^-) and an increase in the acidity of the solution, and explained these interactions on the basis of a two-stage process as follows:

$$\mathrm{(C_2H_4O)_n + nI_2 \rightleftharpoons (C_2H_4OI_2)_n}$$
$$\mathrm{(C_2H_4OI_2)_n \rightleftharpoons (C_2H_3IO)_n + nH^+ + nI^-}$$

The iodide would, of course, affect the free iodine: $I_2 + I^- \rightleftharpoons I_3^-$. Similar charge transfer complexes of iodine with ethers have been investigated by others. Yamada and Kozima (1960) suggested from infra-red measurements that diethyl ether formed complexes such as:

Woodward (1962) made a comprehensive study of the interaction of iodine with both non-ionic and betaine-type surface-active agents. The interactions were followed chemically and by ultra-violet spectroscopy. The amount of the immediate reaction depended on the concentration of the non-ionic agent. The graphs of storage time against absorption peaks indicated at least two stages for the other reactions. Below the c.m.c. little change appears to occur with time and the reactions only take place in the presence of micelles. In solutions containing a high concentration of the surface-active agent and a low proportion of iodine, almost all the iodine is converted to I_3^- immediately but otherwise the reaction is slow. It seems unlikely that a quantitative interpretation of the interactions could be made from the results, because not only are all the interactions happening simultaneously but the absorption bands of each species overlap and the absorptions of the ionized iodine are very high compared to those of the unionized species. However, Woodward proposed the following scheme which is similar to that given by Rossetti for the glycols.

1. Micelle + $I_2 \rightleftharpoons$ Micelle: I_2 complex (non-absorbing in the 280–300 mμ region and with a peak at 390 mμ)
2. Micelle: I_2 complex $\rightleftharpoons$ Micelle: $(I^- + I^+)$
3. Micelle: $I^- + I_2 \rightleftharpoons$ Micelle: I_3^- (peaks at 290 and 390 mμ) (from a complexed form or from free iodine)
4. Micelle: I_3^- + Micelle $\rightleftharpoons$ 2 Micelle: $I^- + I^+$.

Although this work indicates that a proportion of the iodine added to form an iodophor is lost, the amount is unlikely to be serious in the case of products containing 1 to 2 per cent of iodine where the ratio of surface-active agent to iodine is not too high.

In the same way as in the solubilized phenol systems it might be expected that removal of the iodine from free solution by the micelles would affect the activity of the solubilized iodine preparations. A study of the antibacterial activity of a solubilized iodine system has been made by Allawala and Riegelman (1953b). They found that the activity of solubilized iodine depended on the amount in free solution which is

TABLE XXIII

Distribution of Iodine between the Micelles and the Aqueous Phase in Solutions Containing an Alkylphenol Polyether and the Antibacterial Activity of the Solution (after Allawala and Riegelman, 1953b)

Concentration surface-active agent	*Iodine in solution, mg/100 cc* Total	Free (aqueous phase)	*Total saturation %*	*Aqueous saturation %*	*99% Killing time, min.*
0·0	28·8	28·8	87	87	5·1
0·0	14·8	14·8	45	45	9·0
0·0	6·7	6·7	20	20	18
0·0	3·5	3·5	10	10	33
0·0	1·2	1·2	3·7	3·7	58
0·085	49	33	100	100	3·6
0·5	165	33	100	100	3·5
9·3	1200	33	100	100	3·5
0·085	42	24	89	73	4·4
1·2	390	26	83	79	4·2
0·085	6·92	0·7	1·4	2·1	75
2·0	34·4	0·24	0·73	0·73	184

controlled by the proportion of iodine to surface-active agent and the "distribution coefficient" of iodine between the micelles and the aqueous phase. Some of their results are shown in Table XXIII. It can be seen that for maximum activity the preparation must be saturated as much as possible with iodine. In practice this would mean using the smallest proportion of solubilizing agent possible to get the required amount of iodine into solution. Products are sometimes formulated not only with a surface-active agent, but with other solvents as well which do not form micelles, in particular the polyethylene glycols. This enables a larger proportion of iodine to be incorporated into the solution than could be achieved with the surface-active agent alone, which means that less of it is removed into the micelles. On dilution, the saturation of the solution will be maintained but solid iodine may be thrown out if insufficient surface-active agent has been used.

C. VITAMIN PREPARATIONS

Regular administration of the oil-soluble vitamins using fish-liver oils or solutions of concentrates in oils is unpleasant for many adults and unsatisfactory for infants and children. Aqueous solutions may be prepared by solubilizing the vitamins, which are then much more pleasant to take and are particularly suitable for adding to the milk feeds of infants. There is also evidence that absorption is better with solubilized preparations, especially where fat digestion is deficient (Kramer *et al.*, 1951). Non-ionic agents are used as solubilizers because of their low oral toxicity. Products containing vitamin A from different sources affect the amount of surface-active agent required to solubilize it, and since inert oily material is just as difficult as the vitamin, it is usual to use pure vitamin A alcohol, or one of its esters, or a high potency concentrate, to enable a dose to be dissolved in the minimum quantity of solubilizing agent. This is done to avoid unnecessary use of the surface-active agents, which are expensive and which have a bitter taste.

As an example of the requirement for a suitable vitamin A product the following calculation is given. Assuming a dose of 10,000 units, this would correspond to about 6·5 mg of vitamin A palmitate ($1{\cdot}5 \times 10^6$ units/g). From the solubilities recorded by Nakagawa (1958b) this would require about 0·12 g of 20 per cent solution of Tween 80 to solubilize it. It has been pointed out earlier that, qualitatively speaking, the solubilizing power of surface-active agents of the non-ionic type is approximately related to the weight or volume of the hydrocarbon in the interior of their micelles when the agents are of the *n*-alkyl chain type. Whether this criterion may be applied to the Tweens is uncertain, but it should be possible to translate solubilities on the same basis from one solubilizing agent to another, and the solvent power per unit weight of the solubilizing agent should be independent of the concentration of the solution over a considerable range (up to 20 per cent). Many formulae for solubilized vitamin preparations have been described in the patent literature, and data on the effect of the structure of the non-ionic agent, particularly its HLB number on solubility, are also scattered in the literature, though much is rather inaccessible because it is in Japanese journals.

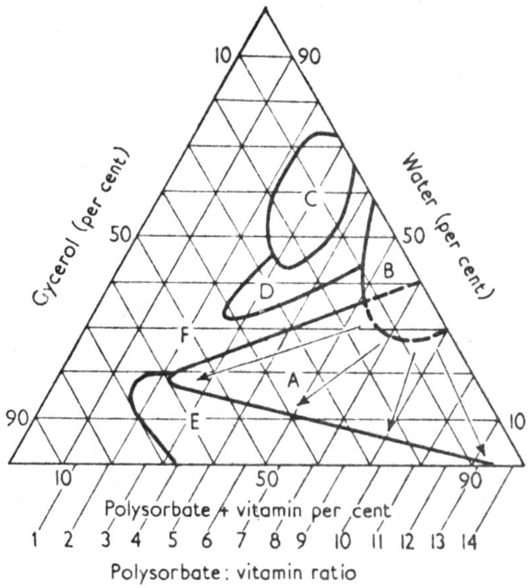

FIG. 60. The Vitamin A + Polysorbate 80 + glycerol + water system. A, transparent single phase; B, semi-solid; C, faintly opalescent; D, markedly opalescent; E, two transparent phases; F, emulsions (from Boon and co-workers, 1961).

Boon *et al.* (1961) have cut down the amount of solubilizing agent necessary by using glycerin as a co-solvent. They also found considerable variation in the solubilizing properties of different samples of Polysorbate 80 (Tween 80). Their data are shown in Figs. 60 and 61. Although Fig. 60 is not a complete phase diagram it appears, in relation to the three component systems described in Section V, that the transparent zone A, at least on the right-hand side of the diagram, is an oily solution (S_2 or L_2). Other regions may also be comparable with three-component systems. Zone B is probably liquid crystal, and the heterogeneous regions emulsions of isotropic liquid or liquid crystal phases. The relation of the clear regions on this diagram to solubilized vitamin A in three-component systems containing less than 30 per cent surface-active agent is probably as L_2 to aqueous L_1 solutions (see Lawrence, 1958, and earlier papers for phase nomenclature). The increased solvent power these workers find with increasing polyglycol chain length (Fig. 61) probably does not apply to the L_1 solutions.

Further data on the solubility of α-tocopheryl acetate, vitamin A palmitate and other vitamins have been published by Nakagawa and his co-workers (1956). Some of this information is collected in the solubility tables at the end of the article. A later series of papers by Mima (1958)

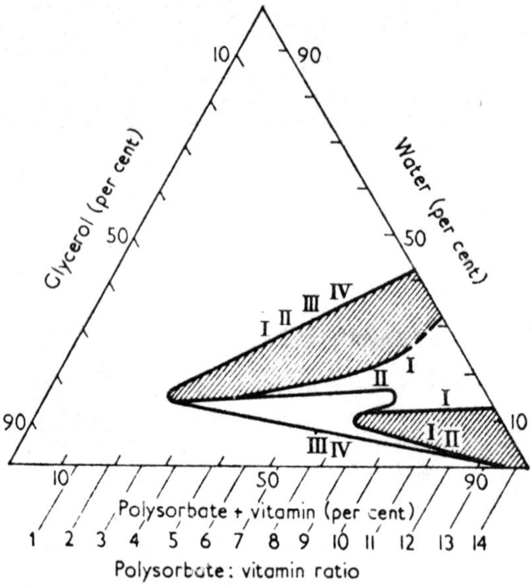

FIG. 61. Variations in the zone of transparent, single-phase preparations with different samples of Polysorbate 80 (I–IV). The shaded areas show where the samples of Polysorbate 80 all gave transparent, single phase preparations (from Boon *et al.*, 1961).

gives data for vitamin A, D_4, D_5, D_2, D_3 and E acetate solubilized by various non-ionic materials including the sucrose esters.

Vitamin preparations, especially vitamin A, are liable to oxidation and several workers have found that solubilized vitamin is more stable than oily solutions (e.g. Coles and Thomas, 1952). More comprehensive studies of a number of readily oxidized materials solubilized by anionic, cationic and non-ionic surface-active agents also show solubilized preparations to be less readily oxidized than emulsions of the material or simple dispersions in water with no emulsifying agent (Carless and Nixon, 1960). The stability of water-soluble vitamin A preparations has been reviewed by Dal Bollo *et al.* (1958).

D. HORMONE SOLUTIONS

Many hormones are administered in oily solution by subcutaneous injection and solutions of anti-inflammatory hormones are also required for external application. Many of these compounds are almost insoluble in water. Production of solutions by preparing derivatives is one way of bringing them into aqueous solution, but frequently the activity of the water-soluble derivatives is low. Oily solutions may be used, but modern dermatological practice is to use aqueous or water-miscible preparations

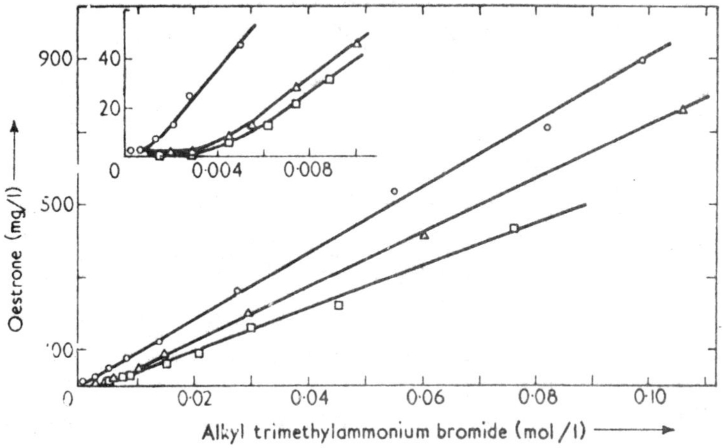

FIG. 62. The solubility of oestrone in aqueous solutions of tetradecyl trimethylammonium bromide at 20°C (squares), and 40° C (triangles). Solubility in hexadecyl trimethylammonium at 40° C (circles) (from Sjöblom, 1956).

as far as possible. For this reason solubilized preparations are attractive alternatives.

A very extensive study of the solubility of oestrone in many different types of surface-active agent has been made by Sjöblom (1956). He found in almost every case that the solubility was directly proportional to the surface-active agent concentration over a wide range. Some of his solubility curves are shown in Figs. 62 and 63. The solubility was found to begin at colloid concentrations not far, in most cases, from the known c.m.c.'s of the solubilizing agents. Sjöblom also compared the percutaneous activity of the solubilized hormone with solutions in ordinary solvents using the activity of the hormone in oil injected subcutaneously as a standard (activity 1·0). The test animals were mice. He found the potency of solutions in oils to be 0·13, that of solutions in surface-active agents 0·36 (averaged over a number of solubilizing agents) and in volatile solvents such as benzene it was 0·84. There was also a prolongation of activity in all solutions applied percutaneously compared with the injected solutions. The activity was not affected over a wide range

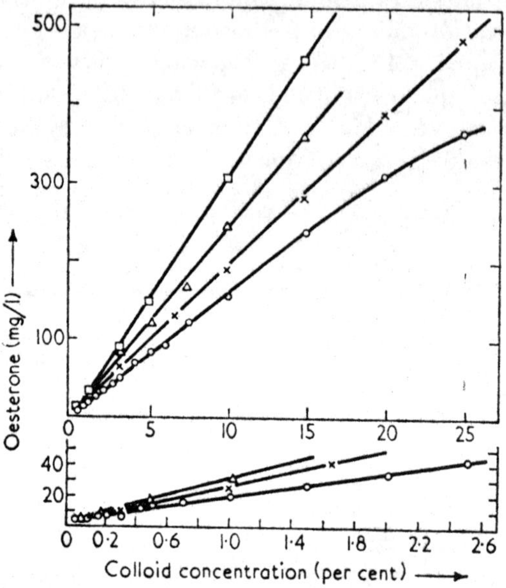

FIG. 63. Solubility of oestrone in solutions of some non-ionic association colloids. Atlas G-2152 at 20° C (crosses) and 40° C (squares). Tween 20 (circles) and Tween 60 (triangles) at 20° C (from Sjöblom, 1956).

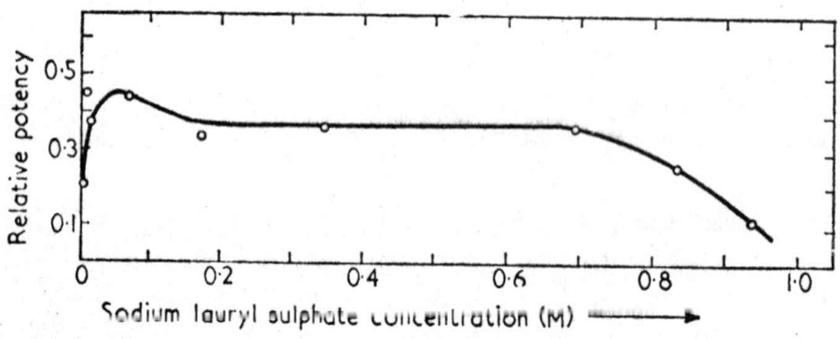

FIG. 64. Variation in the apparent relative potency of oestrone applied percutaneously in aqueous sodium lauryl sulphate solutions of different concentrations (from Sjöblom, 1956).

by the concentration of the surface-active agents (Fig. 64). There is a very extensive survey of the literature relating to oestrone, and to the preparation of solutions of oestrone and other hormones in various solvents including solubilized hormones, in this paper (more than 450 references). In earlier work from the same laboratory Ekwall and co-workers (1949, 1950, 1951, 1953) made less extensive measurements, often at only one or two surface-active agent concentrations, on the solubility of desoxycorticosterone, and its acetate, testosterone, progesterone, oestradiol, oestrone, and testosterone propionate, and in a number of soaps and other surface-active agents. These results show that solubility is proportional to the concentration of the surface-active agent. In a more recent paper, Sjöblom (1958) measured the solubility of oestradiol-17 in tetradecyl trimethyl ammonium bromide, sodium

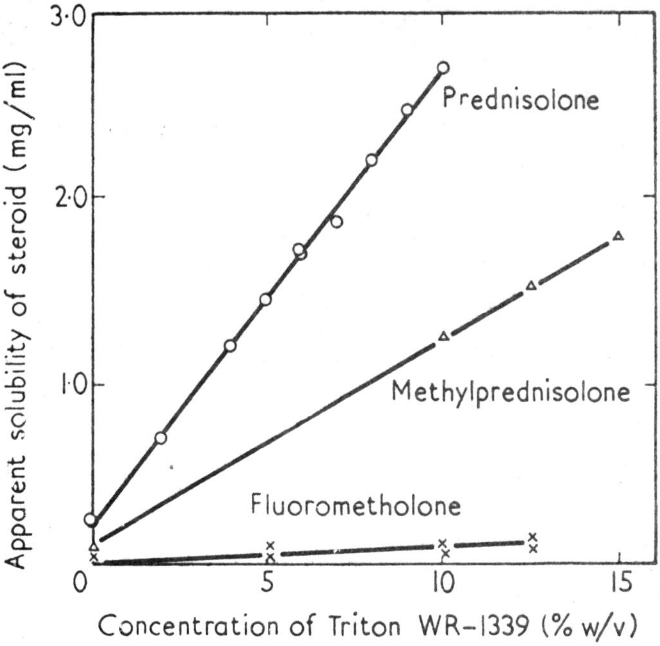

FIG. 65. Solubilities of some steroids in aqueous solutions of Triton WR-1339 (from Guttman *et al.*, 1961).

caprate, Tween 20 and sodium lauryl sulphate. This compound is more readily solubilized than oestrone, probably because it contains an extra hydroxyl group instead of the ketone grouping. The activity (subcutaneously in oil, 1·0) of oestradiol-17β in solubilized preparations was found to be 0·36 in 10 per cent sodium lauryl sulphate; 0·62 in 7 per cent sodium caprate; 0·43 in 2·7 per cent of a quaternary compound and 0·36 in 10 per cent Tween 20. It was more active in oily solution but less than when dissolved in a volatile solvent. These results paralleled those for oestrone. Nylander (1953) has measured the solubility of desoxycorticosterone in Tween 60 and a polyethylene glycol stearate ester. The solubilizing power for a number of hormones of the non-ionic compound polyethylene glycol sorbitan monolaurate containing 12 ethylene oxide units at 20 per cent concentration has been reported by Nakagawa (1953). Nakagawa has also made measurements for the same solubilizing agent at high concentrations which show that the solvent power increases considerably above 65 per cent. In addition, he has made (1954) measurements on the solubility of dienestrol, hexestrol and diethyl stilbestrol and their esters and ether-type derivatives in non-ionic, anionic and cationic surface-active agents. A number of the solubility values have

TABLE XXIV

Solubility of Oestradiol-17β and Oestrone in Some Surface-active Agents (calculated from Sjöblom's results (1956))

Solute	*Solubility* (*g solute per g of hydrocarbon in the non-ionic surface-active agent; values for ionic materials and those in brackets for the non-ionic compounds are in g solute per g of total surface-active agent*)			
	Sod. caprate (0·5 M)	$C_{14}H_{29}N(CH_3)_3Br$ (0·05 M)	Tween 20 (20%)	Tween 60 (15%)
Oestradiol	0·015	0·046	0·021 (0·0029)	—
Oestrone	0·0069 (0·6 M)	0·017 (0·08 M)	0·014 (0·0019)	0·012 (0·0024)

been collected in the table at the end of the article. Preparations of anti-inflammatory steroids intended for application to the eyes, throat, etc., using an alkyl phenol type detergent where the alkyl part of the molecule is cross-linked (Triton WR-1339), have been studied by Guttman and co-workers (1961). Their solubility curves are shown in Fig. 65. Apparently this agent is sufficiently non-toxic to be applied to eye tissue. References to the patent literature and other work on solubilized hormone preparations are given in this paper.

In accordance with the general view taken in this article some of the above solubility data is presented (Table XXIV) in the form used previously in Table XVII. It can be seen that the solubilizing power of the different classes of surface-active agent is quite closely related to the proportion of hydrocarbon that they contain. Thus for the non-ionic compounds the solvent power is poor compared with that of ionic compounds when using a total weight basis, but similar when compared

TABLE XXV

Solubility of Some Materials of Medicinal Importance

Solute	*Surface-active agent and concentration or concentration range*	*Solubility*[a] *(g solute per g surface-active agent)*	*Temperature*[b] *(°C)*	*Reference*
Acetomenapthone (Vitamin K_4)	Polyoxyethylene sorbitan mono-oleate (Tween 80) (20%)	0·027	30	1
21-Acetoxypregnolone	Polyoxyethylene sorbitan monolaurate (20%)	0·0035	—	2
d, 1-α-*trans*-Allesthrin	Polyoxyethylene sorbitan mono-oleate (Tween 80) (20%)	0·053	30	1
Butylparben	Polyoxyethylene sorbitan mono-oleate (Tween 80) (20%)	0·153	30	1
γ-BHC	Polyoxyethylene sorbitan mono-oleate (Tween 80) (20%)	0·034	30	1
Calciferol (Vitamin D_2)	Polyoxyethylene sorbitan mono-oleate (Tween 80) (20%)	0·057	30	1
Calciferol (Vitamin D_2)	Polyoxyethylene sorbitan mono-oleate (Tween 80) (20%)	0·077	—	4
Calciferol (Vitamin D_2)	Polyoxyethylene sorbitan monolaurate (Tween 20)	0·12	—	4
Calciferol (Vitamin D_2)	Polyoxyethylene sorbitan monostearate (Tween 60)	0·09	—	4
Calciferol (Vitamin D_2)	Polyoxyethylene glycol monolauryl Ether (Brij 35)	0·20	—	4
Calciferol (Vitamin D_2)	Sucrose monoester (C_8)	0·13	—	3
Calciferol (Vitamin D_2)	Sucrose monoester(C_{10})	0·13	—	3
Calciferol (Vitamin D_2)	Sucrose monoester (C_{12})	0·10	—	3
Calicferol (Vitamin D_2)	Sucrose monoester (C_{14})	0·071	—	3
Calciferol (Vitamin D_2)	Sucrose monoester (C_{16})	0·05	—	3
Chlorotrianisene	Polyoxyethylene sorbitan mono-oleate (Tween 80)	0·0039	30	1
Chloroxylenol	Polyoxyethylene glycol monocetyl Ether (Cetomacrogol 1000) (0·1 M)	0·24	20	5
Chloroxylenol	$C_6H_{13}(CH_2.CH_2.O)_6OH$ (13%)	0·26	20	6
Chloroxylenol	Potassium laurate (0·134 M)	0·60	20	7
Cortisone acetate	Polyoxyethylene sorbitan mono-oleate (Tween 80) (20%)	0·0054	30	1
Cortisone acetate	Polyoxyethylene sorbitan monolaurate (20%)	0·0022	—	2
Cyclocoumarol	Polyoxyethylene sorbitan mono-oleate (Tween 80) (20%)	0·0029	30	1

TABLE XXV—*continued*

Solute	*Surface-active agent and concentration or concentration range*	*Solubility[a] (g solute per g surface-active agent)*	*Temperature[b] (°C)*	*Reference*
Desoxycorticosterone Acetate	Polyoxyethylene sorbitan mono-oleate (Tween 80) (20%)	0·005	30	1
Desoxycorticosterone Acetate	Polyoxyethylene sorbitan mono-oleate (Tween 80) (5–20%)	0·0082	40	10
Desoxycorticosterone Acetate	Polyoxyethylene stearate	0·0055	—	8
Desoxycorticosterone Acetate	Polyoxyethylene sorbitan monostearate (Tween 60)	0·0039	—	8
Desoxycorticosterone Acetate	Polyoxyethylene sorbitan monolaurate (Tween 20)	0·0045	—	8
Desoxycorticosterone Acetate	Sodium cholate (20%)	0·070	—	9
Desoxycorticosterone Acetate	Sodium cholate (10%)	0·10	—	9
Desoxycorticosterone Acetate	Sodium oleate (10%)	0·015	—	9
Desoxycorticosterone Acetate	Sodium myristate (10%)	0·018	—	9
Desoxycorticosterone Acetate	Potassium myristate (0·5–8%)	0·151	40	10
Desoxycorticosterone Acetate	Sodium lauryl sulphate (0·5–20%)	0·11	40	10
Dicoumarol	Polyoxyethylene sorbitan mono-oleate (Tween 80) (20%)	0·0013	30	1
Dienestrol	Polyoxyethylene sorbitan mono-oleate (Tween 80) (20%)	0·068	30	1
Diethylstilbestrol	Polyoxyethylene sorbitan mono-oleate (Tween 80) (20%)	0·083	30	1
Diethylstilbestrol dipropionate	Polyoxyethylene sorbitan mono-oleate (Tween 80) (20%)	0·004	30	1
Digitoxin	Polyoxyethylene sorbitan mono-oleate (Tween 80) (20%)	0·0085	30	1
Estradiol	$C_{14}H_{29}N(CH_3)_3Br$(0·05 M)	0·046	—	12
Estradiol	Polyoxyethylene sorbitan monolaurate (Tween 20) (20%)	0·0029	—	12
Estradiol	Sodium oleate (10%)	0·007	—	9
Estradiol	Sodium myristyl sulphate (10%)	0·008	—	9
Estradiol	Sodium lauryl sulphate (0·1 M)	0·0146	—	11
Estradiol benzoate	Polyoxyethylene sorbitan mono-oleate (Tween 80) (20%)	0·0053	30	1
Estrone	$C_{14}H_{29}N(CH_3)_3Br$ (0·08 M)	0·017	—	12
Estrone	Polyoxyethylene sorbitan monolaurate (Tween 20) (20%)	0·0019	—	12
Estrone	Polyoxyethylene sorbitan monolaurate (20%)	0·0021	—	2
Estrone	Polyoxyethylene sorbitan monostearate (Tween 60) (15%)	0·0024	—	12
Estrone	Sodium myristyl sulphate (20%)	0·0065	—	9

Ethylbiscoumacetate	Polyoxyethylene sorbitan mono-oleate (Tween 80) (20%)	0·0093	30	1
Ethylparaben	Polyoxyethylene sorbitan mono-oleate (Tween 80) (20%)	0·156	30	1
Ethynyl estradiol	Polyoxyethylene sorbitan mono-oleate (Tween 80) (20%)	0·085	30	1
Ethynyl estradiol	Polyoxyethylene sorbitan monolaurate (20%)	0·053	—	2
Fluorometholone	Triton WR-1339 (Rohm and Haas Co.) (0–12·5%)	0·00093	25	13
Gitoxin	Polyoxyethylene sorbitan mono-oleate (Tween 80) (20%)	0·0021	30	1
Hexestrol	Polyoxyethylene sorbitan mono-oleate (Tween 80) (20%)	0·078	30	1
Hexestrol	Sodium oleate (10%)	0·12	—	9
Hexestrol	Sodium myristyl sulphate (10%)	0·05	—	9
Hexestrol	Sodium cholate (10%)	0·12	—	9
Hydrocortisone	Polyoxyethylene sorbitan mono-oleate (Tween 80) (20%)	0·049	30	1
Hydrocortisone Acetate	Polyoxyethylene sorbitan mono-oleate (Tween 80) (20%)	0·002	30	1
Methyl androstenediol	Polyoxyethylene sorbitan mono-oleate (Tween 80) (20%)	0·0013	30	1
Methyl androstenediol	Polyoxyethylene sorbitan monolaurate (20%)	0·0015	—	2
2-Methyl-1,4-naphthoquinone (Vitamin K_3)	Polyoxyethylene sorbitan mono-oleate (Tween 80) (20%)	0·019	30	1
Methylparaben	Polyoxyethylene sorbitan mono-oleate (Tween 80) (20%)	0·18	30	1
Methylprednisolone	Triton WR-1339 (Rohm and Haas Co.) (0–15%)	0·011	25	13
Methyl testosterone	Polyoxyethylene sorbitan mono-oleate (Tween 80) (20%)	0·014	30	1
Methyl testosterone	Polyoxyethylene sorbitan monolaurate (20%)	0·011	—	2
Phenindione	Polyoxyethylene sorbitan mono-oleate (Tween 80) (20%)	0·041	30	1
Prednisolone	Polyoxyethylene sorbitan mono-oleate (Tween 80) (20%)	0·049	30	1
Prednisolone	Triton WR-1339 (Rohm and Haas Co.) (0–10%)	0·025	25	13
Progesterone	Polyoxyethylene sorbitan mono-oleate (Tween 80) (20%)	0·011	30	1
Progesterone	Polyoxyethylene sorbitan mono-oleate (Tween 80) (5–20%)	0·005	40	10
Progesterone	Polyoxyethylene sorbitan monolaurate (20%)	0·011	—	2
Progesterone	Sodium lauryl sulphate (0–20%)	0·20	40	10, 11
Progesterone	Sodium cholate (0·5–20%)	0·022	40	10
Propylparaben	Polyoxyethylene sorbitan mono-oleate (Tween 80) (20%)	0·15	30	1
Quercetin	Polyoxyethylene sorbitan mono-oleate (Tween 80) (20%)	0·023	30	1
Rutin	Polyoxyethylene sorbitan mono-oleate (Tween 80) (20%)	0·017	30	1
Santonin	Polyoxyethylene sorbitan mono-oleate (Tween 80) (20%)	0·0085	30	1
Testosterone	Sodium oleate (10%)	0·05	—	9
Testosterone	Sodium myristyl sulphate (20%)	0·05	—	9
Testosterone	Sodium cholate	0·01	—	9
Testosterone	Polyoxyethylene sorbitan monolaurate (20%)	0·0065	—	2
Testosterone propionate	Polyoxyethylene sorbitan mono-oleate (Tween 80) (20%)	0·017	30	1
Testosterone propionate	Polyoxyethylene sorbitan mono-oleate (Tween 80) (5–20%)	0·012	40	10

TABLE XXV—*continued*

Solute	*Surface-active agent and concentration or concentration range*	*Solubility*[a] *(g solute per g surface-active agent)*	*Temperature*[b] *(°C)*	*Reference*
Testosterone propionate	Polyoxyethylene sorbitan monolaurate (20%)	0·021	—	2
Testosterone propionate	Sodium oleate (10%)	0·15	—	9
Testosterone propionate	Sodium oleate (0·05–5%)	0·27	40	10
Testosterone propionate	Sodium myristyl sulphate (20%)	0·175	—	9
Testosterone propionate	Sodium myristyl sulphate (0·5–20%)	0·22	40	10
Testosterone propionate	Sodium lauryl sulphate	0·22	—	11
α-Tocopherol (Vitamin E)	Polyoxyethylene sorbitan mono-oleate (Tween 80) (20%)	0·066	30	1
α-Tocopheryl acetate	Polyoxyethylene sorbitan mono-oleate (Tween 80) (20%)	0·18	30	1
α-Tocopheryl acetate	Sucrose monoester (C_{10})	0·10	—	3
α-Tocopheryl acetate	Sucrose monoester (C_{12})	0·13	—	3
α-Tocopheryl acetate	Sucrose monoester (C_{14})	0·071	—	3
α-Tocopheryl acetate	Sucrose monoester (C_{16})	0·05	—	3
Tyrothricin	Polyoxyethylene sorbitan mono-oleate (Tween 80) (20%)	0·026	30	1
Vitamin A acetate (c $1{\cdot}7 \times 10^6$ u/g)	Polyoxyethylene sorbitan monolaurate (Tween 20)	0·29	—	4
Vitamin acetate (c $1{\cdot}7 \times 10^6$ u/g)	Polyoxyethylene sorbitan monostearate (Tween 60)	0·077	—	4
Vitamin A acetate (c $1{\cdot}7 \times 10^6$ u/g)	Polyoxyethylene sorbitan mono-oleate (Tween 80)	0·12	—	4
Vitamin A acetate (c $2{\cdot}0 \times 10^6$ u/g)	Sucrose monoester (C_8)	0·05	—	3
Vitamin A acetate (c $2{\cdot}0 \times 10^6$ u/g)	Sucrose monoester (C_{10})	0·17	—	3
Vitamin acetate c $2{\cdot}0 \times 10^6$ u/g)	Sucrose monoester (C_{12})	0·083	—	3
Vitamin A acetate (c $2{\cdot}0 \times 10^6$ u/g)	Sucrose monoester (C_{14})	0·05	—	3

Vitamin A acetate (c 2·0 × 10⁶ u/g)	Sucrose monoester (C_{16})	0·05	—	3
Vitamin A alcohol (c 2 × 10⁶ u/g)	Polyoxyethylene sorbitan monolaurate (Tween 20)	0·12	—	4
Vitamin A alcohol (c 2 × 10⁶ u/g)	Polyoxyethylene sorbitan monostearate (Tween 60)	0·077	—	4
Vitamin A alcohol (c 2 × 10⁶ u/g)	Polyoxyethylene sorbitan mono-oleate (Tween 80)	0·077	—	4
Vitamin A alcohol (c 2 × 10⁶ u/g)	Polyoxyethylene glycol monolauryl Ether (Brij 35)	0·20	—	4
Vitamin A alcohol (c 2·1 × 10⁶ u/g)	Sucrose monoester (C_8)	0·10	—	3
Vitamin A alcohol (c 2·1 × 10⁶ u/g)	Sucrose monoester (C_{10})	0·12	—	3
Vitamin A alcohol (c 2·1 × 10⁶ u/g)	Sucrose monoester (C_{12})	0·10	—	3
Vitamin A alcohol (c 2·1 × 10⁶ u/g)	Sucrose monoester (C_{14})	0·077	—	3
Vitamin A alcohol (c 2·1 × 10⁶ u/g)	Sucrose monoester (C_{16})	0·05	—	3
Vitamin A palmitate (1·7 × 10⁶ u/g)	Polyoxyethylene sorbitan mono-oleate (Tween 80) (20%)	0·28	30	1
Vitamin A palmitate (1·4 × 10⁶ u/g)	Polyoxyethylene sorbitan monolaurate (Tween 20)	0·042	—	4
Vitamin A palmitate (1·4 × 10⁶ u/g)	Polyoxyethylene sorbitan monostearate (Tween 60)	0·25	—	4
Vitamin A palmitate (1·4 × 10⁶ u/g)	Polyoxyethylene sorbitan mono-oleate (Tween 80)	0·25	—	4
Vitamin A palmitate (1·4 × 10⁶ u/g)	Polyethylene glycol monolauryl Ether (Brij 35)	0·042	—	4
Vitamin A palmitate (1·2 × 10⁶ u/g)	Sucrose monoester (linoleate)	0·042	—	3
Vitamin K_1	Polyoxyethylene sorbitan mono-oleate (Tween 80) (20%)	0·31	30	1

[a] Calculated from literature values which were expressed in various units. The density of surface-active agent solutions has been taken as one. In most cases solubility is approximately proportional to the concentration of the surface-active agent (above its c.m.c.) and therefore a solubility at a single concentration should be valid at others up to 10–20% of surface-active agent. The effect of non-micellar surface-active agent may be neglected unless a solubility is required near the c.m.c. or the c.m.c. is exceptionally high.

[b] The temperature was not always reported. However it seems reasonable to assume that where unspecified the solubility is at "room temperature".

References: 1, Nakagawa (1958b); 2, Nakagawa (1953); 3, Mima (1957); 4, Mima and co-authors (1957); 5, Mulley and Metcalf (1956); 6, Mulley and Metcalf (1961); 7, Berry and Bean (1953); 8, Nylander (1953); 9, Ekwall and Sjöblom (1949); 10, Ekwall and co-workers (1951); 11, Ekwall and co-workers (1953); 12, Sjöblom (1956); 13, Guttman and co-workers (1961).

on the amount of hydrocarbon micellar material they both contain. Shorter chain non-ionic compounds are better than long glycol chain compounds on a weight basis because they contain a high proportion of hydrocarbon. The usual effect of long alkyl chain length of giving efficient solubilization is also shown because, for example, sodium caprate is relatively ineffective. The good performance of cationic materials is also shown by these results.

References

Alexander, A. E. (1942). *Trans. Faraday Soc.* **38**, 248–254.

Alexander, A. E., and Johnson, P. (1950). "Colloid Science", p. 682. Oxford University Press, London.

Alexander, A. E., and Trim, A. R. (1946). *Proc. roy. Soc.* **133***B*, 220–234.

Allawala, N. A., and Riegelman, S. (1953a). *J. Amer. pharm. Ass., Sci. Edn.* **42**, 267–275.

Allawala, N. A., and Riegelman, S. (1953b). *J. Amer. pharm. Ass., Sci. Edn.* **42**, 396–401.

Anacker, E. W. (1953). *J. Colloid Sci.* **8**, 402–413.

Bailey, C. R. (1923). *J. chem. Soc.* **123**, 2579–2590.

Balmbra, R. R., Clunie, J. S., Corkill, J. M., and Goodman, J. F. (1962). *Trans. Faraday Soc.* **58**, 1661–1667.

Barail, L. C. (1954). *Soap, N.Y.* **30**, 52–55; 51–53 and p. 109.

Bean, H. S., and Berry, H. (1951). *J. Pharm., Lond.* **3**, 639–655.

Bean, H. S., and Berry, H. (1953). *J. Pharm., Lond.* **5**, 632–639.

Bean, H. S., Richards, J. P., and Thomas, J. (1961). *Proc. 21st Intern. Congr. Pharmaceutical Sciences, Pisa*, 174–181.

Becher, P., and Clifton, N. K. (1959). *J. Colloid Sci.* **14**, 519–523.

Beckett, A. H., and Woodward, R. J. (1963). *J. Pharm., Lond.* **15**, 422–431.

Bergeron, J. (1954). *Proc. 1st Intern. Congr. Surface Activity, Paris*, **1**, 24–30.

Berry, H., and Bean, H. S. (1948). *Nature, Lond.* **161**, 396–397.

Berry, H., and Briggs, A. (1956). *J. Pharm., Lond.* **8**, 1143–1154.

Berry, H., and Stenlake, J. B. (1942). *Pharm. J.* **148**, 112–113.

Boffey, B. J., Collison, R., and Lawrence, A. S. C. (1959). *Trans. Faraday Soc.* **55**, 654–661.

Boon, P. F. G., Coles, C. L. J., and Tait, M. (1961). *J. Pharm., Lond.* **13**, 200–204T.

Brost, G. A., and Krupin, F. (1957). *Soap and Chem. Spec.* **33**, 93.

Campbell, A. N., and Smith, N. O. (1951). Alexander Findlay "The Phase Rule", 494 pp. Dover Publications, New York.

Cantor, A., and Shelanski, M. V. (1956). *J. Soc. cosmet. Chem.* **7**, 419–427.

Carless, J. E., and Mitchell, A. G. (1962). *J. Pharm., Lond.* **14**, 46–55.

Carless, J. E., and Nixon, J. R. (1960). *J. Pharm., Lond.* **12**, 348–359 and earlier papers.

Carless, J. E., Challis, R. A., and Mulley, B. A. (1964). *J. Colloid. Sci.* **19**, 201–212.

Chakovskoy, N. (1956). *Bull. Soc. chim. Belg.* **65**, 474–493.

Chow, B. F., Burnett, J. M., Ling, C. T., and Barrows, L. (1953). *J. Nutr.* **49**, 563–577.

Cohen, M. (1952). *Mémor. Serv. chim. État*, **37**, 85–89.

Coles, C. L. J., and Thomas, D. F. W. (1952). *J. Pharm., Lond.* **4**, 898–901.

Copp, J. L., and Everett, D. H. (1953). *Disc. Faraday Soc.* **15**, 174–188.

Corkill, J. M., Goodman, J. F., and Ottewill, R. H. (1961). *Trans. Faraday Soc.* **57**, 1627–1636.

Corrin, M. L., and Harkins, W. D. (1947). *J. Amer. chem. Soc.* **69**, 679–683 and earlier papers.

Dal Bollo, F., Polasek, G., and Rossi, G. (1958). *Boll. chim. farm.* **97**, 727–737.

Davies, D. G., and Bury, C. R. (1930). *J. chem. Soc.* 2263–2267.

Davis, J. G. (1962) *J. appl. Bact.* **25**, 195–201.

Debye, P. (1949). *J. phys. Chem.* **53**, 1–8.

Dervichian, D. G. (1954). *Disc. Faraday Soc.* **18**, 302.

Dervichian, D. G. (1957). *Proc. 2nd Intern. Congr. Surface Activity, London*, **1**, 327–333 and earlier papers.

Donbrow, M., and Jan, Z. A. (1963). *J. Pharm. Lond.* **15**, 825–830.

Ekwall, P. (1954). *Extrait de Acta Un. int. Cancr.* **10**, No. 3.

Ekwall, P., and Sjöblom, L. (1949). *Acta chem. scand.* **3**, 1179–1180.

Ekwall, P. and Sjöblom, L. (1950). *Acta Endocrinol.* **4**, 179–191.

Ekwall, P., Lundsten, T., and Sjöblom, L. (1951). *Acta chem. scand.* **5**, 1383–1392.

Ekwall, P., Sjöblom, L., and Olsen, J. (1953). *Acta chem. scand.* **7**, 347–351.

Ekwall, P., Danielsson, I., and Mandell, L. (1960). *Kolloidzschr.* **169**, 113–124.

Elworthy, P. H. (1960). *J. Pharm., Lond.* **12**, 293–299.

Elworthy, P. H., and MacFarlane, C. B. (1962a). *J. chem. Soc.* 537–541.

Elworthy, P. H., and MacFarlane, C. B. (1962b). *J. Pharm., Lond.* **14**, 100–102T.

Finch, W. E. (1953). *Pharm. J.* **170**, 59–60.

Finch, W. E. (1958). "Disinfectants", pp. 179. Chapman and Hall, London.

Fitzhugh, O. G., and Nelson, A. A. (1948). *J. Amer. pharm. Ass., Sci. Edn.* **37**, 29–32.

Fournet, G. (1951). *Disc. Faraday Soc.* **11**, 121–125.

Gonick, E., and McBain, J. W. (1946). *J. Amer. chem. Soc.* **68**, 683–685.

Goodhart, F. W., and Martin, A. N. (1962). *J. pharm. Sci.* **51**, 50–54.

Goto, R., Sugano, T., and Koizumi, N. (1953). *Bull. Inst. chem. Res., Kyoto Univ.* **31**, 305–311.

Green, A. A., and McBain, J. W. (1947). *J. phys. Chem.* **51**, 286–298.

Guttman, D. E., Hamlin, W. E., Shell, J. W., and Wagner, J. G. (1961). *J. pharm. Sci.* **50**, 305–307.

Harkins, W. D., and Oppenheimer, H. (1949). *J. Amer. chem. Soc.* **71**, 808–811.

Harris, L. F. (1956). *Pharm. J.* **176**, 130.

Hartley, G. S. (1936). "Paraffin-Chain Salts", Herman et Cie, Paris.

Hartley, G. S (1938). *J. chem. Soc.* 1968–1975.

Hartley, G. S. (1941). *Trans. Faraday Soc.* **37**, 130–133.

Hartley, G. S. (1949). *Nature, Lond.* **163**, 767.

Hartley, G. S. (1955). *In* "Progress in the Chemistry of Fats and Other Lipids" (R. T. Holman, W. O. Lundberg, and T. Malkin, Eds.), Vol. III. Pergamon Press, London and New York.

Harva, O. (1956). *Rec. Trav. chim. Pays-Bas* **75**, 112–116.

Hedley, T. and Co. Ltd. (1955). "A Study of the Effect of the New Detergents on the Skin". Newcastle upon Tyne, England.

Heller, W., and Klevens, H. B. (1946). *J. chem. Phys.* **14**, 567.

Herzfield, S. H., Corrin, M. L., and Harkins, W. D. (1950). *J. phys. Chem.* **54**, 271–283.

Hsiao, L., Dunning, H. N., and Lorenz, P. B. (1956). *J. phys. Chem.* **60**, 657–660.

Hyde, A. J., Langbridge, D. M., and Lawrence, A. S. C. (1954). *Disc. Faraday Soc.* No. **18**, 239–258.

Jones, E. R., and Bury, C. R. (1927). *Phil. Mag.* **4**, 841–848.

Jones, C. M., Culver, P. J., Drummey, C. D., and Ryan, A. E. (1948). *Ann. int. Méd.* **29**, 1–10.

Klevens, H. E. (1947). *J. phys. Chem.* **51**, 1143–1154.
Klevens, H. B. (1948). *J. phys. Chem.* **52**, 130–148.
Klevens, H. B. (1950). *Chem. Revs.* **47**, 1–74.
Klevens, H. B. (1953). *J. Amer. Oil Chem. Soc.* **30**, 74.
Kling, W., and Lange, H. (1957). *Proc. 2nd Intern. Congr. Surface Activity, London*, **1**, 295–303.
Kolthoff, I. M., and Graydon, W. F. (1951). *J. phys. Chem.* **55**, 699–712.
Kolthoff, I. M., and Stricks, W. (1948). *J. phys. Chem.* **52**, 915–941.
Kolthoff, I. M., and Stricks, W. (1949). *J. phys. Chem.* **53**, 425–454.
Kramer, B., Gordon, S. M., Berger, M., and Sobell, A. E. (1951). *Amer. J. Dis. Child*, **82**, 17–27.
Krehl, W. A., Cowgill, G. R., and Whedon, A. D. (1955). *J. Nutr.* **55**, 35–61.
Kushner, L. M., and Hubbard, W. D. (1954). *J. phys. Chem.* **58**, 1163–1167.
Kushner, L. M., Hubbard, W. D., and Doan, A. S. (1957). *J. phys. Chem.* **61**, 371–373.
Lange, H. (1957). *Kolloidzschr.* **153**, 155–156.
Lange, H. (1959). *Kolloidzschr.* **163**, 9–11.
Lange, H. (1960). *Proc. 3rd Intern. Congr. Surface Activity, Cologne*, **1**, 279–288.
Lawrence, A. S. C. (1937). *Trans. Faraday Soc.* **33**, 815–820.
Lawrence, A. S. C. (1958). *Disc. Faraday Soc.* **25**, 51–58. Part 10 of a series.
Lawrence, A. S. C., and Stenson, R. (1957). *Proc. 2nd Intern. Congr. Surface Activity, London*, **1**, 388–394.
Lester-Smith, E. (1932). *J. phys. Chem.* **36**, 1401–1418; 1672–1684; 2455–2473.
Lottermoser, A., and Puschel, F. (1933). *Kolloidzschr.* **63**, 175–192.
Lumb, E. C. (1951). *Trans. Faraday Soc.* **47**, 1049–1055.
Luzzatti, V., Mustacchi, H., and Skoulious, A. (1957). *Nature, Lond.* **180**, 600–601.
Luzzatti, V., Mustacchi, H., and Skoulious, A. (1958). *Disc. Faraday Soc.* **25**, 43–50.
Marsden, S. S., and McBain, J. W. (1948). *J. phys. Chem.* **52**, 110–130.
Martin, A. N. (1960). "Physical Pharmacy", p. 570. Henry Kimpton, London.
Mattoon, R. W., Stearns, R. S., and Harkins, W. D. (1948). *J. chem. Phys.* **16**, 644–658.
McBain, J. W., and Field, M. C. (1933). *J. Amer. chem. Soc.* **55**, 4776–4793.
McBain, J. W., and McBain, M. E. L. (1936). *J. Amer. chem. Soc.* **58**, 2610–2612.
McBain, J. W., Brock, G. C., Vold, R. D., and Vold, M. J. (1938). *J. Amer. chem. Soc.* **60**, 1870–1876.
McBain, J. W (1942). *In* "Advances in Colloid Science" (E. O. Kraemer, F. E. Bartell, and S. S. Kistler, Eds.), Vol. I. Interscience Publishers, New York.
McBain, J. W. (1950). "Colloid Science", pp. 450, D. C. Heath and Co., Boston.
McBain, J. W., and Green, A. A. (1946). *J. Amer. chem. Soc.* **68**, 1731–1736.
McBain, J. W., and Huff, H. (1948). *J. Amer. chem. Soc.* **70**, 3838–3840.
McBain, J. W., and Johnson, K. E. (1944). *J. Amer. chem. Soc.* **66**, 9–13.
McBain, J. W., Wilder, A. G., and Merrill, R. C. (1948). *J. phys. Chem.*, **52**, 12–22.
McBain, M. E. L., Dye, W. B., and Johnston, S. A. (1939). *J. Amer. chem. Soc.* **61**, 3210–3216.
McBain, M. E. L., and Hutchinson, E. (1955). "Solubilization", pp. 259. Academic Press, New York.

McDowell, M. J., and Kraus, C. A. (1951). *J. Amer. chem. Soc.* **73**, 2173–2176 and earlier papers.

Mima, H. (1957). *Pharm. Bull. (Tokyo)* **5**, 496–497.

Mima, H. (1958). *J. pharm. Soc. Japan* **78**, 988–992; *Chem. Abs.* **53**, 1636g.

Mima, H., Asaki, Y., and Kanzawa, T. (1957). *J. pharm. Soc. Japan* **77**, 1201–1203; *Chem. Abs.* **52**, 4106*h*.

Moilliet, J. L., Collie, B., and Black, W. (1961). "Surface Activity", 2nd Edn., E. and F. N. Spon, London.

Moore, C. D., and Bell, M. (1959). *Pharm. J.* **182**, 171–173.

Moore, Q., and Walker, J. N. (1939). *Pharm. J.* **143**, 507–509.

Mukerjee, P., and Mysels, K. J. (1955). *J. Amer. chem. Soc.* **77**, 2937–2943.

Mulley, B. A. (1958). *J. chem. Soc.* 2065–2066.

Mulley, B. A. (1959). *Drug Standards*, **27**, 108–109.

Mulley, B. A. (1960). *Proc. 3rd Intern. Congr. Surface Activity, Cologne* **1**, 31–34.

Mulley, B. A. (1961). *J. Pharm., Lond.* **13**, 205–206T.

Mulley, B. A., and Metcalf, A. D. (1956). *J. Pharm., Lond.* **8**, 774–779.

Mulley, B. A., and Metcalf, A. D. (1961). *Proc. 21st Intern. Congr. Pharmaceutical Sciences, Pisa*, 718–724.

Mulley, B. A., and Metcalf, A. D. (1962). *J. Colloid Sci.* **17**, 523–530.

Murray, R. C. (1935). *Trans. Faraday Soc.* **31**, 206–207.

Murray, R. C., and Hartley, G. S. (1935). *Trans. Faraday Soc.* **31**, 183–189.

Nakagawa, T. (1953). *J. pharm. Soc. Japan* **13**, 469–475; *Chem. Abs.* **47**, 9563*g*.

Nakagawa, T. (1954). *J. pharm. Soc. Japan* **74**, 1116–1119; *Chem. Abs.* **49**, 2033*a*.

Nakagawa, T. (1956). *J. pharm. Soc. Japan* **76**, 1113–1115; *Chem. Abs.* **51**, 2231*h*.

Nakagawa, T. (1958a). *Annu. Rep. Shionogi Res. Lab.*, pp. 805–914. No. 8, Shionogi and Co. Ltd., Amagasaki, Japan.

Nakagawa, T. (1958b). *Yakugaku Saikin no Shimpô*, No. 2, 75–92; *Chem. Abs.* **53**, 3601*g*.

Nakagawa, T., Kuriyama, K., and Inoue, H. (1960). *J. Colloid Sci.* **15**, 268–277.

Nixon, J. R. (1958). "Studies on Oxidation of Emulsified and Solubilised Oils". Ph.D. thesis, Univ. London.

Nylander, A. (1953). *Farm. Notisbl.* **62**, 183–190.

O'Malley, W. J., Pennati, L., and Martin, A. N. (1958). *J. Amer. pharm. Ass., Sci. Edn.* **47**, 334–337.

Palit, S. R., Moghe, V. A., and Biswas, B. (1959). *Trans. Faraday Soc.* **55**, 463–476.

Paquette, R. G., Lingafelter, E. C., and Tartar, H. V. (1943). *J. Amer. chem. Soc.* **65**, 686–692.

Patel, N. K., and Kostenbauder, H. B. (1958). *J. Amer. pharm. Ass., Sci. Edn.* **47**, 289–293.

Pethica, B. A. (1960). *Proc. 3rd Intern. Congr. Surface Activity, Cologne*, **1**, 212–226.

Pethica, B. A., and Schulman, J. H. (1953). *Biochem. J.* **53**, 177–185.

Phillippoff, W. (1950). *J. Colloid Sci.* **5**, 169–191.

Phillips, J. N., and Mysels, K. J. (1955). *J. phys. Chem.* **59**, 325–330.

Powney, J., and Addison, C. C. (1937). *Trans. Faraday Soc.* **33**, 1243–1253.

Riegelman, S. (1960). *J. Amer. pharm. Ass., Sci. Edn.* **49**, 339–343.

Riegelman, S., Allawala, N. A., Hrenoff, M. K., and Strait, L. A. (1958). *J. Colloid Sci.* **13**, 208–217.

Robinson, N. (1960). *J. Pharm., Lond.* **12**, 193–218.

Ross, S., and Olivier, J. P. (1959). *J. phys. Chem.* **63**, 1671–1674.

Ross, S., and Silverstein, A. M. (1954). *J. Colloid Sci.* **9**, 157–165.

Rossetti, V. (1959). *Ann. Chim. appl., Roma* **49**, 923–943.

Saxen, E., and Ekwall, P. (1950). *Extrait de Acta Un. int. Cancr.* **7**, No. 1.

Schönfeldt, N. (1959). "Oberflachenaktive Anglagerunsprodukte des Äthyleneoxyds", pp. 452. Wissenschaftliche Verlagsgesellschaft M.B.H., Stuttgart.

Schwartz, A. M., Perry, J. W., and Berch, J. (1958). "Surface-active Agents and Detergents", Vol. II, pp. 368–384. Interscience Publishers, New York.

Shelanski, H. A. (1952). *Soap, N.Y.* **28**, 32–33.

Sjöblom, L. (1956). *Acta Acad. åbo. Math. Phys.* **20**, pp. 164.

Sjöblom, L. (1958). *Acta Acad. åbo. Math. Phys.* **21**, No. 7.

Smyth, H. F., Carpenter, C. P., and Weil, C. S. (1955). *J. Amer. pharm. Ass., Sci. Edn.* **44**, 27–30.

Soehring, K., Scriba, K., Frahm, M., and Zaellner, G. (1951). *Arch. int. Pharmacodyn* **87**, 301–320.

Stearns, R. S., Oppenheimer, H., Simon, E., and Harkins, W. D. (1947). *J. chem. Phys.* **15**, 496–507.

Stüpel, H. (1955). *Soap Perfum. Cosm. Tr. Rev.* **28**, 58–62 and 300–304.

Swarbrick, J., and Carless, J. E. (1963). *J. Pharm., Lond.* **15**, 507–517.

Sykes, G. (1958). "Disinfection and Sterilization", pp. 396. E. and F. N. Spon, London.

Tartar, H. V. (1955). *J. phys. Chem.* **59**, 1195–1199.

Tartar, H. V., and Lelong, A. L. M. (1955). *J. phys. Chem.* **59**, 1185–1190.

Tartar, H. V., and Wright, K. A. (1939). *J. Amer. chem. Soc.* **61**, 539–544.

Van Abbe, N. J. (1955). *Pharm. J.* **175**, 163.

Vold, M. J. (1941). *J. Amer. chem. Soc.* **63**, 1427–1432.

Waldstein, S. S., and Schoolman, H. M. (1952). *J. Lab. clin. Med.* **40**, 958–959.

Ward, A. F. H. (1940). *Proc. roy. Soc.* **176A**, 412–427.

Ward, A. F. H., and Chitale, A. G. (1957). *Proc. 2nd Intern. Congr. Surface Activity, London* **1**, 319–326.

Weisberger, A. (1959). "Physical Methods of Organic Chemistry", 3rd Edn., Part I, Determination of Solubility by Mader, W. J. Vold, R. D., and Vold, M. J., pp. 655–683. Interscience Publishers, New York.

Weston, C. D. (1953). "Hexagon Digest", I.C.I. Dyestuffs Division, Manchester, England, January pp. 3–15.

Williams, R. J., Phillips, J. N., and Mysels, K. J. (1955). *Trans. Faraday Soc.* **51**, 728–737.

Winsor, P. A. (1948). *Trans. Faraday Soc.* **44**, 463–471.

Winsor, P. A. (1954). "Solvent Properties of Amphiphilic Compounds", pp. 217. Butterworths, London.

Woodward, R. J. (1962). "The Preparation and Properties of Some Surface-active Agents", Ph.D. thesis, University of London.

Wright, K. A., Abbott, A. D., Sivertz, V., and Tartar, H. V. (1939). *J. Amer. chem. Soc.* **61**, 549–554.

Yamada, H., and Kozima, K. (1960). *J. Amer. chem. Soc.* **82**, 1543–1547.

PRESERVATION OF EMULSIONS AGAINST MICROBIAL ATTACK[1]

DOREEN L. WEDDERBURN

Unilever Research Laboratory, Isleworth, Middlesex, England

I. INTRODUCTION

Before the late nineteen-thirties almost all cosmetic and pharmaceutical emulsions were stabilized with soaps. These emulsions did not provide a particularly favourable environment for microbial growth, and although it was necessary to add a preservative to most soap emulsified systems, microbial spoilage was a rare problem.

After the Second World War a large number of new emulsifiers and

[1] MS submitted January 1963.

other ingredients became available and their use resulted in new preservation problems. The apparent incompatibility between the new materials and the conventional preservatives attracted the attention of scientists of many different disciplines and a large literature has accumulated. This has resulted in an interchange of ideas between microbiologists, physical chemists, pharmacists and pharmacologists and although many of the reasons for the failure of preservatives in modern systems are now known, the prevention of microbial growth in the presence of the newer materials is far more complex than it was previously.

It is tempting to think that if the experimental methods and results described in every work published on this subject could be fed into a suitably programmed computer, a set of rules for preserving all kinds of emulsions could be drawn up. This may be possible in the future but there are still too many gaps in our knowledge of the physical structure of emulsions, the metabolism of micro-organisms and the action of preservatives on bacteria and fungi to permit this approach at present. Until such time as our knowledge of the factors governing the action of preservatives in all usable systems is complete, the best we can do is to understand the main principles which contribute to microbial growth and those which enhance or limit the effectiveness of growth inhibitors.

In almost all systems there are factors which favour microbial growth —water and molecules which can be metabolized—and at the same time there are usually hostile elements such as adverse pH conditions, osmotic pressure effects or toxic molecules which may suppress growth. The balance between these factors determines whether micro-organisms flourish or gradually die out.

The efficiency of the preservative is likewise subject to favourable and unfavourable influences, the keys to which lie in the ingredients and structure of the emulsion.

Knowledge of these balancing and counterbalancing factors enables suitable compromises to be made in preservative selection, but in the absence of complete understanding of all the forces at work, it is foolish to rely on predictions of how preservatives will function in new systems without subjecting them to thorough testing.

Numerous publications recommend various concentrations of different preservatives as being effective, without considering the multiplicity of factors in particular systems which may make the recommendations valueless. The important factors bearing on preservative efficiency are highlighted in this chapter so that those confronted with preservation problems may make their own choice with an understanding of some of the factors which operate in their particular emulsion systems.

This review has been written from the standpoint of the microbiologist, and inevitably certain aspects which are important to those of other disciplines will have been omitted or dealt with inadequately. It is hoped, nevertheless, that it will fulfil three limited objectives; first, to indicate to those who encounter problems of microbial spoilage in existing formulae where they might look for the cause, second to help the formulator of new emulsions in the selection of the most suitable preservative, and to point the way to its evaluation, and third to highlight some of the deficiencies in our knowledge and indicate where further research is necessary.

A. CHEMICAL ACTIVITY OF BACTERIA AND FUNGI

Living organisms propagate at the expense of their environment and in considering any spoilage problem created by the presence of micro-organisms, the variety of chemical reactions they can carry out and the rate at which these occur should be taken into account.

Bacteria and fungi have a wide distribution in nature and there are few places on or near the surface of the earth that are free from them. Some of the more unlikely places in which they occur are Arctic snows, effluents from gas works, stagnant salt lakes, hot mineral springs and in essentially anhydrous diesel fuel. They are absent only in those places where a sterilizing influence prevails or in the interior tissues of healthy animals and plants.

The metabolism of bacteria and fungi, if uninhibited by any sterilizing influence, often results in a rapid and profound change in the chemical environment, and in the synthesis of new protoplasm many complex chemical reactions are accomplished within a remarkably short period of time. These chemical reactions are made possible by a wide variety of enzymes secreted by micro-organisms and the following are some of the basic reactions which can be carried out.

Hydrolysis: the addition of H_2O to the molecule. The next step in molecular breakdown is often thus facilitated so that molecules are split at the hydrolysed link.

Dehydration: the removal of H_2O from the molecule.

Oxidation: the removal of hydrogen or the addition of oxygen to the molecule; also a process which involves an increase in the number of positive charges on an atom, or a decrease in the number of negative charges.

Reduction: the removal of oxygen or the addition of hydrogen; the reverse reactions to those of oxidation.

Decarboxylation: the removal of CO_2 from —COOH.

Deamination: the removal of $-NH_2$.

Phosphorylation: the esterification of the molecule with phosphoric acid. This is usually accomplished by the transfer of the phosphate radicle from some substance other than phosphoric acid itself.

Dephosphorylation: the removal by hydrolysis of phosphoric acid from phosphorylated compounds.

Different bacteria and fungi utilize different methods to attack the same substrate depending on their complement of enzymes, and in an environment supporting the growth of several different micro-organisms, a variety of end-products will be produced.

In a mixed population there is often a certain amount of competition for essential nutrients between the different flora, and those which can convert the environment more rapidly and efficiently survive, while the less fortunate die out, providing a further source of convertible substrate for those that remain.

The metabolic pathways employed by bacteria differ not only between different genera and species and between different strains of the same species, but can vary in one strain according to the environmental conditions. For example, *Aerobacter aerogenes* will attack pyruvic acid at pH 8 to give acetic and formic acids.

$$CH_3.CO.COOH + H_2O = CH_3.COOH + H.COOH$$

At pH 6 the same organism will attack pyruvic acid by decarboxylation.

$$2CH_3.CO.COOH = CH_3.CO.CHOH.CH_3 + 2CO_2$$

By decomposing the environment many of these metabolic processes result in the formation of acid end-products which have a limiting effect on the growing organisms, and in some instances the changes brought about are sufficient to inhibit growth altogether. Most organisms are, however, capable of carrying out neutralizing reactions which have alkaline end-products and in this way some degree of stabilization of the environment can be achieved.

In order to synthesize new protoplasm, the organism has to change the environment which supplies the material for the growth process. Since the elements for growth are rarely in an assimilable form, the organism has to degrade complex molecules into a utilizable form. This involves the expenditure of energy, which the organism obtains by the degradation of energy-rich substances in the environment. If, during the process, the physico-chemical properties of the environment are significantly changed, the organism reacts by carrying out further processes which stabilize the environment.

The variety of reactions which can be accomplished by micro-organisms and the speed with which they can be carried out—one organism can give rise to over 1,000,000 organisms in 5 h—shows how necessary it is to inhibit microbial growth in products whose form we wish to remain unchanged.

B. EMULSION STRUCTURE

Emulsions can be simply defined as two phase systems consisting of two immiscible liquids, one being dispersed in the other in the form of small droplets. In simple systems, one phase is always aqueous and the other lipid or fatty in nature. The phases are separated by definite boundary surfaces, and the film which is adsorbed at the boundary is often regarded as a separate third phase.

Dispersions of the aqueous phase in the lipid phase are water-in-oil emulsions and the converse are oil-in-water. Both phases usually contain a number of different substances, either in solution or suspension. Multiple emulsions also occur, with a separate phase dispersed within an already dispersed phase.

The constituents of the aqueous phase and those which are adsorbed at the interfacial boundary are important in the context of emulsion preservation for two reasons. First, because micro-organisms depend on the presence of water for growth, they will exist in the aqueous phase or at the interfacial boundary on the aqueous side of the interface. The substances present in the aqueous phase and the physical properties of this phase will therefore determine whether organisms survive in a quiescent state, thrive and multiply or are inhibited. Secondly, preservatives, which interfere with the metabolism of micro-organisms and ultimately destroy them, are only effective in aqueous solution, and consequently the constituents of the aqueous phase and those at the interface will influence the thermodynamic activity of the preservative by affecting its solubility, dissociation and partition coefficient.

Humectants such as glycerol, sorbitol and various glycols are frequent constituents of the aqueous phase, and are used primarily to prevent moisture loss from the product and to provide desirable flow properties. A variety of hydrocolloids such as cellulose derivatives, gums and other thickening agents are also often present in the aqueous phase to regulate rheological properties and stabilize emulsions.

II. THE NEED FOR PRESERVATION

Many of the materials used in the preparation of emulsions are susceptible to biological degradation and Barr and Tice (1957d) have reported the splitting of the ester linkages of certain nonionic surfactants by *Pseudomonas aeruginosa*, *Aspergillus niger*, *Penicillium notatum* and *Monilia albicans*. Table I shows their findings.

Results indicated that the organisms were capable of growing in the surfactant esters and splitting them, and the rate of growth and ester splitting was dependent on the number of organisms in the inoculum.

TABLE I

The Growth of Micro-organisms in 1 and 5 per cent W/V Solutions and Dispersions of Non-ionic Surfactants of the Sorbitan Partial Ester and Polyoxyethylene Ester Types (from Barr and Tice, 1957d)

Surfactant	*Control*	*Pseudomonas aeruginosa*	*Monilia albicans*	*Aspergillus niger*	*Penicillium notatum*
Polyoxyethylene 20 sorbitan monolaurate	—[a]	+[b]	+[b]	+[b]	+[b]
Polyoxyethylene 20 sorbitan monopalmitate	—	+[b]	+[b]	+[b]	+[b]
Polyoxyethylene 20 sorbitan monostearate	—	+[b]	+[b]	+[b]	+[b]
Polyoxyethylene 20 sorbitan mono-oleate	—	+[b]	+[b]	+[b]	+[b]
Sorbitan monolaurate	—	+	+	+	+
Sorbitan monopalmitate	—	+	+	+	+
Sorbitan monostearate	—	+	+	+	+
Sorbitan mono-oleate	—	+	+	+	+
Polyoxyl 40 stearate	—	+[b]	+[b]	+[b]	+[b]

[a] No inoculum.
[b] Splitting of ester observed.
\+ Growth of micro-organisms observed.

Micro-organisms are also capable of utilizing anionic surfactants as sources of energy. The chemical structure of surfactants controls their susceptibility to attack and certain bacteria are capable of oxidizing terminal methyl groups to carboxyl groups. The alkyl sulphates, sulphonated fatty acids, amides and esters and the low molecular weight polyethylene glycol derivatives are rapidly broken down according to Sawyer and Ryckman (1957) while the alkyl aryl sulphonates, alkyl phenoxypolyoxy ethanols and high molecular weight polyethylene glycol derivatives are attacked more slowly. Dodecyl benzene sodium sulphonate is readily attacked by many Gram negative bacteria but similar compounds with branched side chains are less susceptible.

The author has studied the respiration rate of *Pseudomonas fluorescens* in the presence of 2 per cent solutions of various surfactants as the sole energy source. Actively growing cells freed from residual nutrients by thorough washing were studied in a Warburg microrespirometer when suspended in 2 per cent surfactant solutions at 30° C. Their respiration rate was followed over a period of 3 h in comparison with that of cells in the absence of any surfactant.

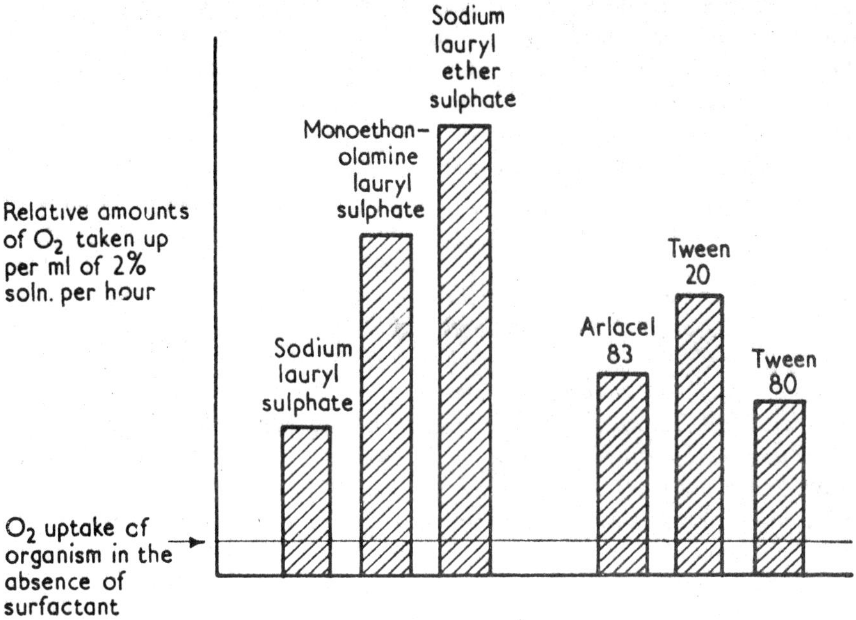

FIG. 1. Relative effect of 2 per cent solutions of surfactants on oxygen uptake of *Pseudomonas fluorescens*.

Figure 1 shows the relative amounts of O_2 taken up per ml of surfactant solution per hour by sodium lauryl sulphate, monoethanolamine lauryl sulphate, sodium lauryl ether sulphate, Arlacel 83 (sorbitan sesqui-oleate), Tween 20 (polyoxyethylenes orbitan monolaurate) and Tween 80 (polyoxyethylene sorbitan mono-oleate). The line across the diagram indicates the rate of respiration of cells in the absence of any surfactant.

Baker (1959) has reported the hydrolysis of polyhydric alcohol-fatty acid sulphates by *Pseudomonas aeruginosa*, and it is also known that the fatty alkanolamides are susceptible to attack by bacteria.

Various humectants, at concentrations below those at which they exert an adverse osmotic pressure on cell walls, are also utilized as sources of energy, and glycerin and sorbitol can be broken down.

The nutritive value of the many vegetable gums utilized as thickeners is too well known to be stressed here and it need hardly be pointed out that the presence of proteins, amino acids, protein hydrolysates, carbohydrates or other readily fermentable substances in an emulsion will contribute to its deterioration unless steps are taken to prevent microbial growth.

Sokolski *et al.* (1962) have shown that *Cladosporium resinae* is capable of hydrolysing methyl *p*-hydroxybenzoate to *p*-hydroxybenzoic acid even though in certain circumstances this preservative is fungicidal to the mould. The hydrolysis of the preservative is attributable to an esterase produced by the organism, and in experiments where 0·2 per cent aqueous solutions of methyl *p*-hydroxybenzoate were inoculated with *C. resinae*, only 50 per cent of the preservative remained unchanged after 4 days at 25° C.

Other micro-organisms probably produce similar esterases, and when the conditions are such that the organisms are not overcome by the preservative, changes in the preservative can be expected.

It has been known for many years that phenols are often oxidized by bacteria, and Wagner (1914) found that cresol was broken down. Since that time *p*-cresol, *o*-cresol, *m*-cresol and 4,6-dinitro-*o*-cresol have been reported to be oxidized by certain bacteria within the pH range 7·0–8·0 under aerobic conditions.

Walker (1954) noted that soil bacteria were able to oxidize some chlorinated phenols, and Gundersen and Jensen (1956) found that traces of certain inorganic salts, notably calcium carbonate, were necessary for the oxidation of 4,6-dinitro-*o*-cresol by *Corynebacterium simplex*.

These few examples of the chemical activities of bacteria provide a glimpse of the tremendous range of reactions which can be carried out, and serve to show that unless their propagation is inhibited in some way, micro-organisms will change their environment to suit their own purposes.

Most of the materials used in the manufacture of pharmaceutical and cosmetic emulsions are contaminated to some extent with bacteria and fungi, and even if the degree of contamination is low initially, the addition of water, which probably contains more organisms, will provide a favourable environment for growth.

Emulsions prepared for topical application to the skin, and even those intended for oral administration, need not necessarily be entirely free from micro-organisms, but because of the changes which viable and propagating organisms can bring about in an emulsion, steps must be taken to ensure that active growth does not occur. Quite apart from the unaesthetic appearance of products supporting mould growth on their surface or pack, the presence of viable bacteria can lead to separation of emulsions, discoloration, the formation of gas and of odours, and changes in rheological properties. These effects on the product can be brought about quite quickly if large numbers of organisms are present, or if the product possesses properties which favour rapid multiplication. Decomposition might, however, only reveal itself after many months if

TABLE II

Some of the Micro-organisms Isolated from Pharmaceutical and Cosmetic Emulsions

Fungi	*Bacteria*	*Yeasts*
Absidia	*Achromobacter*	*Candida*
Alternaria[a]	*Aerobacter*	*Monilia*
Aspergillus[a]	*Bacillus*[a]	*Torula*
Citromyces	*Enterococcus*	*Zygosaccharomyces*
Cladosporium[a]	*Escherichia*	
Dematium	*Micrococcus*	
Fusarium	*Proteus*	
Geotrichum	*Psuedomonas*[a]	
Helminthosporium	*Sarcinia*	
Hormodendrum	*Serratia*	
Mucor[a]	*Staphylococcus*[a]	
Paecilomyces	*Streptococcus*[a]	
Penicillium[a]		
Phoma		
Pullularia		
Rhizopus[a]		
Stemphylium		
Thamnidium		
Trichothecium		
Verticillium		

[a] Several different species of these genera have been reported.

the conditions are such that growth can only take place after the organisms have adapted themselves to the environment. The process of adaptation may involve the organism in altering the pH gradually to a level at which growth can take place at greater speed, or could necessitate the use of metabolic processes not normally employed by the organism under optimum conditions.

Rapid spoilage of emulsions during the development of new products can be, and often is, confused with faulty formulation because initial storage tests are frequently carried out on prototype formulae without either preservative or perfume. Breakdown of unpreserved emulsions at temperatures approaching 30–37° C within a few days of manufacture is frequently caused by bacterial attack of the emulsifier, and if this possibility is taken into account much unnecessary reformulation can be avoided.

The sale of inadequately preserved products can lead to large-scale financial loss on the part of the manufacturer, and apart from visible product deterioration in the form of mould growth or other kinds of spoilage due to bacteria, invisible contamination can constitute a toxicity hazard.

Many kinds of fungi, yeasts and bacteria have been identified in cosmetic and pharmaceutical emulsions, and there must be many more which have never been characterized.

Some of the various genera reported by Sagarin (1957), Manowitz (1961), Babicka (1957), de Navarre (1962) and Tice and Barr (1958) are given in Table II.

A. SOURCES OF CONTAMINATION

Raw materials and the water used in manufacture are obvious sources of contamination. Most refined oils, fats and waxes contain relatively few organisms per gram, as shown by Herbold (1943), but Hall (1938), in examining dried natural materials such as gums and herbs, found counts of up to 16 million bacteria per gram and a variety of fungi and yeasts as well. The natural gums, tragacanth, karaya and acacia, are always very heavily contaminated, as are talc, kaolin, chalk and rice starch. The degree of contamination of synthetic materials varies, and while the number of organisms is usually lower than in natural products, they are seldom sterile.

Distilled and demineralized water are very seldom free from bacteria, and filter beds and storage tanks are frequently responsible for harbouring a rich flora. Baker (1959) describes several cases of serious product deterioration which were traced to heavy contamination in the resin beds of ion exchangers or water storage tanks.

Other sources of contamination prior to manufacture are the air, raw material containers such as drums, sacks, cartons, etc., and the hands of operatives.

In the study of preservation problems, much has been written about the cleanliness and design of manufacturing plant, and steam or chemical sterilization is frequently recommended. Pieces of equipment which have inaccessible joints, pipes and pumps are often difficult to clean properly, and washing with detergent solutions can simply lead to dilution of the remains of the product and the formation of stagnant foci where bacteria and fungi thrive.

Sokolski *et al.* (1962) described a case where a pharmaceutical preparation containing clay and pectin, and preserved with methyl *p*-hydroxybenzoate was hydrolysed when large numbers of *Cladosporium resinae* were present. The preservative was effective against the normal number of organisms present in the product, but failed when the number increased when an occasional batch of clay was heavily contaminated. Use of contaminated clay resulted in the accumulation of clumps of *C. resinae* in a trap in the production pipe-line. These clumps occasionally broke loose and entered the product. The problem was solved by cleaning the plant more frequently and thoroughly.

Deeley (1962), describing the problems of preserving emulsions used in the textile industry, advocates the "education of those concerned in manufacture" and describes procedures for good-housekeeping.

Some of the detergent sanitizers containing quaternary ammonium compounds, or detergent/iodine mixtures, formaldehyde or sodium hypochlorite solutions are suitable for use during the cleaning of manufacturing plant, but before flushing with any of these it is essential to remove as much product residue as possible and to rinse with plenty of hot water after the treatment.

Comprehensive details of the best methods of plant cleaning and disinfection are given by Davis (1960) who states that 150 to 200 p.p.m. of hypochlorite will sanitize clean metal and glass in 2 min, and sterilize completely in 10 min. He points out the corrosive nature of chlorine as being a disadvantage of its use and stresses the significance of thorough removal of product residues in the plant before sterilization.

According to Davis "one of the most important lessons which has been learned by industry and manufacturers of food equipment is the necessity for a smooth finish to, and absence of crevices and dead ends in, all items which come into contact with food, because they are difficult to free from traces of organic matter, and may escape contact with cleaning and sterilising solutions by reason of air-locks. Losses to the food industry from these causes alone must have been great in the past; fortunately the lesson has now been well learned." These comments apply equally well to the pharmaceutical and cosmetic industries, but in the latter particularly, the lesson is still being learned painfully.

After manufacture most products are exposed to further contamination from filling machinery, and the containers, caps and cap linings. The latter are notorious for their abundant fungal flora and much of the growth on the surface of cosmetic creams is directly attributable to this source. On many occasions creams containing preservatives, able to control the growth of micro-organisms from all other sources, have broken down following the introduction of large numbers of fungal spores from the cap lining. These usually germinate initially in the micro-film of water on the lining and spread gradually to areas of slight separation around the edge of the cream.

Products packed in wide-mouthed jars and flexible bottles which draw air back into them are liable to contamination in use and even if the number of micro-organisms in the product is small when it leaves the factory it is necessary to ensure that the preservative will deal effectively with organisms introduced by the consumer. de Navarre (in a private communication) described how a cleansing cream containing a non-ionic surfactant had been contaminated by *Monilia albicans* thought to have been introduced by the consumer returning unused portions of the cream to the jar from the palm of the hand. Products packed in collapsible tubes and bottles with small orifices are less prone to contamination in use, but are often susceptible to spoilage because these packs are difficult to clean properly before the product is filled.

Many pharmaceutical and cosmetic emulsions, in addition to having a long shelf life, are often in the possession of the consumer for many months, and even if spoilage does not become apparent until the contents are more than half used, any form of decomposition will reflect unfavourably on the manufacturer.

B. FACTORS AFFECTING GROWTH IN EMULSIONS

The following factors influence the need for preserving emulsions and determine the type of micro-organisms which will survive and the rate at which they will propagate if preservation is inadequate:

—the ratio of oil to water and the type of emulsion, i.e. oil-in-water or water-in-oil;
—the pH of the aqueous phase, its surface tension, oxygen tension and osmotic pressure;
—the nutritive value of the emulsion;
—the degree of aeration of the emulsion and the availability of oxygen;
—the amount and type of perfume or flavour present;
—the type of container in which the product is to be packed.

Since micro-organisms depend on water for the synthesis of their cellular components the physical and chemical characteristics of the water phase are the dominant factors in determining whether growth occurs. It has frequently been stated that because of their dependence on water, organisms will only survive in the water phase of an emulsion, but Eisman (1954), in studying the preservation of parenteral vegetable oils, found that self-sterilizing conditions for vegetative bacteria only prevailed in completely anhydrous oils, and even in the total absence of moisture the spores of *Bacillus subtilis* survived.

Bullock and Keepe (1951) reported the viability of dried *Streptococcus faecalis* cells and *Bacillus subtilis* spores in peanut oil for more than 6 months, and De Gray and Killian (1962) maintain that "certain bacteria and fungi can survive for extended periods of time in hydrocarbons free of any separate aqueous phase".

In emulsions there is likely to be migration of organisms from the oil phase to the water phase and since the oil phase will not be entirely "anhydrous", migration in the opposite direction cannot be ruled out. The relative volumes of the phases influence the degree to which organisms will survive and, in general terms, the less water the less growth. Bennett (1962), in a study of the preservation of emulsions used in the metal-working industry, found that the oil–water ratio had a significant effect upon the magnitude of growth. By inoculating equal numbers of *Pseudomonas aeruginosa* cells into a series of emulsions with different oil–water ratios it was found that the amount of growth increased with an increase in water content.

Tice and Barr (1958) state that preservation of oil-in-water emulsions is more necessary and important than that of the water-in-oil type. Where oil is the external and continuous phase, they believe that the spread of organisms throughout the product will be hindered and hence visible growth will seldom be seen. Spores falling on the surface of oil-continuous emulsions, while not killed, find themselves in an arid environment which is not conducive to growth. Although some cosmetic and pharmaceutical emulsions of the water-in-oil type have been distributed without a preservative, this is not to be recommended because even slight growth can produce oxidase enzymes which may cause rancidity and odour changes if natural oils and fats are present.

The presence in the aqueous phase of molecules which can be utilized by micro-organisms will obviously contribute to the amount of growth which will occur, but this in turn will be influenced by the pH, osmotic pressure, surface tension and oxygen tension of the solution.

The pH of the aqueous phase will affect the degree of ionization of utilizable materials, influence the electrical charge at the cell walls, determine enzyme production and activity and hence regulate the availability of nutrients and the ease with which they are assimilated into the cell. The growth tolerance limits for pH differ widely for various organisms as can be seen from a few examples quoted in Table III.

In general, fungi grow more abundantly in acid environments, but have been known to flourish on unpreserved creams with an aqueous phase of pH 8·5.

If bacteria manage to survive at a pH that is less than optimum, they try to alter the environment in their favour. This is sometimes achieved by the breakdown of amino acids. In conditions which are too alkaline deaminases are produced which, in the attack on amino acids, liberate ammonia leaving behind an acid end-product, the corresponding keto acid. In acid environments the decarboxylases are produced which liberate carbon dioxide leaving an alkaline end-product, the amine.

Since cosmetic and pharmaceutical emulsions seldom, if ever, have an aqueous phase with pH above or below the very wide tolerance limits for the majority of organisms likely to contaminate them, this factor alone cannot be expected to exert a preserving influence.

TABLE III

pH Tolerance Limits for some Bacteria

Organism	*pH tolerance limits*
Coliforms	3·2– 9·8
Enterococci	4·8–11·0
Pseudomonas species	3·0–11·0
Lactobacillus species	3·0– 6·5
Yeasts	1·5– 8·5

The osmotic pressure of the aqueous phase can, however, have a limiting effect on growth. The bodies of all micro-organisms are surrounded by living semi-permeable membranes, and any sudden and drastic changes in the osmotic pressure or even slow but profound changes in the environment can lead to swelling and rupture of the membrane or shrinkage and dehydration. Although glycerin can be used at low concentrations as a nutrient by many organisms, at concentrations of between 40 and 50 per cent it is inhibitory by reason of its osmotic effect. High concentrations of electrolytes exert a similar limiting action.

Variations in the surface tension of culture media are well known to microbiologists as a means of influencing growth, and thus the surface tension of the aqueous phase of an emulsion is certain to be a factor in determining what organisms will survive in it, quite apart from the nutritive value of some surfactant molecules. Many Gram negative bacteria, and the coliforms in particular, flourish in environments abounding in surfactants while most Gram positive organisms do not grow well at surface tension levels much below 50 dyn/cm. In most emulsions the surface tension is very low and this may account in part for the fact that Gram positive bacteria are comparatively rare contaminants of these systems. Cationic surfactants are toxic to many organisms, anionics to a few and non-ionics to hardly any, thus surface tension *per se* will not be a growth-limiting factor, but will have an effect in association with the presence or absence of toxic groups in the surfactant molecules.

Many of the bacteria and all the fungi which contribute to the spoilage of pharmaceutical and cosmetic emulsions are aerobic, depending on the availability of oxygen for their metabolism. Many other bacteria are facultative anaerobes and can grow either in the presence or absence of oxygen, hence the oxygen tension alone will not limit growth, but may enable particular species to propagate if all other factors are favourable.

Essential oils used in perfumes and flavours inhibit the growth of many bacteria and fungi which thrive in emulsions. Lord and Husa (1954) made an extensive study of the effects on fungi of over 200 essential oils. They found very marked differences between the inhibitory properties of the essences when tested at concentrations between 0·01 and 0·2 per cent. The vapours of essential oils are often more active against bacteria and fungi than the oils in liquid form.

Okazaki *et al.* (1953) tested several essential oils against bacteria and fungi, and reported anti-fungal activity in the following descending order of effectiveness: sandalwood; vetiver; rose; neroli; citronella; geranium; bay; patchouli; jasmin; anise; ylang-ylang and lemon.

Essential oils are rarely used as preservatives because of their cost, coupled with the fact that they are volatile and their effectiveness diminishes with time. Frequently, however, they contribute significantly towards making the environment less favourable to microbial growth.

C. PRESERVATIVE REQUIREMENTS

The wealth of literature over the last decade referring to the failure of many of the well-established and long-used preservatives to inhibit the growth of bacteria and fungi in pharmaceutical and cosmetic emulsions indicates that the whole problem requires a new approach and that some of the well-entrenched attitudes to preserving products should be re-examined.

Boehm (1933a) listed the properties of preservatives for use in cosmetics, and Briggs and Cook (1962) in considering the preservation of bi-phasic systems used in the pharmaceutical and cosmetic industries outlined the properties of the "ideal" preservative before describing some of the complexities of inhibiting the growth of micro-organisms in emulsions. Having studied the many factors involved, they agreed with Wedderburn

(1958) that the preservative should be selected early in the development of any new formula and be considered an integral part of it, not merely an *ad hoc* addition.

In the light of the experience of pharmaceutical and cosmetic chemists during the last 15 years, this conclusion must be correct, although judging by the many surprised and almost aggrieved observations in the literature that the erstwhile "ideal" preservatives failed in the presence of many of the newer materials used in formulation, it seems that there is a general reluctance to accept it. This reluctance is understandable because in the days when most emulsions were made with ingredients which did not present a favourable environment to micro-organisms, the formulator could rely on the effectiveness of one of the "old favourites" to preserve it and did not have to call in the microbiologist to carry out elaborate tests on the compatibility of individual components and the preservative, or even on the finished product itself. The microbial decomposition of his product was one of his lesser problems, and he knew how to deal with it if it arose.

The advent of new emulsifiers, thickeners, solubilizers, opacifiers, suspending agents and "active ingredients" has complicated matters and has led to what has amounted to an almost frenzied search on the part of physico-chemists, microbiologists and chemists for preservatives which would be effective in products containing the new materials. Much of the literature on the compatibility between preservatives and other materials used in emulsions has been contradictory, partly because of a wide divergence of test techniques, but mainly because different workers have investigated systems, which although often broadly similar, have differed in some minor respect.

At the present time no single antimicrobial agent has emerged as the universally applicable preservative for emulsions, and study of the principles involved in preventing growth in these systems shows clearly that this is highly unlikely to occur.

The number of compounds suitable for use as preservatives in pharmaceutical or cosmetic emulsions is limited by the essential requirements, which are:

1. Freedom from toxic or irritant effect at the concentrations used on the skin, mucous membranes and, in the case of orally administered products, on the gastro-intestinal system.
2. Stability to heat and prolonged storage.
3. Freedom from gross incompatibility with other ingredients in the formula resulting in loss of antimicrobial action.

Several other requirements, as follow, have been specified by Boehm

(1933b), Gershenfeld and Pearlstein (1939), Manowitz (1961), Briggs and Cook (1962) and de Navarre (1962).

A preservative for pharmaceutical and cosmetical emulsions should: be active at low concentration; retain its effectiveness over a wide range of pH; be effective against a wide range of micro-organisms; be readily soluble at its effective concentration; have no odour or colour; be non-volatile; retain its activity in the presence of the metallic salts of aluminium, zinc, iron and alloys such as tin foil; be non-corrosive to collapsible metal tubes, and rubber.

TABLE IV

Some Preservatives used in Cosmetic and Pharmaceutical Emulsions

p-hydroxybenzoic acid	phenol
benzoic acid	cresol
sorbic acid	chlorothymol
dehydroacetic acid	methylchlorothymol
formic acid	chlorbutanol
salicylic acid	*o*-phenylphenol
boric acid	dichlorophene
vanillic acid	hexachlorophene
p-chlorobenzoic acid	parachlormetaxylenol
o-chlorobenzoic acid	parachlormetacresol
propionic acid	dichlormetaxylenol
sulphurous acid	*p*-chlorphenylpropanediol
trichlorphenylacetic acid	β-phenoxyethylalcohol
	β-*p*-chlorphenoxyethylalcohol
methyl *p*-hydroxybenzoate	β-phenoxypropylalcohol
ethyl *p*-hydroxybenzoate	potassium hydroxyquinolin sulphate
propyl *p*-hydroxybenzoate	8-hydroxyquinolin
butyl *p*-hydroxybenzoate	*p*-chlorphenylglyceryl ether
benzyl *p*-hydroxybenzoate	formaldehyde
	hexamine
benzethonium chloride	monomethylol dimethyl hydantoin
benzalkonium chloride	
cetyltrimethyl ammonium bromide	
cetylpyridinium chloride	phenyl mercury acetate
dimethyldidodecenyl ammonium chloride	phenyl mercury borate
	phenyl mercury nitrate
tetramethylthiuramdisulphide	
	tetrachlorsalicylanilide
vanillin	trichlorsalicylanilide
ethyl vanillin	trichlorcarbanilide

These, and the three essential requirements, are descriptive of the "ideal" preservative which would be suitable for all types of emulsion, all conditions of use and varieties of pack, and if slavishly adhered to would make preservation of some individual emulsions containing the newer materials almost impossible.

For many years the esters of *p*-hydroxybenzoic acid appeared to fulfil all these requirements and were widely used in the cosmetic industry. It was seldom necessary even to test their efficiency in most formulae since they were compatible with almost all the materials used in emulsions, but with the advent of non-ionic emulsifiers and a variety of other useful substances, it became apparent that the customary 0·1 to 0·2 per cent of these esters was inactive in many formulae. These findings led to the examination of a far wider range of antimicrobial agents than had ever before been considered for preserving emulsions.

Table IV lists some of the preservatives used in cosmetic and pharmaceutical emulsions.

Compounds closely related to those above have also been used, and inspection of the variety of preservatives available shows that a thorough understanding of the factors which can influence their efficiency in a particular system is necessary before a selection can be made.

III. Influence of Specific Factors on Preservatives

A. PRESERVATIVE DISSOCIATION AS A FUNCTION OF pH

Weak acids often act as preservatives in their undissociated form, the equilibrium between undissociated acid and anion being a function of pH.

Kostenbauder (1962) expresses this succinctly as follows:

$$K_a = \frac{(H^+) \quad (A^-)}{(HA)}$$

The fraction of total acid in undissociated form can be expressed as:

$$\text{Fraction undissociated} = \frac{(HA)}{(HA)+(A^-)} = \frac{(HA)}{(HA)+\dfrac{K_a(HA)}{(H^+)}} = \frac{(H^+)}{(H^+)+K_a}$$

The concentration of undissociated acid present at any pH would be given by:

$$\text{Undissociated acid} = (\text{Total})\frac{(H^+)}{(H^+)+K_a}$$

If the inhibitory concentration of undissociated acid is known, the total concentration of acid required in the aqueous phase can be calculated.

$$\begin{matrix}\text{Total required}\\ \text{preservative}\end{matrix} = \frac{(\text{Inhibitory conc. of undissociated acid})\,((H^+)+K_a)}{(H^+)}$$

The proportions of benzoic acid remaining undissociated at various pH levels are given in Table V.

Thus at pH 6 approximately sixty times as much benzoic acid is required as at pH 3.

TABLE V

Proportion of Benzoic Acid Undissociated at Various pH Levels

pH	*Undissociated Benzoic acid* %
2	99·4
3	94·3
4	62·5
5	13·7
6	1·6

pK_a Benzoic acid = 4·2.

TABLE VI

Preservative Activity of Sorbic Acid (from de Navarre, 1959)

Organism	*Concentration to inhibit growth* %	*pH*
Candida albicans	0·1	4·5
Penicillium chrysogenum	0·15	3·5
Aspergillus niger	0·05	2·5
	0·15	3·5
Escherichia coli	0·12	5·0–5·5
Bacillus subtilis	0·15	5·6–7·0
Staphylococcus aureus	0·12	5·0–5·5

Sorbic acid has a similar pH-concentration dependence, and Bell *et al.* (1959), in studying the effect of sorbic acid on the growth of various species of bacteria, yeasts and filamentous fungi found it was most effective at the highest concentration of undissociated acid. At pH 4·8 they reported that 50 per cent of the acid was undissociated. This finding supports statements by de Navarre (1959) in presenting data produced by manufacturers of sorbic acid. In this work 70 per cent of sorbic acid is said to be undissociated at pH 4·4. Table VI shows the concentration and pH of solutions of sorbic acid found to inhibit certain micro-organisms.

Wolf and Westveer (1950), in a study of the antimicrobial activity of several substituted pyrones, state that dehydroacetic acid enolizes to give a weak acid, and hence at pH 9 the compound exists primarily as the sodium salt. They tested dehydroacetic acid at pH 5, 7 and 9 against *Micrococcus pyogenes* var. *aureus* and *Salmonella typhosa* and found no

Table VII

Dissociation Constants of Acids used as Preservatives

		Dissociation constant
Sulphurous acid	H_2SO_3	$1{\cdot}70 \times 10^{-2}$
o-Chlorbenzoic acid	$O\text{-}Cl.C_6H_4.COOH$	$1{\cdot}20 \times 10^{-3}$
Salicylic acid	$O\text{-}HOC_6H_4COOH$	$1{\cdot}06 \times 10^{-3}$
Formic acid	$H.COOH$	$1{\cdot}80 \times 10^{-4}$
p-Chlorbenzoic acid	*p*-$Cl.C_6H_4.COOH$	$1{\cdot}05 \times 10^{-4}$
Benzoic acid	$C_6H_5.COOH$	$6{\cdot}30 \times 10^{-5}$
p-Hydroxybenzoic acid	*p*-$OH.C_6H_4.COOH$	$3{\cdot}00 \times 10^{-5}$
Sorbic acid	$CH_3CH{:}CHCH{:}CHCOOH$	$1{\cdot}73 \times 10^{-5}$
Propionic acid	$C_2H_5.COOH$	$1{\cdot}40 \times 10^{-5}$
Dehydroacetic acid	$OCOCH(COCH_3)$— $COCH{:}C(CH_3)$	$5{\cdot}30 \times 10^{-6}$

change in the minimum bactericidal concentration at the three pH levels. From this they concluded that the anion must be as active as the undissociated acid, in contrast to the true organic acids which are more active in the acid pH range.

These findings are at variance with those of Von Schelhorn (1953) who found that 100 times as much dehydroacetic acid was required to inhibit *Aspergillus niger* at pH 7 as at pH 3·5, and that 200 times as much was needed for *Willia anomala* at the same pH levels.

Von Schelhorn (1952) in extensive studies on preservatives for foods, examined the dissociation constants of various acids and found dehydroacetic acid to have the lowest. This indicated that it would retain its activity at higher pH values than most other organic acids and, therefore, would command a wider usage. Table VII gives dissociation constants for some of the acids used as preservatives.

The esters of *p*-hydroxybenzoic acid do not appear to dissociate even in the neutral pH range and Bandelin (1958) in examining the effect of twelve different compounds at pH 3, 5, 7 and 9, found their activity only slightly influenced by pH. Vanillin and ethyl vanillin were unaffected by changes in pH, and thought by Bandelin to be worthy of further study as preservatives.

Similar investigations of the relationship between pH and preservative effectiveness have been made by Entrekin (1961) who studied a wide range of preservatives and supported many of Bandelin's findings.

Many other preservatives, such as the bis-phenols and salicylanilides, are weak acids which dissociate to varying extents depending on the pH of the environment. Simon (1952) has shown that the biological activities of weak acids are influenced in a regular manner by changes in pH. Figure 2, which is based on a study of ninety pH experiments involving a wide range of acids (pK_a [1] 4–6), and many test organisms and responses, illustrates the the importance of pH, and represents a relationship between pH and activity which is quite general for this type of preservative. Since the dissociation constant of different preservatives varies, their behaviour in different pH conditions will vary, and some will be inactivated by small increases in pH while others may not be influenced at all. When the pH of the environment is below the pK_a, changes of pH are of little consequence, but as the pH is increased above the pK_a the rising curve shows that higher concentrations are required to produce a standard response.

Albert (1957) reported that salicylic acid is more active at pH 5·0 than at any higher pH, and that at pH 5·0 a larger proportion is non-ionized than at any higher pH. The neutral molecule of salicylic acid is the only toxic form. The case of benzoic acid is rather different since a constant concentration of undissociated molecules does not produce the same response at different pH levels and this indicates that the anions are also slightly toxic. Other phenols such as phenylacetic acid, chlorinated phenols, and nitro- and amino-nitrophenols exhibit similar effects, where the neutral molecules are more toxic although the anions are active to some extent.

Many cases are known where ionization is essential to toxic action, and a classic example of a positive correlation between ionization and biological activity is found in the acridine antibacterials. Albert (1945) has found that the most important factor in the action of the acridines at any pH is the amount of drug present as cation. This depends on both the pH of the medium and the dissociation constant of the drug, and not

[1] pK_a = the negative logarithm of the dissociation constant K_a. Numerically the pK_a is equivalent to the pH at which 50 per cent of the acid is dissociated.

the total amount of drug, i.e. cations and neutral molecules. This relationship between cationic ionization and antibacterial activity holds not only for the acridine series, but also for the three series of benzacridines, the three series of benzquinolines and the phenanthridines.

In order to utilize a preservative economically and effectively it is necessary to know whether there is a correlation between pH and activity, and if this aspect of formulation had been studied more closely in the past a great deal of money could have been saved by the many manufacturers who used preservatives which could not possibly be effective under the pH conditions in their products.

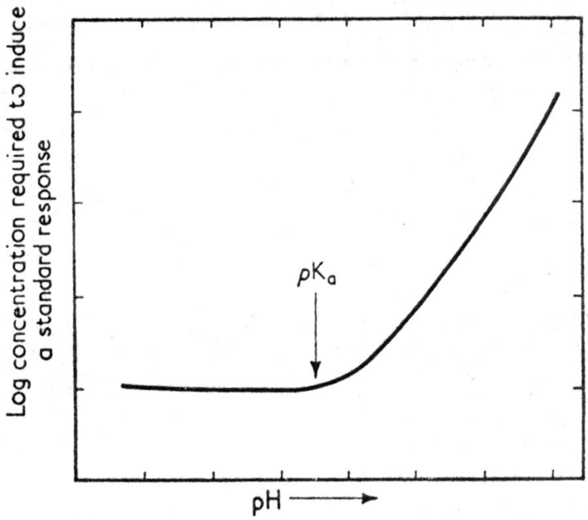

FIG. 2. Effect of pH on the concentration of a weak acid that is required to give a standard response from a test organism.

B. CONCENTRATION OF PRESERVATIVE

To be effective a sufficient concentration of preservative must be in solution in the aqueous phase. The amount required in this phase will depend mainly on the kind of micro-organisms likely to contaminate the emulsion, their number, and the rate at which it is necessary to kill them. In the case of parenteral preparations or those used for ophthalmic purposes, sterility is essential and hence the rate of kill must be high. In emulsions used externally, however, a slow rate is all that is required. Provided those organisms which survive are non-pathogenic, and as long as their survival does not ultimately lead to vigorous growth involving metabolism of their environment, their presence can be tolerated.

The classic work of Ferguson (1939) related the activity of structurally non-specific antimicrobial agents to the thermodynamic activity of the toxic substance, and described their chemical potentials as indices of toxicity. The rate of kill is a kinetic process and Allawala and Riegelman (1953) have shown that this is dependent on the "availability" of the preservative. The availability is defined in accordance with the mechanism of action of the particular preservative, and may be the permeability across the cell wall, if this is the mechanism, the flux, if diffusion rate is important, or degree of adsorption if the preservative acts by coating the surface of the organism. Although the rate is determined by these factors the thermodynamic activity of the toxic agent will determine the magnitude of the effect.

Price (1950) in an elegant piece of work has examined "bacteriostatic" and "bactericidal" effects and his experimental observations have indicated that when these terms are applied to agents acting on a group of bacteria, time is the only factor which distinguishes them. He maintains that sensitivity to inhibition and sensitivity to death cannot be separated; they seem to run parallel, but inhibition precedes death. "Every antibacterial agent is both inhibitory and lethal, often for the individual cell and certainly for a bacterial group as a whole. It is a matter of time."

This concept is interesting in the context of preservation in that it conflicts with the views of many who distinguish inhibitory from lethal effects in terms of the concentration of a particular agent, claiming a low concentration to be inhibitory and a high one lethal, and others who believe certain agents to be either, but not both. Price believes that even weak antimicrobial agents which cause prolonged inhibition will eventually kill individual cells, but does not deny that certain resistant cells will recover from their injury and give rise to descendants which are much less affected by the inhibitor.

Figure 3 illustrates schematically the effect of an acid on a group of bacterial cells which vary in their resistance to the particular acid. The difference in sensitivity of the cells influences the time at which they are killed. If a neutralizing factor is introduced into the environment during inhibition, but before the cells die, the more resistant organisms will recover. The stages of inhibition illustrated in Fig. 3 show that, in testing for the effect of an inhibitor, different results will be obtained in samples taken at different intervals of time, and that the number of surviving organisms in any culture will depend on the sensitivity of the cells as well as upon the duration of exposure to the test substance.

In emulsions where sterility is not an essential requirement, the concentration of preservative should be such that the organisms present initially gradually decrease in number until none survive. If viable organisms are found in products after several months, it is probable that resistant cells have given rise to descendants which in time could bring about changes in the emulsion.

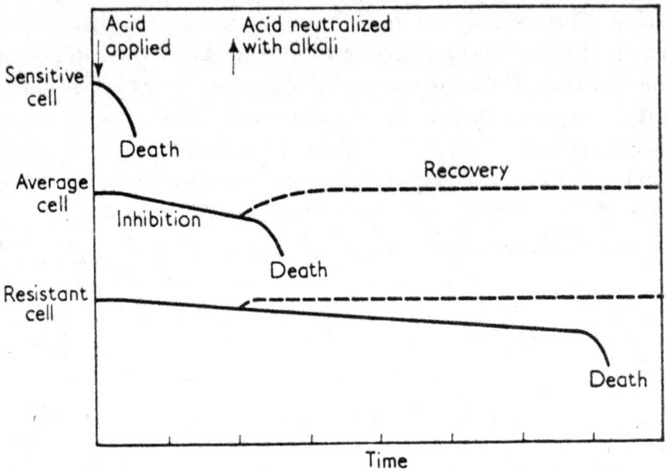

FIG. 3. Schematic representation of effects of acid on bacterial cells which vary in sensitivity (from Price).

C. DISTRIBUTION OR PARTITION OF PRESERVATIVE BETWEEN PHASES

The dissolved substances in the aqueous phase of an emulsion may take a considerable time to come to equilibrium with the other phases and during this time some of the preservative may migrate from the water. Conversely agents which reduce its efficiency may enter the aqueous phase and influence its thermodynamic activity even though the original concentration remains constant.

Knowing that a minimum concentration of preservative is necessary in the aqueous phase, the question of transfer of agents which are preferentially soluble in other materials must be considered. Some preservatives, as pointed out by Atkins (1950) are much more soluble in oil than in water, and when these are used, additional preservative must be added to maintain the required concentration in the aqueous phase.

The distribution or partition coefficient K between the phases is usually expressed as follows:

$$\mathrm{K} = \frac{C_{\mathrm{oil}}}{C_{\mathrm{water}}} \qquad C_{\mathrm{oil}} = (\mathrm{K})\,C_{\mathrm{water}}$$

Knowing the concentration required in the aqueous phase, and knowing the volume of each phase and the partition or distribution coefficient, the total preservative required in the system can be calculated.

C_{water} = required preservative in aqueous phase.

$C_{oil} = (K) C_{water}$

Total preservative $= (C_{water} V_{water} + C_{oil} V_{oil})$

Bean *et al.* (1962) examined the activity of phenol against *Escherichia coli* in oil–water dispersions and determined the distribution of phenol between oil and water in liquid paraffin and arachis oil dispersions. In liquid paraffin–water dispersions the partition coefficient is less than one and thus a fixed overall concentration of phenol is partitioned so that as the ratio of oil to water is increased, the concentration in both phases increases. In the case of arachis oil–water systems, for which the partition coefficient is greater than one, an increase in the oil–water ratio leads to a reduction of phenol concentration in each phase, although the overall concentration is maintained constant. Determination of the extinction times of *E. coli* in these systems showed that the bactericidal activity was governed by the concentration of phenol in the aqueous phase and the proportion of oil to water. The latter influences the oil–water interfacial area and this was shown to contribute to the total activity of the phenol. The formation of an interface was shown to be associated with increased bactericidal activity and thus the interface appeared to be the site of increased phenol action.

Kamakaka (1956) has shown that bacteria are adsorbed at oil–water interfaces and Bean *et al.* found that in their systems bacteria were accommodated at the interface.

These investigations were carried out in systems without emulsifiers, the addition of which would undoubtedly have altered the conditions, but they nevertheless highlight the importance of the relationship between preservative activity, oil–water ratio and the distribution of the preservative between phases.

Hibbott and Monks (1961) studied the solubility of methyl *p*-hydroxybenzoate in a number of oils, waxes and non-ionic surfactants and correlated their findings with the partition coefficient of the preservative between oil and aqueous phases. Table VIII is taken from their paper.

This work shows that in the case of mineral oil, very little methyl *p*-hydroxybenzoate is lost to the oil phase whereas with the range of esters, the partition coefficients are very much higher. With approximately 5 per cent of isopropyl myristate to 95 per cent of water only half the preservative will remain in the aqueous phase. Methyl *p*-hydroxybenzoate is very soluble in propylene glycol and addition of this to the aqueous phase was found to reduce the partition coefficient and thus

TABLE VIII

Partition Coefficient and Solubility of Methyl *p*-hydroxybenzoate in Oils, Waxes and non-ionic Surface-active Agents (from Hibbott and Monks)

Oil	*Solubility of methyl* p-*hydroxybenzoate g/100 g solvent*	*Partition coefficient oil/water*
Mineral oil	0·2	0·3
Tallow	0·6	1·3
Stearic acid	0·9	2·4
Almond oil	1·4	6
Lanolin	1·8	7
Oleic acid	2·9	7
Oleyl oleate	3·9	10
Isopropyl stearate	6·3	18
Butyl stearate	6·5	12
Isopropyl oleate	6·7	16
Butyl oleate	7·0	16
Cyclo hexanol stearate	8·0	13
Isopropyl myristate	8·2	18
Cetyl acetate	9·3	18
Ricinoleic acid	11·9	24
Acetoglyceride	12·5	27
Cetyl alcohol	13·6	23
Oleyl alcohol	15·8	31
Nonex 59 (a polyethylene glycol ester)	18·0	30
Castor oil	18·8	47
Nonex 43 (a polyethylene glycol ester)	23·0	45
Diethyl phthalate	25·8	56
Diethyl sebacate	31·2	86
Ethyl hexane diol	39·0	159
Diethyl adipate	41·0	204
Nonex 32 (a polyethylene glycol ester)	13·1	
Arlacel 83 (a sorbitan ester)	14·9	
Lanbritol (a polyethylene glycol ether)	20·4	
Tween 80 (a polyethylene glycol ester)	44·7	
Lubrol W (a polyethylene glycol ether)	54·3	

make more preservative available in the water. Hibbott and Monks found propylene glycol more effective in this respect than glycerol.

Barr and Tice (1957a, b) in studying the effect of glycerin–sorbitol and propylene glycol–sorbitol combinations on the growth of microorganisms found that glycerin and sorbitol supplement each other in their inhibition of both bacteria and moulds. This effect they attribute purely to the osmotic effect of high concentrations of the humectants. Propylene glycol, however, appeared to have a specific inhibitory effect in addition to its effect on the osmotic pressure of aqueous solutions, and it was concluded that, on these grounds propylene glycol would have a significant and useful preservative effect. de Navarre (1962) has found propylene glycol to be a reliable preservative at 16 per cent vol./vol. in many cosmetic products and states its anti-microbial properties to be three or four times the equivalent amount of glycerin. Poprzan and de Navarre (1959) have also found that propylene glycol at 10 per cent prevented interaction between methyl *p*-hydroxybenzoate and Tween 80.

These findings, when viewed in the light of those of Hibbott and Monks, indicate that propylene glycol is a useful addition to the aqueous phase of emulsions because it has functions other than those of reducing the partition coefficient of some preservatives and making them more readily available to act on micro-organisms.

The solution of surfactants in the aqueous phase has a profound effect on the availability of the preservative, and Allawala and Riegelman (1953) pointed out that changes in the concentration of preservative are not an index of their activity when surfactants are present. They also noted that changes in the concentration of surfactant modify the thermodynamic activity, which is the real measure of activity, of an antimicrobial agent. These findings are supported by extensive work by Bean and Berry, Kostenbauder, Briggs, Cook, Guttman and Higuchi, Beckett and Robinson, de Navarre, and others, and will be discussed in detail in Section V, A.

D. VULNERABILITY OF ORGANISMS TO PRESERVATIVE

It is possible that in some circumstances, even though a normally active concentration of preservative is present in the aqueous phase of an emulsion, it will not be fully effective because the micro-organisms are protected from its action.

Judis (1962) has studied the mechanism of action of phenolic disinfectants by measuring the release of radioactivity from cells of *Escherichia coli* labelled with C^{14}. The cells were grown in media containing C^{14} glutamate, and leakage of cell contents was determined after exposure to a variety of phenolic disinfectants. Tween 80 was found to protect *E. coli* from the lethal effects of *p*-chloro-*m*-xylenol and to prevent in part the leakage of the cell contents as indicated by release of radioactivity.

In the earlier work of Beckett and Robinson (1958) a similar phenomenon was observed using different experimental techniques. The addition of extremely low concentrations of polyethylene glycol 1000 monocetyl ether (Cetomacrogol) was found to reduce the amount of hexylresorcinol taken up by *E. coli* at several different concentrations. The amount of Cetomacrogol present was too small to have interfered with the availability of hexylresorcinol to the bacteria, and it was therefore concluded that the non-ionic interfered with the interaction of the drug at the cytoplasmic membrane of the organism.

The author's own work, using cells of several different bacteria which were suspended in non-ionic solutions and then washed thoroughly in saline before exposure to a medium containing 0·1 per cent of mixed esters of *p*-hydroxybenzoate, is in agreement with these findings. Tween 80 and polyethylene glycol 400 laurate protected the cells of *E. coli*, *Pseudomonas fluorescens* and *Streptococcus bovis* from the inhibitory effects of the preservative.

IV. Mechanism of Action of Preservatives

No attempt will be made here to examine in detail the mechanism of action of the many substances which can be used as preservatives, since the exact mechanisms of few antimicrobial agents are fully understood, and a great deal of research on the subject is still in progress.

The mode of action of any antimicrobial substance is closely related to the specific resistance of a particular organism. When exposed to a potently toxic substance, many modifications to the delicately organized and highly reactive substance of the living cell will occur. Destruction of the organism will be brought about when the most essential function necessary to the growth of the cell is modified, and many toxic substances inhibit or modify several cellular activities simultaneously.

Cruickshank (1956) in reviewing the mechanisms involved in microbiocidal action, concluded that no single factor is responsible for the death of micro-organisms. Amongst the factors influenced by chemical substances he lists:

1. Modification of membrane permeability.
2. Action on enzymes and other proteins.
3. Oxidation and reduction of cellular constituents.
4. Hydrolysis.
5. Interference with essential metabolites.

In the case of acids, the effect of pH itself is a consideration; the relationship between the effects of dissociated and undissociated acid relative to pH is also of account, in addition to certain specific effects. Many of the actions of acids involve two or more of the above factors and it is only possible to make valid comparisons between the inhibitory powers of different acids when allowance has been made for their dissociation.

Different acids have different specific effects as shown by Von Schelhorn (1953). Benzoic acid is roughly equally effective against yeasts and the true fungi, while dehydroacetic acid is as effective as benzoic acid against yeasts, much more toxic to fungi and much less so to bacteria. Specific effects of this kind depend on the differences in molecular structure of the acids which influence the ease with which they penetrate the cell, the part of the cell they attack, or the chemical nature of the attack.

TABLE IX

Possible Modes of Action of some Acid Preservatives (from Wyss)

Benzoic derivatives	Membrane action and competition with co-enzymes
Boric acid	Inhibition of phosphate enzymes
Fatty acids:	
Long chain	Interference with cell membranes
Short chain	Competitive inhibition of enzymes
Salicylic acid	Membrane action: competition with cozymase and with amino acid metabolism
Sorbic acid	Suppression of fumarate oxidation in catalase positive organisms

Ingram *et al.* (1956) have reviewed the preservative action of acid preservatives and state that the hope of finding radically better preservatives lies in a clearer understanding of the specific effects attributable to different molecules.

The possible modes of action of some acid preservatives on the intracellular mechanisms of micro-organisms are given by Wyss (1948) in Table IX.

The esters of *p*-hydroxybenzoic acid and of vanillic acid are thought to act in the same way as benzoic acid.

The mechanism of action of phenol has been extensively studied. Gale and Taylor (1947) found that a 1 per cent solution of phenol caused leakage of glutamic acid from cells of *Streptococcus faecalis* and Maurice (1952) observed that phenol promoted the penetration of basic dyes through the cell walls of *E. coli*. It can be concluded that phenol renders the cell wall permeable to essential cell constituents. This has been confirmed more recently by Judis (1962) who used a radio-tracer method to investigate phenol, *p*-chloro-*m*-xylenol, *p*-chloro-*m*-cresol, *p*-chloro-*o*-cresol, 2,4-dichlorophenol, 2,4,6-trichlorophenol, and 2,4-dichloro-*m*-xylenol. Leakage of cell contents was caused by all the above and similar effects were caused by ethanol, mercuric chloride, acriflavine, and merthiolate.

Beckett *et al.* (1959) in an extensive study of the mechanism of action of hexylresorcinol on *Escherichia coli* have demonstrated the release of cellular constituents and have also shown that sodium chloride has a potentiating effect on the activity of hexylresorcinol.

These findings for phenols indicate that their effect is due to physical damage of the cell membrane, but in view of the fact that different organisms differ markedly in their susceptibility to phenol there are obviously other factors to be considered.

The mechanism of action of 8-hydroxyquinoline has received much attention because it furnishes an outstanding example of biological specificity. Of seven possible isomers, 8-hydroxyquinoline is the only one with antimicrobial properties, and its action is attributable to its ability to form weakly dissociated chelate complexes with trace metals essential to the functioning of vital cellular enzymes. Albert and co-workers (1953) have studied this mechanism extensively and more recent contributions to a fuller understanding of the specificity of this compound have been made by Block (1956) and Beckett *et al.* (1958a).

Hotchkiss (1946) has shown that certain surface-active antimicrobial agents such as quaternary ammonium compounds, tyrocidin, tricresol, and hexylresorcinol disrupt the permeability barrier of the cell, and confirmed that when the concentration of surface-active agents were adequate to kill bacteria, leakage of compounds containing nitrogen and phosphorus occurred.

Alcohol and strong mineral acids coagulate albumins and globulins, phenolic compounds denature proteins, heavy metals form proteinates and these combinations or reactions contribute to the destruction of enzymes vital to metabolism. Substances which are capable of oxidizing —SH groups to —S—S groups, such as the halogens and peroxides, disrupt the function of many enzymes which contain sulph–hydryl groups, and the action of silver, mercury, copper and arsenic is associated with this mechanism. Formaldehyde is a strong protein denaturant and owes its effect to a reaction with the protein fraction of enzymes and also to its effect on —SH groups.

The quaternary ammonium compounds interfere with the respiration and glycolysis of bacteria and inhibit the oxidation of certain carbohydrates (Miller *et al.*, 1939). The mode of action of quaternaries has been reviewed by Lawrence (1950) but the wide differences in the specific effects on various organisms and the differences between the effects of quaternaries themselves have not yet been satisfactorily evaluated. It has been postulated by Hauser (1950) in studying the mechanism of penicillin, that substances bearing an electric charge opposite to the charge on bacteria will cling to the cell surface, and Albert (1942) attributed the action of cationic antiseptics to their basic ions which react with the acidic ions of micro-organisms. Organisms with an excess of acidic groups over basic radicals are affected to a greater extent, and this may account for the greater activity of quaternary ammonium compounds on Gram positive bacteria which contain a high ratio of acidic over basic groups, while the Gram negative bacteria, with a reversed ratio, are much less affected.

The mechanism of action of surface-active compounds, both anionic and cationic, has been reviewed by Newton (1960). Evidence for several different modes of action is presented, amongst which are:

disorganization of cell permeability barriers,
indirect disorganization through the dissolution of the cell wall,
direct disorganization of the protoplast membrane.

The inhibition of enzymes located in and involved in the maintenance of the membrane is also a possibility and it is therefore true to say that the mode of action of the ionic surface-active agents is extremely complex.

The non-ionic surface-active agents do not inhibit the growth or metabolism of micro-organisms to any significant extent and Glassman (1950) found that they do not precipitate proteins nor inactivate bacterial toxins on either side of the protein isoelectric point. In this respect they differ radically from the ionic surfactants.

V. Interaction Between Emulsion Ingredients and Preservatives

A. SURFACE-ACTIVE AGENTS

The structure of surfactants plays an important part in the mechanism by which they influence the effectiveness of antimicrobial agents. The molecules of surface-active agents have a hydrophilic and a hydrophobic part and in most cases the hydrophobic part is a hydrocarbon chain while the hydrophilic group may be cationic, anionic, ampholytic or non-ionic. At very low concentrations, the molecules of surfactants occur singly, but with increasing concentration there is a tendency for association between molecules and the formation of aggregates or micelles. The concentration of surfactant at which extensive formation of micelles begins is known as the critical micelle concentration, and it depends on several factors, most prominent of which is the length of the hydrocarbon chain. The nature of the hydrophilic group also has an effect, as has the presence of electrolytes in the solution which neutralize the repulsive charges between surfactant ions.

1. *Soaps and Anionic Surface-Active Agents*

Soaps are used to produce oil-in-water and water-in-oil emulsions. The monovalent water-soluble soaps such as the stearate, oleate and higher fatty acid soaps of sodium, potassium, ammonium and substituted amine bases form oil-in-water systems. These are frequently stabilized with oil-soluble polar materials such as the fatty alcohols and partial higher fatty acid esters. The polyvalent soaps are used in water-in-oil systems, often stabilized with fatty polar materials such as cholesterol.

Apart from soaps, the alkyl sulphates and the synthetic phosphoric acid esters are also used as emulsifiers.

It has been known for many years that soaps modify the activity of certain antimicrobial agents, but the adverse modification of the action of those used as preservatives has not caused much concern in the past because emulsions made with soaps do not generally present very favourable conditions for growth of bacteria and fungi.

Because of the mildly inhibitory properties of most soap-stabilized emulsions, preservation has traditionally been effectively accomplished by use of the *p*-hydroxybenzoate esters although failures have been known to occur. These may have been due to a variety of causes, such as loss of the preservative from the aqueous to the oil phase because of unsuitable solubility characteristics, the use of insufficient concentrations relative to optimal dissociation, or physical incompatibility between the preservative and the soap emulsifier. Evidence of the latter type of incompatibility has been given by many, including Hampil (1928), who found that sodium oleate reduced the activity of phenol, *m*-cresol, and hexylresorcinol, and Bean and Berry (1951, 1953) who studied the effect of potassium laurate on chloroxylenol and benzyl-chlorophenol. Alexander and Trim (1946) studied the anthelminthic activity of hexylresorcinol-soap mixtures and Agar and Alexander (1949) measured the extinction times of *Escherichia coli* when exposed to phenol and chlorinated phenols dissolved in aqueous solutions of anionic and cationic surface-active agents.

Enhanced germicidal activity is usually found as the soap concentration is increased up to the critical micelle concentration (c.m.c.) followed by a decrease in activity as the soap concentration is increased above the c.m.c. The increased activity of soap–phenol mixtures below the c.m.c. is thought to be due to a decrease in interfacial tension which will favour an increase in the adsorption of soap and phenol, causing the concentration of phenol at the bacterial or fungal surface to be much higher than in bulk solutions. Above the c.m.c. the phenol is solubilized in the soap micelles, and reduction in antimicrobial activity is due to phenol depletion of the aqueous phase. At very high soap concentrations, nearly all the phenol is dissolved in the micellar phase and the activity of the mixture is then due to the activity of the soap itself, and to those portions of the phenol molecule projecting into the aqueous phase. The work of Bean and Berry (1951, 1953) shows that the activity of systems containing phenols solubilized by soaps is independent of the total concentration of phenol in the system, but is related to the concentration in solution in the water.

Allawala and Riegelman (1953) have made a detailed study of the release of antimicrobial agents from solutions of surface-active agents and have reviewed and explained some of the controversial findings in the earlier literature. They relate the effects of surfactants to well known thermodynamic quantities and explain many of the observed activation–inactivation phenomena by calculated solubilization data.

The weight of evidence in this field supports the theory that many preservatives have far higher activity in aqueous solutions of surface-active agents at concentrations of surfactant below and up to the c.m.c., and that activity decreases dramatically beyond this point. However, despite the evidence and the theory which supports it, unusual and unexplained observations have been reported. Shafiroff (1961) has reviewed the subject of germicide-surfactant synergism and describes the potentiating effects of a variety of surface-active agents on antimicrobial agents. Some of his statements are at variance with the generally accepted views on the subject indicating that forces other than solubilization phenomena may play a part. Experimental techniques obviously influence the conclusions to be drawn from work of this nature, and in using death times of bacteria as a criterion of synergism or inactivation it is important to consider the volume, growth phase and susceptibility of the organism used. These aspects are too frequently omitted from publications on this subject and may well be responsible for some of the divergent observations reported.

The preservation of emulsions stabilized with either soap or anionic surface-active agents has not, in general, presented as many problems as might be expected from examination of the theoretical considerations. As mentioned previously, the environment in these emulsions is usually mildly hostile to microbial growth, and this might conceivably permit concentrations of preservative, which theoretically would be ineffective, to have a certain effectiveness. Many soaps have a non-specific effect on bacterial growth, particularly at the concentrations used to stabilize emulsions, and the pH of the aqueous phase is often sufficiently alkaline to discourage some fungal growth. The alkali metal soaps, when used as emulsifiers, often present conditions unfavourable to fungal growth, while the amine soaps, such as triethanolamine oleate are less alkaline, and emulsions made with these often present spoilage problems.

2. *Cationic Surface-active Agents*

Quaternary nitrogen compounds can be used as emulsifiers although their value for this purpose is limited and the presence of a non-ionic as an auxiliary emulsifier is often necessary.

Certain cationic surface-active agents have strong antimicrobial properties of their own and when they are used in combination with other antiseptics or preservatives it is difficult to separate the action of the two. Alexander and Trim (1946) reported that the addition of small amounts of cetyl trimethyl ammonium bromide (CTAB) caused enhancement of the uptake of hexylresorcinol by the Ascaris worm. This enhancement continued until the c.m.c. of CTAB was reached, at which point there was a rapid decrease in the rate of uptake of hexylresorcinol by the organism. Analysis of these results, together with surface-tension data, indicates that the presence of small amounts of the surfactant favoured an increase in adsorption of hexylresorcinol. Alexander and Trim also pointed out that small amounts of CTAB appeared to change the permeability of Ascaris.

This type of enhancement of activity of antimicrobial agents by cationic surfactants below the c.m.c. followed by a depressant action above that point, is probably associated with similar solubilization phenomena to those described for soaps and anionic detergents.

Cationic surface-active agents are far less frequently used as emulsifiers than are soaps, anionic or non-ionic surfactants since they are less versatile and frequently irritant to the skin and mucous membranes at the concentrations at which they would be useful as emulsion stabilizers. However, in those instances where they are used they are unlikely to present problems of preservation, provided there is a sufficient concentration of free cationic in the aqueous phase to exert an inhibitory effect. The antimicrobial effectiveness of cationics varies according to the length of the hydrophobic chain, the most effective compounds having an alkyl chain length of about C_{12} to C_{14}. They are more effective against Gram positive bacteria than against the Gram negatives and fungi, and when cationics are used as emulsifiers it is sometimes necessary to add low concentrations of two or even three different compatible cationics to ensure adequate preservation.

3. *Non-ionic Surface-active Agents*

During the past decade non-ionic surfactants have become increasingly useful as emulsifiers and are gradually replacing the more conventional soaps and anionic materials. Their rise in popularity has not, however, been without tribulation owing to the fact that despite their many advantages in formulation, they have one serious disad[illegible] in the form of a suppressant action on the efficacy of preserv[illegible] added antiseptics.

It will not be possible, or indeed desirable, to mention [illegible] investigations which support this statement as the fi[illegible] covered by many workers reporting qualitative and qua[illegible] about numerous structurally different non-ionic surfact[illegible]y wide variety of antimicrobial agents.

a. *Effects of non-ionics on esters of* p-*hydroxyben*[illegible]aps because of their very widespread use as pharmace[illegible]metic preservatives, most attention has been paid to th[illegible]-ionics on the esters of *p*-hydroxybenzoic acid. There c[illegible]ubt that these materials resemble the "ideal preservati[illegible]sely than many others, and before the discovery that n[illegible] an adverse effect on their activity, they enjoyed almost [illegible] in cosmetic emulsions. It will be seen from later sections of this [illegible]r that despite a reduction in their efficacy in the presence of non-ionics, the esters of *p*-hydroxybenzoic acid are by no means rendered useless as preservatives as a result, and they will no doubt continue to be used successfully in many preparations. For this reason it is worth mentioning at least some of the work which describes them. Sabalitschka and Boehm (1929) described their use in foods, medicaments and cosmetics, and from that time to the present day there has been a wealth of further evidence of their usefulness. The further works of Boehm (1933) and Boehm and Jones (1957) describe the advantages of using combinations of two or more esters to protect certain types of system and Aalto *et al.* (1953) have reviewed their uses and given details of effective concentrations. The methyl, ethyl, propyl and butyl esters are the derivatives most commonly used and it has been shown by Huppert (1957) that antimicrobial activity rises with increased chain length. Neidig and Burrell (1944) have reviewed their usefulness in a wide variety of preparations and Schimmel and Husa (1956) and Littlejohn and Husa (1955) have shown the advantages of using mixtures over the individual components. Matthews *et al.* (1956), having studied the pharmacology of the esters of *p*-hydroxybenzoic acid, found a low order of acute toxicity and concluded that they could be used in foods and drugs with safety. In concentrations below 5 per cent none of the esters produce primary irritation on intact human skin. Further toxicity studies have been carried out by Jones *et al.* (1956) who showed that topical application of ointments containing 10 per cent methyl and 10 per cent propyl *p*-hydroxybenzoate produced no primary irritation on rabbit skin during 48 h contact. Hjorth and Trolle-Lassen (1962) have reported the sensitization of patients with eczema who had been treated with ointments containing above 10 per cent of *p*-hydroxybenzoate esters. When used at the levels normally employed as preservatives, however, sensitization appears to be rare.

A method of separating and determining mixtures of *p*-hydroxybenzoate esters in pharmaceutical preparations was given by Higuchi *et al.* (1952), and recently Prickett *et al.* (1961) have shown that the addition of propylene glycol to simple pharmaceutical syrups potentiates the effect of the methyl and propyl esters of *p*-hydroxybenzoate thus enabling their effective concentration to be reduced.

None of the above works, however, relates to the efficacy of these esters in the presence of non-ionic surface-active agents, and during the last 15 years a considerable literature has described their diminished effectiveness when used to preserve preparations containing non-ionic emulsifiers.

Bolle and Mirimanoff (1950) were not the first to note the reduced effect of methyl *p*-hydroxybenzoate in the presence of several structurally different non-ionic surfactants, but because they pointed out the importance of their findings to the pharmaceutical and cosmetic industries, their paper stimulated widespread interest. They found that the surface-active sorbitan esters and polyoxyethylene sorbitan esters reduced the effect of methyl *p*-hydroxybenzoate, oxyquinoline sulphate and dioxydichlorodiphenyl-methane, whereas the non-surface active Carbowax 1500, a polyethylene glycol polymer, had no inactivating effect. de Navarre followed up this work and in 1957 remarked that practically all non-ionics based on ethylene and propylene oxide condensed, with each other, or with fatty esters, alcohols or acids, inactivate all the preservatives currently considered suitable for drug and cosmetic preparations.

Wedderburn (1958) assessed the effect of thirty-six different non-ionics on twenty-six antimicrobial agents and found that although all the surface-active non-ionics exerted some depressant effect, those which were not surface-active had negligible effects. The extent of the adverse effect was different for different combinations of non-ionic surfactant and preservative, and appeared to be related not only to the hydrophile–lipophile balance (see page 234) of the surfactant but also to the chemical structure of the preservative.

A mixture of methyl, ethyl, propyl and butyl esters of *p*-hydroxybenzoic acid was amongst the preservatives shown to be affected.

More recently Blaug and Ahsan (1961b) examined the interaction of the methyl, ethyl, propyl and butyl esters with several non-ionic macromolecules and reported that the higher molecular weight esters of *p*-hydroxybenzoic acid were influenced to a greater extent than those of lower molecular weight. In determining the binding tendencies of the esters with Tween 80 (polyoxyethylene sorbitan mono-oleate), Myrj 52 (polyoxyethylene monostearate), polyethylene glycol 4000 and 6000, and Pluronic F-68 (polyethylene polypropylene glycol), they confirmed that the hydrophile–lipophile balance strongly influenced the effect: those compounds with greater lipophilic tendencies reduced the effectiveness more than the more hydrophilic macromolecules.

b. *Effects of non-ionics on other phenolic antiseptics.* Most of the papers describing the effects of non-ionics on the *p*-hydroxybenzoate derivatives have also mentioned adverse effects on other antimicrobial agents and naturally the phenolics have been thoroughly examined in this connection.

In seeking a bacteriological growth medium which would inhibit the action of hexachlorophene carried over from solutions in which the antiseptic had been in contact with test organisms, Lawrence and Erlandson (1953) discovered that Tween 80 was more satisfactory as a "quenching agent" than serum, globulin or serum albumin. Further work by Erlandson and Lawrence (1953) showed that media containing Tween 80 inhibited the action of many other substituted phenolic antiseptics. Einola (1955) confirmed these findings and endorsed similar observations made by Bouchardy and Mirimanoff (1951) and Engler and Mirimanoff (1951).

Earlier, Gregg and Zopf (1951) had noted an increase in the effectiveness of hexachlorophene in the presence of Tween 80, but in view of the weight of evidence to the contrary, their findings must be attributed to the experimental conditions which involved the use of an agar diffusion technique. It is well known that the presence of a surface-active agent in a test solution can increase the diffusion rate of an antiseptic, but the formation of a larger zone of growth inhibition does not necessarily indicate improved antiseptic action within the test system.

c. *Effects of non-ionics on quaternary ammonium compounds.* In testing the potency of quaternary ammonium compounds and other antiseptics it is often desirable to stop or "quench" their action at a particular point in an experiment. Serum and the other conventional inactivators often inadequately quench the quaternary ammonium compounds, and Baker *et al.* (1941) and Hotchkiss (1946) reported that non-ionics could serve this purpose. By 1950 Tween 80 had become established as a useful addition to bacteriological media, but it was not realized until 2 or 3 years later that creams and ointments containing non-ionics and quaternary ammonium compounds as preservatives, or active antiseptics, often possessed far less antimicrobial action than expected. Non-ionics are often listed by the manufacturers of quaternaries as "compatible" because, when solutions of the two are mixed, a precipitate does not form as occurs with anionic–cationic mixtures. This lack of visible complex formation does not, however, necessarily indicate unimparied antimicrobial activity. Quaternaries of differing structure possess widely different biological activity, and are more selective in their action than the phenolics. For this reason the test organism, and the test method used to assess their effect in the presence of non-ionics, have a marked effect on the result.

All surface-active agents influence the solubility and hence the availability of antimicrobial agents, and in examining the effects of non-ionics on quaternary ammonium compounds it should be remembered that both are highly surface-active. Even more important is the fact that the quaternaries are ionized and strongly polar, while the non-ionics are non-polar.

Gershenfeld and Stedman (1949) reported on the activity of several cationics including cetylpyridinium chloride and cetyltrimethylammonium bromide in the presence of varying concentrations of a non-ionic of the polyethylene glycol ether type. They used *Escherichia coli*, *Pseudomonas aeruginosa* and *Staphylococcus aureus* as test organisms and found that a lower molar ratio of non-ionic to cationic was inhibitory to *Ps. aeruginosa* than was effective against *E. coli*. In testing against *S. aureus* they found that the non-ionic had virtually no influence on the bacteriostatic effect of the quaternaries at high concentrations of non-ionic, but as this was reduced the cationics became increasingly more effective. These findings highlight the differing response of the three test organisms to these particular quaternaries (the two Gram negative bacteria being in general more resistant to cationics than the Gram positive staphylococcus) and also reveal the importance of the molar ratio of non-ionic to cationic.

Moore and Hardwick (1956) confirmed in tests on staphylococci that at very low molar ratios of non-ionic surfactant to quaternary ammonium compound, the activity of the latter was enhanced. At a ratio of one non-ionic to four quaternary they found increased effectiveness.

Davies (1949) showed that polyethylene glycol cetostearyl ether neutralized the effect of cetyltrimethylammonium bromide and Ritter

(1956) found that Tween 80 reduced the effect of cetylpyridinium chloride.

All these studies show that non-ionic surface-active agents behave in a similar way to soaps and anionic surfactants in as much as they increase the activity of certain antimicrobial agents at very low concentrations and considerably diminish their effect at higher concentrations.

d. *Effects of non-ionics on acids and other preservatives*. Many other classes of preservatives have been found to be similarly affected by non-ionic surface-active agents, and Barr and Tice (1957e) carried out an extensive screening programme on solutions of forty-eight preservatives in the presence of 5 per cent polyoxyethylene 20 sorbitan monostearate. All the preservatives were tested at concentrations known to be inhibitory to the three test organisms *Pseudomonas aeruginosa*, *Monilia albicans* and *Aspergillus niger*. Prior to this comprehensive study they had observed, like several other workers, that other non-ionic surfactants had effects similar to those of polyoxyethylene 20 sorbitan monostearate.

In addition to confirming a depressant effect on the various esters of *p*-hydroxybenzoic acid, several substituted phenols, and quaternary ammonium compounds, they noted similar effects on sorbic acid, benzoic acid and organic mercurials.

Blaug and Ahsan (1961a) have also reported an interaction between sorbic acid and non-ionic surfactants and Deeb and Boenigh (1958) noted that chlorbutanol was inactivated by Tween 20 at a ratio of 1:4. Okabayashi (1953) investigated the effect on the activity of several preservatives, antibiotics and vitamins. All exhibited varying degrees of inactivation in the presence of non-ionic surfactants, and in his study of the effects on dehydroacetic acid, Okabayashi found that the usual correlation between antiseptic action and dissociation of dehydroacetic acid was almost non-existent in the presence of a non-ionic detergent.

The organic mercury compounds, phenyl mercury borate, acetate and nitrate are extremely effective preservatives, and very low concentrations inhibit most micro-organisms. Their activity is, however, markedly reduced in the presence of non-ionic surfactants as shown by Barr and Tice (1957e) and Wedderburn (1958).

The inactivating effects of non-ionic surface-active agents are of greater significance than those of soaps, anionic and cationic agents, because not only is the order of their inactivation much higher, but, unlike the other surfactants, non-ionics have no growth-inhibiting properties, making the necessity for adequate preservation of systems containing them much greater. Non-ionics have no denaturing effect on bacterial proteins, many can be utilized by bacteria and fungi as sources of energy, and because of this the absence of an effective preservative in non-ionic emulsified creams often becomes unpleasantly apparent in a remarkably short time.

There is no universal solution to the problem, and it is of fundamental importance to understand the mechanisms of interference, so that reasonable predictions of preservative efficiency can be made in the early stages of product formulation.

B. MECHANISM OF INACTIVATION OF PRESERVATIVES BY NON-IONIC SURFACE-ACTIVE AGENTS

A very wide range of non-ionic compounds is used in modern emulsions. Of particular value as emulsifiers are the partial fatty acid esters of the polyhydric alcohols ranging from propylene glycol to the anhydrides of sorbitol. Polyoxyethylene derivatives of these partial esters, and polyoxyethylene fatty acid or fatty ether condensates are also used. The fatty portion of these compounds is usually derived from naturally occurring fats and waxes.

Griffin (1954) has provided a system of classifying non-ionic surfactants related to their behaviour and their solubility in water. Numerical values, called the Hydrophile Lipophile Balance (HLB), denote the relative affinity for oil and water. Oil soluble materials have low values while water soluble compounds have high numbers. Commonly used emulsifiers nave HLB values ranging from 1 to 40. Table X gives HLB values of some of the non-ionic and anionic surfactants mentioned in this review.

The more oil soluble compounds, having HLB values of about 3 to 6, are used in water-in-oil emulsions and those with values near the range 7 to 20 are used in oil-in-water systems.

Until recently, the chemical structure of non-ionics was not well defined, because in the case of the commercially available products it was difficult to classify similar compounds having only slightly different chain lengths. Fundamental work on the structure and physical properties of non-ionic surfactants is now appearing more frequently in the literature, and the availability of more pure compounds of known structure should help those trying to elucidate the mechanism of interaction with preservatives and other biologically active substances. Gingras (1957) and Chakovskoy *et al.* (1956) have described the preparation of some pure compounds of the alkyl polyoxyethylene glycol ether type, and Schick *et al.* (1962) have studied the micellar structure of ethylene oxide condensates of nonylphenol, *n*-dodecanol, and *n*-octadecanol. Schick and his co-workers have reported that the critical micelle concentration of non-ionic surface-active agents is much lower than that of ionic surfactants with comparable hydrophobic groups, and that consequently the aggregate molecular weights are much larger than those of ionic surfactants. The aggregation of the non-ionics they studied was dependent on the length of both the hydrophobic and hydrophilic groups and they showed that aggregation increased with increasing

TABLE X

HLB Values of some Non-ionic Surfactants (data from Griffin, 1954)

Name	*Chemical designation*	*HLB*
Arlacel 83	Sorbitan sesquioleate	3·7
Span 60	Sorbitan monostearate	4·7
Span 20	Sorbitan monolaurate	8·6
PEG 400 laurate	Polyoxyethylene monolaurate	13·1
Tween 60	Polyoxyethylene sorbitan monostearate	14·9
Tween 80	Polyoxyethylene sorbitan mono-oleate	15·0
Tween 40	Polyoxyethylene sorbitan monopalmitate	15·6
Tween 20	Polyoxyethylene sorbitan monolaurate	16·7
Myrj 52	Polyoxyethylene monostearate	16·9

HLB Values of Some Anionic Surfactants

		HLB
Glycerol monostearate (self emulsifying)		5·5
Alkyl aryl sulphonate		11·7
Triethanolamine oleate		12·0
Sodium oleate		18·0
Potassium oleate		20·0
Pure sodium lauryl sulphate	Approx.	40·0

hydrophobic group lengths and decreased when the hydrophilic group was longer.

Since micellar solubilization of preservatives by non-ionic surfactants has been widely postulated as the predominant factor in the mechanism of inactivation, this work is of fundamental importance because it provides a sound foundation for some of the previous hypotheses.

Non-ionic surfactants are soluble in water and there has been considerable speculation about their interaction with water and the influence of a preservative upon this interaction. Beckett and Robinson (1958) in an excellent review of the subject, discussed the possibility of the formation of insoluble complexes between preservative and non-ionic surfactant molecules, and also the likelihood of solubilization within non-ionic micelles.

The formation of water-insoluble complexes between certain non-ionics and pharmaceutical compounds has been described by Higuchi and co-workers in several papers. Higuchi and Lach (1954) studied the complexing behaviour of high molecular weight polyethylene glycols with a number of biologically active materials. By means of solubility measurements they found that pentobarbital formed stable and stoichiometric molecular compounds with polyethylene glycols. Phase analysis indicated that one pentobarbital molecule is bound by two ethylene oxide units of the polyether chain, and it was also shown that phenolic compounds are bound by the polyethylene glycols in the same way. Similar studies on various preservative acids showed that these are only weakly bound.

Guttman and Higuchi (1955) showed that complexes could be formed between iodine and polyethylene glycols, and in 1956 the same authors found that the interaction of various phenols with polyethylene glycols resulted in the formation of water-insoluble oily liquids even at very low dilutions of the non-ionic. Mulley and Metcalf (1956) also showed that water-insoluble complexes occurred using various monohydric phenols at similar ratios of phenol to non-ionic, and they produced evidence for the formation of hydrogen bonds between phenolic hydroxyl groups and the ether chains of non-ionic surfactants. Their experimental evidence suggested that a hydrogen-bonded complex of the phenol, non-ionic surfactant and water is precipitated at the limit of solubility, due to a reduction in the hydrophilic character of the non-ionic micelles.

Hall and de Navarre (1957) used chromatographic and chemical titration techniques to study the formation of complexes between methyl *p*-hydroxybenzoate, sorbic and benzoic acids, and a non-ionic made by adding twenty moles of ethylene oxide to stearyl alcohol. They found that pH and the composition of the solvent system were important factors, and that between pH 4·0 and 6·0 complexes were formed between the non-ionic surfactant and the three different preservatives.

The formation of such complexes in emulsions containing non-ionic emulsifiers often leads to instability of the emulsion, quite apart from the fact that the preservative is rendered inactive.

Marcus *et al.* (1956) demonstrated that an interaction between certain phenolic preservatives and non-ionics of the polyethylene polypropylene glycol type resulted in physical changes in emulsions, and similar observations have been reported by Goldstein (1952) and Meyers *et al.* (1950).

Hadgraft (1954) made a systematic examination of the pharmaceutical uses and limitations of a series of polyethylene glycol ethers of ceto-stearyl alcohol, and determined the physical compatibility of one of these non-ionics with a range of dermatological medicaments in an ointment base. Using Cetomacrogol 1000 (polyethylene glycol monocetyl ether) he found that all preparations containing phenolic compounds such as salicyclic acid, resorcinol and phenol itself, showed separation on storage at room temperature, and based on experiments with resorcinol and Cetomacrogol 1000, he postulated the formation of addition compounds.

Further evidence for the formation of complexes between non-ionic surfactants and phenol can be deduced from the findings of Karabinos *et al.* (1955) who reported that phenol has a detrimental effect on the detergent properties of non-ionic surfactants.

From the evidence of complex formation, many workers have postulated the existence of a non-micellar interaction by hydrogen bonding between the phenolic hydroxyl group in certain preservatives and the basic oxygen in the ether group of the ethylene oxide adducts. This undoubtedly occurs in many circumstances but the fact that some preservatives have reduced activity in the presence of high molecular weight polyethylene glycols but not to the same extent with carboxymethyl cellulose or gum tragacanth, indicates that the interaction is not purely a matter of hydrogen bonding since equal opportunities for this exist with carboxymethyl cellulose and tragacanth as with the other hydrocolloids.

There is abundant evidence in the literature to support the view that the mechanism of interaction is attributable to micellar solubilization of preservatives by non-ionic surfactants, and a wide variety of techniques of demonstrating this have been used.

Kostenbauder and his co-workers have perhaps contributed most to a fuller understanding of the nature of the physico-chemical interaction between phenols and non-ionic surfactants and other macromolecules, and Kostenbauder (1960) maintains that it is unnecessary to distinguish between the mechanisms of complex formation and micellar solubilization. "Micellar solubilization and, indeed micelle formation itself, can be considered to fall within the broad scope of the complex formation described by Higuchi." Kostenbauder (1962) reasons that micelle formation is a type of complex formation since it obeys the law of mass action.

The juxtapositioning of preservatives and non-ionic surfactants is inevitable in emulsified systems since both, to be of use, must be in solution in the aqueous phase. Non-ionics form micelles in aqueous solutions at very low concentrations, and Hsiao *et al.* (1956) report the critical micelle concentration of the condensation products of alkyl phenols and ethylene oxide to be of the order of 10^{-4} M, while Higuchi and Lach (1954) report the c.m.c. of Cetomacrogol to be 10^{-6} to 10^{-7} M.

Non-ionic surfactants used either as emulsifiers or solubilizers will always be present at concentrations well above their c.m.c., thus, from the point of view of the emulsion chemist, their behaviour in non-micellar solutions is only of academic interest. Attempts to overcome the practical difficulties associated with the interaction, and to make reasonable predictions as to the amount and type of preservative required can, however, only be made if the nature and magnitude of the binding between preservatives and non-ionic surfactants can be assessed.

Patel and Kostenbauder (1958) employed a semi-permeable nylon membrane to evaluate the degree of intermolecular association between esters of *p*-hydroxybenzoic acid and Tween 80. Data obtained by means of an equilibrium dialysis study facilitated the calculation of the quantity of preservative which must be added to an aqueous system containing a known concentration of Tween 80 in order to have the desired concentration of unbound preservative. The dialysis method permits an estimation of the degree of binding irrespective of whether the association between the preservative and the non-ionic surfactant is attributable to the type of complex formation postulated previously or to some other mechanism such as preferential solubilization of the preservative within a micelle. During this careful study it was found that the nylon used for the dialysis bag had a tendency to bind some of the *p*-hydroxybenzoate, but this loss was taken into account in the calculations and did not invalidate the findings. Both the methyl and propyl esters of *p*-hydroxybenzoate were investigated, and a relatively high degree of interaction with Tween 80 was observed for both. The binding was seen to be a function of both the concentration of unbound *p*-hydroxybenzoate and the concentration of Tween 80.

The propyl ester was found to have a far greater affinity for Tween 80 than the methyl ester. At a concentration of 5 per cent Tween 80, only 22 per cent of the total methyl *p*-hydroxybenzoate existed as free preservative and at 10 per cent Tween 80 only 12 per cent existed as free methyl *p*-hydroxybenzoate. In the case of the propyl ester, with 5 per cent Tween 80 only 4·5 per cent existed as free propyl *p*-hydroxybenzoate.

These findings highlight the importance of the hydrophile–lipophile characteristics of the preservative in its relationship with the non-ionic. The more lipophilic propyl ester is bound to a greater extent than the more water-soluble methyl ester. This points to a partitioning effect which depends upon the solubility of the preservative as well as the HLB of the non-ionic surfactant.

Pisano and Kostenbauder (1959) later proceeded to correlate the binding data for *p*-hydroxybenzoates and Tween 80, with the amounts required to inhibit the growth of *Aerobacter aerogenes* and *Aspergillus niger*. Their results indicated that the concentrations of preservative in Tween 80 which could be predicted as likely to be inhibitory by the dialysis method, were in good agreement with the actual inhibitory concentrations found by microbiological experiments.

These investigations suggest that the required concentration of *p*-hydroxybenzoate can be estimated by multiplying the usual preservative concentration by the ratio of total to free preservative at any given Tween 80 concentration. This approach to emulsion preservation assumes, however, that other factors such as the oil–water ratio, pH and electrolyte content of the water phase, do not contribute to the efficacy of the preservative. Since it is known that these factors can exert powerful influences it would be wrong to rely on this kind of prediction to the exclusion of other considerations, but a knowledge of the binding data will undoubtedly indicate whether the use of a particular preservative in a non-ionic-containing formula is at all feasible on grounds of cost, toxicity, odour, etc.

Deluca and Kostenbauder (1960) used the dialysis technique described previously to investigate the association and accompanying inhibition of quaternary ammonium compounds with non-ionic surfactants.

In studies on cetylpyridinium chloride and Tween 80 an extremely high degree of interaction was observed, and the ratio of total to free cetylpyridinium chloride was found to be a function of the Tween 80 concentration. At a concentration of 1 per cent Tween 80 approximately 95 per cent of the quaternary was bound and thus inactivated, and even at 0·1 per cent of Tween 80, 60 per cent of the total cetylpyridinium chloride was inactivated. Studies with benzalkonium chloride and Tween 80 showed that much less binding occurred and that at 1 per cent Tween 80, only 50 per cent of the total quaternary was bound. Microbiological observations of the activity of the two quaternaries against *Aerobacter aerogenes* in the presence of Tween 80 showed an even higher degree of inactivation than would have been predicted from the dialysis experiments. This was ascribed to the presence of about 0·1 M total electrolyte in the culture medium which would lower the critical micelle concentration of the quaternaries and enhance the interaction between the cationics and Tween 80. These studies illustrate the fallacy of assuming that non-ionic surfactants will not interfere with the activity of cationic antiseptics.

Goodhart and Martin (1962) have studied further the interaction between non-ionic surfactants and a group of solid benzoic acid derivatives. The object of their investigation was to relate the degree of solubilization of closely related solid solubilisates to the hydrophile–lipophile character of certain non-ionic surfactants. Their data strongly support the theory of micellar solubilization of preservatives by non-ionic surfactants. A series of five polyoxyethylene stearates differing only in ethylene oxide content were used to serve as a series for comparing solubilization of related compounds as a function of hydrophile–lipophile balance. The solid benzoic acid derivatives studied included benzoic, *p*-aminobenzoic and *p*-hydroxybenzoic acids as well as the methyl, propyl and butyl esters of *p*-hydroxybenzoic acid. With a few exceptions solubility was greater in the least hydrophilic surfactant solutions, and binding of the esters of *p*-hydroxybenzoate was in the order butyl > propyl > methyl. These observations were in good agreement with those of Blaug and Ahsan (1961b) mentioned previously.

Both sets of findings are again in line with what would be expected of the more lipophilic preservatives in that binding may largely be due to their solubility in the fatty part of the non-ionic.

Surfactant solutions can be regarded as two-phase systems containing hydrophilic and lipophilic fractions. The orientation of the fractions will vary according to the micellar state of the solution, and above the critical micelle concentration the arrangement of the lipophilic chains will favour partitioning of preservatives.

The micelles of non-ionic surfactants appear to provide ideal conditions for association with various preservatives. They afford the possibility for hydrogen bonding and also for partitioning and micellar solubilization. Molecules such as polyethylene glycols of various molecular weights show some degree of binding to preservatives but to a much lesser extent than do the surface-active agents. Wedderburn (1958) showed that reduction in the effect of methyl *p*-hydroxybenzoate by polyethylene glycols at a fixed ratio of 1 to 20, was associated with molecular weight. Polyethylene glycols of molecular weight below 1500 showed little or no adverse effect on the preservative, while those with molecular weights above 2000 reduced the activity to some extent. Polyethylene glycols have an ether function to participate in hydrogen bonding but no large lipophilic group.

Evidence for the contribution of the hydrophobic chain in these interactions can be found in the effects of anionic surfactants which bind preservatives in a similar manner. The relative importance of the dipole–dipole interaction, and Van der Waal attraction forces of hydrophobic chains will vary considerably between different cases of binding, and since both mechanisms probably contribute to reduced preservative activity there is little point in attributing these interactions to one mechanism with the exclusion of other possibilities.

In addition to these mechanisms, the possibility exists that non-ionics prevent or interfere with the uptake of preservatives by bacterial cells. Beckett *et al.* (1958b), Wedderburn (1958) and Judis (1962) have provided evidence to support this hypothesis.

In the complex systems of emulsions the opportunity probably exists for all these mechanisms to operate and the degree to which they do so will depend on the type and concentration of non-ionic, the type and concentration of preservative and the presence of additional substances which might reduce or enhance the interaction between them or with the cells of micro-organisms.

C. EFFECT OF HYDROPHILIC POLYMERS ON PRESERVATIVES

Several workers have reported that macromolecules without surface-active properties reduce the efficacy of certain preservatives, and since many hydrophilic polymers are used in emulsions to provide desired rheological properties, their effects must be considered.

1. *Polyethylene glycols*

The low molecular weight polyethylene glyools do not inactivate preservatives to any great extent, but where the molecular weight is higher than two to three thousand slight effects become apparent. Miyawaki and co-workers (1959) studied the effect of polyethylene glycol 4000 on methyl and propyl *p*-hydroxybenzoate using both solubility and equilibrium dialysis methods. Their results showed that in a solution of 5 per cent polyethylene glycol 4000, approximately 1·6 times as much of the methyl ester would be required to affect adequate preservation as would be needed in the absence of the macromolecule, and that the propyl ester was bound to a greater extent than the methyl.

The binding of the *p*-hydroxybenzoates by polyethylene glycols is of minor importance compared with that exhibited by the polyoxyethylene surfactants, and de Navarre and Bailey (1956) suggest that in practice there is little or no interference with the activity of methyl *p*-hydroxy-benzoate in the presence of 2 per cent polyethylene glycol 4000.

Deluca and Kostenbauder (1960) studied the effects of Polyox, a very high molecular weight linear polymer of ethylene oxide, on quaternary ammonium compounds, and found that neither cetylpyridinium chloride nor benzalkonium chloride were bound.

2. *Gum Tragacanth*

Eisman *et al.* (1957) examined the effectiveness of chlorbutanol, phenylmercuric acetate, merthiolate, a mixture of methyl and propyl *p*-hydroxybenzoates, benzalkonium chloride and phenol in 3 per cent gum tragacanth jellies. By contaminating the variously preserved jellies with a standard number of *Staphylococcus aureus* and determining survival rates, they found the activity of all the above compounds reduced in comparison with their activity in water. Chlorbutanol, the mixed esters of *p*-hydroxybenzoate and benzalkonium chloride were all very much less effective in 3 per cent gum tragacanth than in water, while the effects of phenol and the mercurials were reduced but not to such a high degree. A "neutralizing effect" by gum tragacanth, probably as the result of physical adsorption was suggested by the authors.

Using the dialysis technique, Miyawaki *et al.* (1959) could find no evidence of physical adsorption of methyl *p*-hydroxybenzoate by gum tragacanth, and, in their view, if increased quantities of preservative are required for tragacanth dispersions, the factor responsible for this requirement is other than physical adsorption. Gum tragacanth is itself frequently heavily contaminated with a variety of micro-organisms, and is also an exceptionally favourable medium for growth. These factors are most likely to account for the increased quantities of preservative found to be necessary in protecting tragacanth dispersions, since the number of organisms present may be greater than that which can be influenced by the usual concentrations of preservative.

3. *Methylcellulose*

Tillman and Kuramoto (1957) have reported an interaction between methylcellulose and the methyl, propyl and butyl esters of *p*-hydroxybenzoate. Their evidence, based on solubility measurements, suggested the existence of both soluble and insoluble complexes between the polymer and the preservatives. It is possible that the phenolic group of the *p*-hydroxybenzoates would interact with the ether groups of the methylcellulose in a similar manner to the interaction with polyethylene glycol.

Examination of this interaction by Miyawaki *et al.* (1959) using their dialysis technique, showed that although some degree of binding between methyl *p*-hydroxybenzoate and methylcellulose could be demonstrated, it was unlikely that the interaction would necessitate the addition of supplementary quantities of preservative, at the concentrations in which methylcellulose is normally used.

4. *Carboxymethylcellulose*

Specific interactions between carboxymethylcellulose and preservatives have not been reported in the literature, and Miyawaki *et al.* (1959), who studied its effect on methyl *p*-hydroxybenzoate, could find no evidence of association between the two compounds.

5. *Polyvinylpyrrolidone*

Polyvinylpyrrolidone (P.V.P.) contains an amido group and Kostenbauder and Higuchi (1956) have demonstrated that compounds such as phenols which are capable of acting as proton donors tend to form complexes with amides. Miyawaki *et al.* (1959) again using the equilibrium dialysis technique found that the methyl and propyl esters of *p*-hydroxybenzoic acid were bound to P.V.P. to a greater extent than to the polyethylene glycols, methyl cellulose, carboxymethylcellulose or gum tragacanth. This degree of binding, although of a far lesser order than that which occurs with non-ionic surfactants, might under some conditions necessitate the addition of a supplementary amount of preservative.

D. EFFECT OF SUSPENDED PARTICLES ON PRESERVATIVES

There is little evidence in the literature of adverse effects on preservatives due to the presence of suspended solid particles, but there is every likelihood that in certain circumstances adsorption and an accompanying reduction in activity will occur.

A very wide variety of insoluble solids is used in cosmetic and pharmaceutical emulsions and talc, kaolin, titanium dioxide, zinc oxide and chalk are but a few examples of white materials often added. Many insoluble solids are used to colour emulsions, amongst which are iron oxides, chromium oxides, and various natural and synthetic pigments.

The extent to which adsorption of the preservative on to the suspended solids will occur will depend upon the nature of the solid, the type of preservative and the pH of the system. Consideration of the electrical charge at the surface of the solid under the particular conditions in the emulsion, the total surface area it presents to the aqueous phase and any ion exchange mechanisms which might operate, should enable reasonable predictions of preservative efficiency to be made.

Tamamushi and Tamaki (1959) have examined the adsorption of long-chain electrolytes at solid–liquid interfaces. Cationic and anionic surfactants in aqueous solutions were used, and their adsorption isotherms on alumina, titanium dioxide, barium sulphate, calcium fluoride and carbon black, were determined. Adsorption was found to attain saturation at an equilibrium concentration near the c.m.c. of the surfactant.

In emulsions containing suspended solids, the solid–liquid interface will invariably be saturated with the emulsifier. The degree to which the preservative becomes adsorbed will depend upon its polarity, and on whether it comes into contact with the solid before the emulsifier. The order of addition of ingredients during the manufacture of the emulsion can affect preservative adsorption, in that if the preservative is dissolved in the slurry carrying the suspended solid particles, greater adsorption will occur than if it is added after the particle surfaces have become coated with the emulsifier.

Harris (1961) has shown that cationic antiseptics are inactivated by bentonite suspensions while anionic and non-ionic antiseptics are not affected. The mechanism of inactivation is attributed to a removal from solution of the cationic by a cation exchange process known to be associated with montmorillonite. Harris emphasizes strongly that cationic antiseptics or preservatives ought not to be used with bentonite unless proved by bacteriological tests to be effective.

E. EFFECT OF PACKAGING MATERIALS ON PRESERVATIVES

The physical form of the containers in which emulsions are packed can influence the state of preservation by permitting the loss of volatile preservatives and essential oils which may help inhibit growth. Containers with unsterile cap linings often provide a source of contamination and, when the product is in use, some forms of pack such as wide-mouth jars and polythene tubes allow large numbers of organisms to enter.

Apart from these factors, packaging materials often reduce the efficacy of preservatives by undergoing physico-chemical interactions.

Rubber closures have long been known to bind and inactivate some preservatives and this problem has been particularly apparent in the case of parenteral solutions packed in vials with elastomer seals. Royce and Sykes (1957) studied the loss of phenol, chlorocresol, benzyl alcohol and phenyl mercuric nitrate from vials with rubber closures and found that chlorocresol was absorbed to a much greater extent than phenol. Benzyl alcohol and phenol were also much less affected than phenyl mercuric nitrate. Lachman *et al.* (1962) investigated the effect of natural rubber, neoprene polymer and butyl polymer rubbers on several preservatives including methyl *p*-hydroxybenzoate. The butyl rubber closure was found to be physically incompatible with all the preservatives due to a leaching of an accelerator residue, and in general the natural rubber exerted the least deleterious effect. Distribution studies on *p*-chloro-β-phenylethyl alcohol and phenylethyl alcohol showed that the chlorinated compound is absorbed into rubber to a far greater extent than the non-chlorinated analogue.

A wide variety of materials are now used for tubes, jars and closures, and studies on nylon, polyethylene, and polystyrene have been carried out.

Marcus *et al.* (1959) report that nylon bound *p*-hydroxybenzoic acid, and its methyl and propyl esters, sorbic acid, phenol and 4-chloro-3-methyl phenol, while polyethylene and polystyrene had no such effect. The polar groups in nylon were thought to be responsible for the binding phenomenon. Patel and Kostenbauder (1958) also found that nylon bound methyl *p*-hydroxybenzoate and postulated that the amide groups in nylon would form molecular complexes with certain organic compounds which act as proton donors.

Kim and Autian (1960) examined the effect of polyethylene and polystyrene on benzoic, *m*-hydroxybenzoic, *p*-aminobenzoic and salicyclic acids and found no interference with the activity of these preservatives.

Autian and Shaikh (1960) have suggested that the binding of preservatives to packaging materials might be turned to advantage, since slight leaching of the preservatives from the material to which they are bound might confer bacteriostatic properties to the contents of the pack. Careful practical tests would, however, have to be carried out before such steps could be recommended.

VI. Prediction of Preservative Efficiency

A. THEORETICAL CONSIDERATIONS

During the formulation of new emulsions weeks of work can often be saved by considering, on a theoretical basis, the factors which are likely to influence the preservation of the product. This approach, coupled with simple laboratory tests on various combinations of the formula components, although it cannot substitute for thorough microbiological testing of the finished formula, can quickly put the formulator in the approximate range of effective preservative type and concentration.

The availability of the preservative in the aqueous phase of an emulsion determines the efficiency of inhibition of microbial growth. Because of the complexity of many emulsion formulae, the suitability is often influenced by several factors, some of which act in its favour and others against it, while the relative hostility to micro-organisms or the nutritive value of the formula itself is also a consideration.

The extensive literature on emulsion preservation deals mainly with individual principles and cases, and although it is not possible to abstract a set of "rules" to which the formulator should adhere, some degree of guidance can be obtained by examining any new formula in detail before attempting to decide how to preserve it.

Consideration of the degree of contamination of raw materials and the factors which are likely to encourage or inhibit growth in the emulsion will show whether the product is likely to be resistant or susceptible to decomposition.

TABLE XI

Percentage of Preservative Undissociated Related to pH

	pH					
	2	3	4	5	6	7
Benzoic acid	99	94	60	13	1·5	0·15
Boric acid	100	100	100	100	100·0	100·0
Dehydroacetic acid	100	100	95	65	15·8	1·9
p-Chlorobenzoic acid	99	91	52	9·7	1·06	0·107
Propionic acid	100	99	88	42·0	6·7	0·71
Salicylic acid	90	49	8·6	0·94	0·094	0·0094
Sorbic acid	—	98	86	37	6·0	0·6

A knowledge of the pH of the aqueous phase will indicate which preservatives are worth considering in the light of their dissociation constants. Since dissociation governs the degree of activity of most preservatives, pH is of prime importance in making a selection. Table XI shows the percentage of some preservatives undissociated at various pH.

Apart from boric acid which cannot be recommended as a preservative because of its toxicity, dehydroacetic acid has a higher percentage undissociated at pH 6–7 than the other acids shown. It also has a wide spectrum of action, and low toxicity, making it a useful material.

The ratio of oil to water is another very important factor, and the distribution of preservative between the phases must be known before it is worthwhile testing the effectiveness.

Hibbott and Monks (1961) have examined the partition coefficient of methyl *p*-hydroxybenzoate in a series of oil and fat mixtures and their results are given in Table XII (see also Table VIII).

The same authors found that the addition of propylene glycol to the aqueous phase reduced the partition coefficient and made more methyl *p*-hydroxybenzoate available. Conversely, if a non-ionic surfactant is present, this is likely to increase the partition coefficient and make less available.

In establishing the effects of propylene glycol and glycerol on the partition coefficient of methyl *p*-hydroxybenzoate, Hibbott and Monks used a mixture of 200 g water, 50 g oleyl alcohol and 0·3 g preservative with increasing amounts of either propylene glycol or glycerol. Their results are given in Table XIII.

TABLE XII

Partition of Methyl *p*-Hydroxybenzoate between Oil Mixtures and Water (from Hibbott and Monks, 1961)

		Partition coefficient oil/water
90 ml	isopropyl myristate	20
90 ml	water	
3 g	methyl *p*-hydroxybenzoate	
65 ml	isopropyl myristate	11
25 ml	mineral oil	
90 ml	water	
1·5 g	preservative	
65 ml	isopropyl myristate	10
25 ml	mineral oil	
10 g	stearic acid	
100 ml	water	
1·5 g	preservative	
65 ml	isopropyl myristate	15
25 ml	mineral oil	
3 g	cetyl alcohol	
93 ml	water	
3 g	preservative	

These results indicate that the presence of more than 5 per cent propylene glycol in the aqueous phase changes the solubility of the preservative, making more available than when equivalent amounts of glycerol are present. Poprzan and de Navarre (1959) have reported similar effects for up to 10 per cent additions of ethyl alcohol, 1,3-propanediol, 1,4-butanediol and 2-methyl-2,4-pentanediol in systems containing 0·2 per cent methyl *p*-hydroxybenzoate with 2 per cent Tween 80. Barr and Tice (1957e) in studying the effect of non-ionic surfactants on sorbic acid, showed that the presence of 3 per cent hexylene glycol reduced the inactivating effects of the sorbitan partial fatty acid esters and the polyoxyethylene ester types.

Mechanisms such as these may well account for the fact that preservatives often do not fail as completely as might be expected from the predictions based on compatibility tests on individual formula ingredients.

The stability and general properties of many emulsions would doubtless be adversely affected by the addition of some of the substances mentioned above and data predicting the approximate total concentrations of preservative required when certain macromolecules are present can be of immense value.

Kostenbauder (1960) has summarized some of the work showing the degree of binding of methyl *p*-hydroxybenzoate by various macromolecules, and Fig. 4 shows the relationship.

TABLE XIII

Effect of Propylene Glycol and Glycerol on Partition Coefficient (from Hibbott and Monks, 1961)

Propylene Glycol %	*Partition coefficient oil/aqueous phase*	*Glycerol* %	*Partition coefficient oil/aqueous phase*
0	31	0	31
2	29	2	29
5	22	5	26
10	19	10	26
15	18	15	27
20	16	20	26

Blaug and Ahsan (1961a, b) and Deluca and Kostenbauder (1960) have presented binding data for a variety of preservatives and macromolecules and Table XIV is compiled from their figures and those of Kostenbauder (1960).

The figures in Table XIV are the approximate ratios of total to free preservative and indicate the factor by which the normally required concentration of preservative should be multiplied to obtain the required free concentration in the presence of the various concentrations of the macromolecules shown.

This kind of information can be used as a rough guide in preservative selection, but the other factors influencing the availability of preservative in the aqueous phase cannot be overlooked.

The theoretical considerations covered so far have been concerned with the thermodynamic activity of the preservative, and there is over-

TABLE XIV

Approximate ratios of Total to Free Preservative in the Presence of Macromolecules

	Factor by which normal concentration of preservative should be multiplied							
Preservative	2% *Tween* 80	5% *Tween* 80	2% *Myrj* 52	5% *Myrj* 52	2% *P.E.G.* 4000	5% *P.E.G.* 4000	2% *Methyl cellulose*	5% *Methyl cellulose*
Methyl *p*-hydroxybenzoate	2·5	4·5	2·0	3·0	1·2	1·5	1·05	1·25
Ethyl *p*-hydroxybenzoate	5·0	11·0	3·0	5·0	1·3	1·6	—	—
Propyl *p*-hydroxybenzoate	12·5	27·0	6·0	13·5	1·4	1·7	—	—
Butyl *p*-hydroxybenzoate	30·0	63·0	18·0	40·0	—	—	—	—
Phenol	1·6	2·5	—	—	1·2	1·25	—	—
Sorbic acid	1·8	2·9	1·7	2·7	1·1	1·2	—	—
Cetylpyridinium chloride	38·0	60·0	—	—	—	—	—	—
Benzalkonium chloride	3·0	5·5	—	—	—	—	—	—

whelming evidence that for a given preservative the thermodynamic activity is equivalent to the preservative activity. Allawala and Riegelman (1954) have shown that the thermodynamic activity of a dissolved phenol can be expressed in terms of the per cent saturation by setting the saturated solution as the standard state of reference. They demonstrated

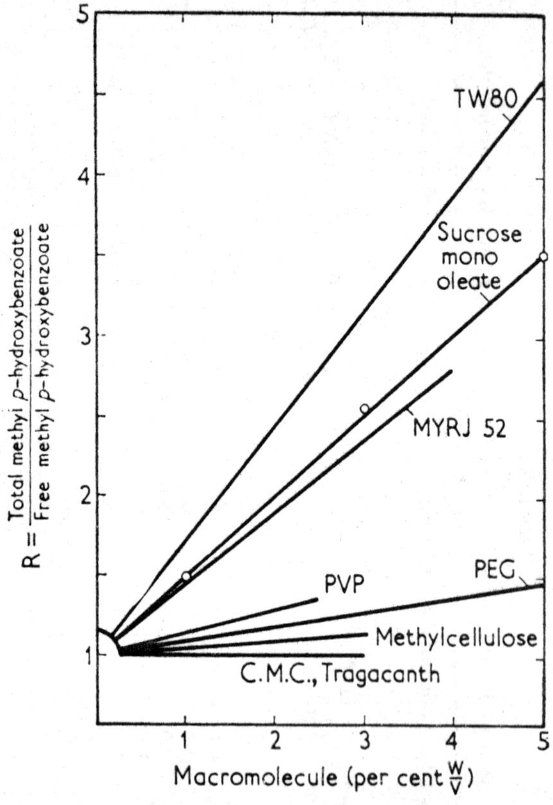

Fig. 4. Ratio of total to free preservative concentration in the presence of varying concentrations of macromolecules (R value of 1·0 corresponds to no measurable binding) (from Kostenbauder).

that the equitoxic solutions of different phenols are those in which the thermodynamic activity or the per cent saturation, and *not* the actual concentration, is the same. In studying twenty-three different phenols they found the phenol coefficients approximately the same as the ratios between the solubility of the unknown disinfectants and the solubility of phenol.

When binding between a preservative and a macromolecule occurs, an equilibrium is set up such that when some of the preservative is adsorbed or otherwise removed by its action on micro-organisms, there will be a change in the equilibrium, making more preservative available. Thus in systems where some of the preservative is bound, the reservoir of preservative may make the system more efficient than a simple aqueous solution of similar theromodynamic activity. This could be particularly important where preservatives of low water solubility are used.

The concentrations of preservative normally used in formulae where there are no materials which dramatically hinder their effectiveness are usually somewhat higher than the actual minimum inhibitory concentrations estimated by microbiological techniques. This is because some degree of interference occurs in most formulae and the minimum inhibitory concentration of any preservative varies widely between different bacteria and fungi.

The differing responses of different bacteria and fungi to various preservatives often makes it necessary to consider the use of two or more inhibitors which together will protect the product from a variety of contaminants, but alone would only inhibit certain organisms. The use of mixtures often permits the use of low concentrations of two or more preservatives instead of a high concentration of one which would have the same effectiveness but might be undesirable on grounds of cost, toxicity to the consumer or its effect on emulsion stability. This approach is particularly useful when a quaternary ammonium compound is used, since these materials inhibit Gram positive bacteria at very low concentrations, but are only effective against Gram negative bacteria and fungi at levels which sometimes interfere with the performance of the emulsifier. In these instances it is helpful to add a preservative which has a high degree of specificity for Gram negative organisms and fungi. In this way a wide-spectrum mixture can be used to good effect.

Deeb and Boenigh (1958) have suggested mixtures of 0·5 per cent chlorbutanol and 0·5 per cent benzylalcohol, and Barr and Tice (1957c) report that a mixture of 0·12 per cent methyl *p*-hydroxybenzoate, 0·02 per cent propyl *p*-hydroxybenzoate and 0·15 per cent sorbic acid was effective in preserving aqueous sorbitol solutions.

Osman and El-Mariah (1960) report that salicylic acid had a potentiating effect on formic acid, sorbic acid, benzoic acid, *o*- and *p*-chlorobenzoic acid and the methyl, ethyl, propyl and butyl esters of *p*-hydroxybenzoic acid.

Boehm and Jones (1957) recommended the use of mixtures of the methyl, ethyl, propyl and butyl esters of *p*-hydroxybenzoic acid and state that although true synergism between the esters is unlikely, the additive effects are so great as to give the impression of an increase in action. In discussing the solubilities of the various esters they mention the possibility that one ester promotes the concentration of another at the emulsion interface or at the bacterial cell surface giving a total action greater than simple addition of each separate ester.

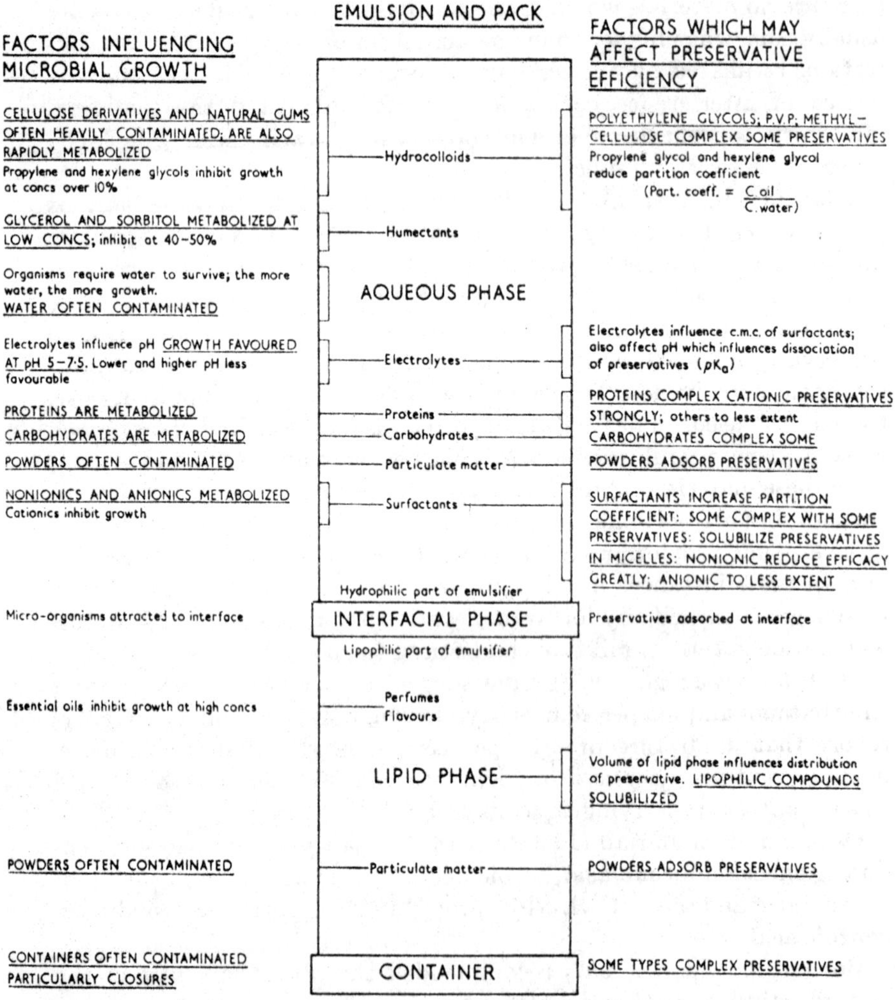

FIG. 5. Schematic representation of the factors in emulsions which influence microbial growth and the efficacy of preservatives.

There are thus three reasons for considering the use of mixtures of preservatives rather than single substances:

(i) True synergism between preservatives—Maccacaro (1961) has written a fascinating review which defines and discusses synergism and, although this work is of limited application to preservation, it gives a clear insight into the effects of the interaction between antibacterial drugs.

(ii) Additive effects which, by influencing the solubility of the preservatives, make mixtures more effective than single substances.

(iii) Broadening the spectrum of activity by using low concentrations of two or more preservatives each of which inhibit different varieties of organisms.

In attempting to solve a spoilage problem in an existing formula or in selecting an appropriate preservative for a new one, the many factors acting in favour of microbial survival, and those which may discourage it should be examined individually. The task is often bewilderingly complex, particularly in some modern formulae which contain a large number of components whose positioning in the emulsion is obscure and their chemical composition ill-defined. Nevertheless, some degree of separation of the many counterbalancing factors can usually be achieved, and those which cannot be postulated, can be tested.

Figure 5 illustrates the important emulsion factors which influence microbial growth and those which determine whether a particular preservative will be effective. This schematic representation summarizes the main points to be considered, but does not pretend to be complete in itself. In studying Fig. 5 it is important to remember that the thermodynamic activity of the preservative in the aqueous phase determines the effectiveness against micro-organisms, and also that bacteria and fungi depend upon water for their survival.

B. TESTS TO AID PRESERVATIVE SELECTION

1. *Microbiological Tests*

The tests which help towards predicting the physico-chemical compatibility between a preservative and the system in which it is to be used can only be usefully applied in practice if the concentration of active preservative required in solution in the aqueous phase is known. This can be decided either by relying on past history and utilizing concentrations which were thought effective in other formulae, or by microbiological testing. The latter is obviously preferable since preservatives are so often used wastefully and because the active and available concentration in the aqueous phase of an existing formula is seldom, if ever, known with certainty.

Assessment of the minimum inhibitory concentrations of several likely preservatives against a selection of Gram positive and Gram negative bacteria, and also yeasts and fungi is a simple matter. The classic serial dilution test is recommended to determine minimum inhibitory concentrations, and the following organisms are numbered amongst those most likely to cause spoilage in emulsions, and therefore worthy of testing.

Gram Positive	Gram Negative
Staphylococcus aureus	*Pseudomonas aeruginosa*
Streptococcus mitis	*Escherichia coli*
Bacillus subtilis	*Aerobacter aerogenes*

Fungi	Yeasts
Aspergillus niger	*Monilia albicans*
Penicillium chrysogenum	*Candida*
Alternaria solani	

Normally a preservative with a wide spectrum of activity against bacteria, fungi and yeasts is required. The lowest concentration of either a single preservative or a mixture which will inhibit all likely contaminants in culture medium for a period of at least 7 days, can be used as the basis for subsequent compatibility testing.

Knowing the minimum inhibitory concentration of preservative required in the aqueous phase of the emulsion, the next step is to measure the effect of other constituents of the phase on the activity of the chosen preservative concentration. This is simply done by setting up two parallel series of preservative dilutions in culture medium, one series containing descending concentrations of the preservative alone and the other containing the preservative with a constant amount of whatever aqueous phase constituent is to be tested. After inoculation of both series with appropriate test organisms, followed by incubation for at least a week, some idea of the activity of the preservative in the presence of other aqueous phase constituents can be obtained. In order to make these tests as informative as possible, synthetic, rather than natural culture media containing peptone and beef extracts should be used, since these substances may bind some preservatives. The pH of the media should be adjusted to simulate that of the aqueous phase of the emulsion as closely as possible.

This kind of test can provide limited yet useful information about the interaction of preservatives with aqueous phase components, but, being performed in the absence of the constituents of the oil phase, important factors such as the partitioning of preservative between the phases are not taken into account. Because of this limitation, component testing in culture media can never be regarded as a substitute for more comprehensive and longer tests on the whole formula.

Agar diffusion tests are quite unsuitable for evaluating the degree of interaction between preservatives and other constituents, and it is interesting to note that the few authors whose conclusions on the effects of non-ionic surface-active agents on preservatives are at variance with the generally accepted views on this topic used this kind of technique. The result of an agar diffusion test indicates the distance through the agar that the antimicrobial agent travelled before growth of unaffected organisms began. The size of the zone of inhibition is directly related to the diffusion characteristics of the inhibitor in agar, and hence a comparison between the size of the inhibition zone produced by a preservative solution alone, and that formed by the preservative in solution with a substance likely to influence its diffusion characteristics is meaningless.

Quisno *et al.* (1946) condemned the agar diffusion test for quaternary ammonium compounds after showing that agar reduces the potency of these materials. Their results suggested that the reduction was due to a physical adsorption on agar, rather than poor diffusion through the medium, but both mechanisms could well mitigate against a valuable result when other antimicrobial agents or combinations are tested in this way.

Wailes (1962) has shown that a manometric method using the Warburg apparatus is a useful technique for screening preservatives more rapidly than the more conventional microbiological tests in culture media. He used baker's yeast as the test organism and measured the effects of preservatives and preservative-surfactant combinations on respiration. His results were in excellent agreement with those obtained by more time-consuming methods using culture media. Similar work carried out in the author's own laboratory using *Pseudomonas aeruginosa* as the test organism supports the view that manometric techniques provide accurate information in a short time and do not involve the disadvantages inherent in adding preservatives to culture media. Any organism with a high respiration rate can be used and, when studying the effects of substances likely to reduce the efficacy of preservatives, useful quantitative data on the inhibitory or stimulatory effect of the substance itself can be obtained at the same time.

2. *Tests for Physico-Chemical Compatibility*

Techniques for determining the partition coefficient or distribution of preservative between emulsion phases are well known and relatively simple to perform. The method used by Hibbott and Monks (1961) in their studies of the partitioning of methyl *p*-hydroxybenzoate can be adapted to the investigation of other inhibitors, and determination of the availability of the preservative in the aqueous phase may be made by either chemical analysis or microbiological assay. Serial dilution tests on the aqueous fraction can be carried out against a suitable test organism, and it is also possible to use manometric assay methods to determine the activity of the preservative in the water after equilibration with the oil phase.

The equilibrium dialysis method described by Patel and Kostenbauder (1958) is convenient for the estimation of the interaction between preservatives and various macromolecules present in the aqueous phase. This technique utilizes a membrane which permits free passage of the preservative but is impermeable to the macromolecule. At equilibrium the activity of the preservative is identical on both sides of the membrane and for dilute solutions the concentration of free preservative on both sides is essentially equal. By placing a solution or suspension of the macromolecule on one side of the membrane and determining the concentration of preservative on the opposite side, it is possible to discover the concentration of free or unbound preservative in equilibrium with the macromolecule. Since the effectiveness of the preservative is related to its thermodynamic activity, which is in turn proportional to the concentration of free or unbound preservative, the concentration of free preservative will provide an index of efficiency.

The dialysis method permits the estimation of the degree of binding between preservative and macromolecule irrespective of whether the association is due to complex formation, some other mechanism such as preferential solubility of the preservative within a micelle, or a simple increase in partition coefficient.

VII. Confirmatory Tests for Preservative Effectiveness

Discrepancies between predicted preservative behaviour and what actually occurs in a finished emulsion formula have often been reported. This state of affairs is inevitable, not only because all the factors governing the efficacy of preservatives are at present incompletely understood, but also because it is extremely difficult to take account of each and every factor, and to predict the various ways in which those acting against preservative efficiency will be counterbalanced by those factors enhancing the chances of its success. (See Fig. 5.)

No two emulsion formulae are identical, and even where the same formula is made with slightly different raw materials, on a different plant and in a new environment, the changed circumstances can lead to preservation problems where none existed before.

Reliable information about emulsion resistance to microbial spoilage can only be obtained by extended testing of the final formula containing perfume or flavour, and made under conditions as close as possible to those to be used in full-scale production.

Several techniques of confirming whether an emulsion is adequately preserved have been reported, and because of the inconvenience of carrying out tests which simulate realistic conditions, shorter and more stringent methods have been suggested. Baker (1959) has described methods which can be completed in 10 to 14 days, but also points out that no laboratory test is infallible in showing whether a product is absolutely immune from invasion by micro-organisms. To test for resistance to bacterial contamination he suggests an inoculation test where 10 g samples of the product are injected with 0·1 ml of various culture suspensions. The number of organisms is usually about 6,000,000/g of product, and the number of survivors in each sample of inoculated product is determined at intervals after storage at room temperature. If the product is effectively preserved there should, according to Baker, be no survivors after 2 to 4 days.

To test for resistance to fungal invasion, Baker used an agar plate method which provided results in about 10 days. This method employed petri dishes containing 30 ml of buffered yeast agar, seeded with spores of selected fungi, in which wells were cut to contain a sample of the test product. The petri dishes were incubated at a high humidity at 28° C for 10 days, during which the product in the wells was examined microscopically for the presence of fungal hyphae on the surface. Products on which the fungi grew within this period were rejected as inadequately preserved, whereas those free from growth were considered satisfactory.

There are obvious dangers in relying on this kind of method to assess preservative efficiency and probably the most important lies in the fact that some of the preservative will diffuse through the agar, leaving a lower concentration in the product in the well. This reduced concentration may be insufficient to prevent fungal growth on the surface of the product, whereas if loss through diffusion had not occurred it might have proved effective.

Preservatives ought not to be used at levels much in excess of their minimum inhibitory concentration, for reasons of economy and safety to the consumer and, in this kind of test, products which do not support growth probably contain an unnecessarily high concentration of preservative. Figure 6 shows the result of tests in the author's own laboratory using the agar plate method. Cream A was an oil-in-water emulsion with aqueous phase pH 5·2 preserved with 0·3 per cent sorbic acid, while Cream B was the same formula with the aqueous phase at pH 6·5 and preserved with 0·2 per cent methyl *p*-hydroxybenzoate. The zones of growth inhibition around Cream A show that neither of the test fungi is likely to grow on the cream in practice, since the lower concentration of sorbic acid which had migrated into the agar was sufficient to suppress growth. Both fungi grew on Cream B although the product could be shown by other techniques to be adequately preserved and had been on sale to the public without signs of microbial spoilage for a considerable time.

Bacteria cause spoilage to an even greater extent than fungi, and since their growth in an emulsion cannot be detected visibly, the agar plate test is not suitable for estimating product resistance to bacterial contamination.

Inoculation techniques, where known numbers of bacteria or fungi are introduced into the product and samples taken at intervals to estimate survival, are by far the most reliable although accurate results cannot be obtained quickly. The slow adaptation of micro-organisms to their environment makes it essential to test for long enough to determine whether inoculated bacteria and fungi will flourish after a prolonged dormant period, and the author's own experience has shown that in some instances even tests lasting 6 months can sometimes be too short.

Charles and Carter (1959) have reported extensive tests on a variety of formulae containing different preservatives. The object of their study was to correlate data on preservative efficiency in finished products with predictions made on the basis of laboratory tests in simplified systems. They found that the *p*-hydroxybenzoate esters were more effective in finished formulae than had been predicted from their performance in component testing, and that sorbic acid appeared to afford adequate protection in most cases where the phenolic esters failed. Their test method involved inoculation of the products with different micro-organisms followed by observation for changes in the emulsions for 3 months.

Rdzok *et al.* (1955) have also described an inoculation method, using a suspension of garden soil with the addition of the spores of nine fungi.

The "Killing Time Test" described by Fotor and Nisonger (1950) for the evaluation of the germicidal efficiency of semi-solid pharmaceuticals

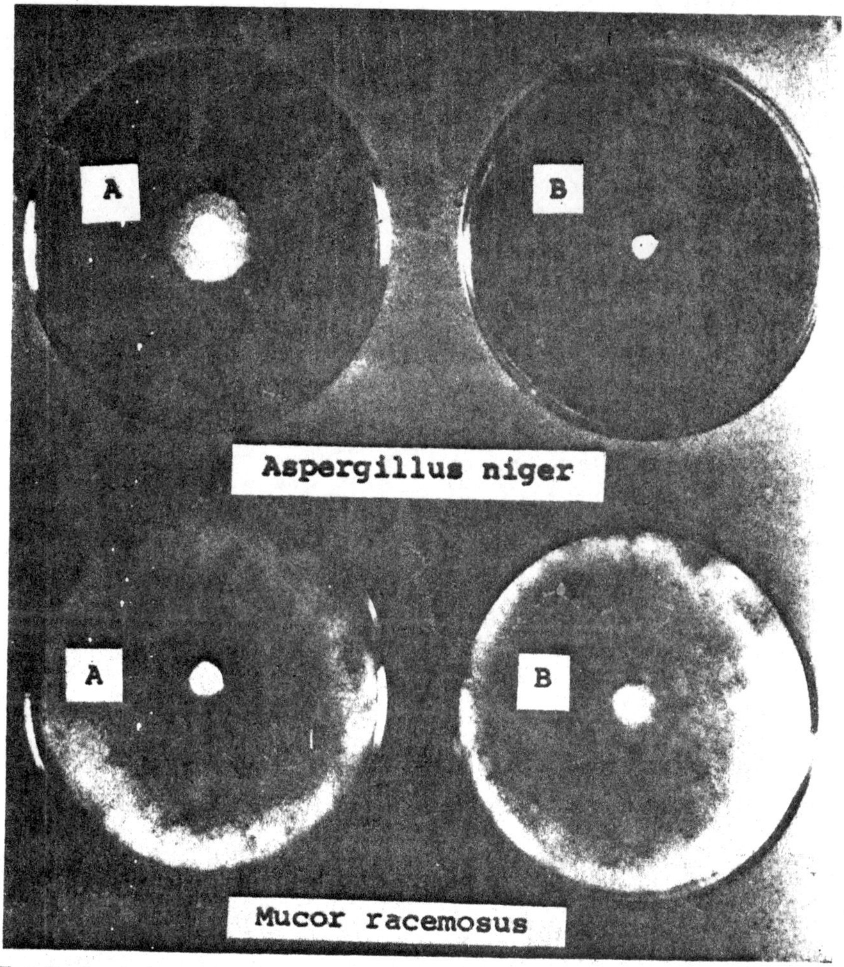

FIG. 6. Agar plate test showing diffusion of preservative into medium. Cream A: Oil-in-water cream containing 0·3 per cent sorbic acid (aqueous phase pH 5·2). Cream B: Oil-in-water cream containing 0·2 per cent methyl *p*-hydroxybenzoate (aqueous phase pH 6·5).

Cream B is known to be adequately preserved. Both fungi grew on the cream as a result of preservative loss into the agar.

could be adapted for the testing of product resistance to bacterial contamination, but would not be suitable for tests with fungi since preservatives do not normally *kill* fungal spores but act by inhibiting development of the mycelium.

Surprisingly little has been written about suitable techniques of assessing the effectiveness of preservatives in finished formulae and most of the published methods appear to contain elements which prevent them from simulating the conditions which prevail in normal practice. This is probably because testing in a realistic way is laborious and very time consuming, and most published methods represent short-cuts. As in the case of storage testing for emulsion stability, "accelerated" tests can provide limited information, but there is no substitute for the long-term test with built-in realism.

In devising a realistic test method, consideration ought to be given to whether spoilage is likely to occur as the result of microbial contamination in the raw materials and water, through organisms introduced during manufacture and packaging, or at some later time when the product is in the hands of the consumer. The growth of organisms from all three sources must be prevented, and because their distribution within the product will vary according to when and how they are introduced, the test method should allow for these variables. This will mean preparing special batches of the emulsion to be tested, with appropriate bacteria and fungi artificially introduced during manufacture as well as after processing.

It is difficult to predict which types of bacteria and fungi are likely to flourish in a particular emulsion. Some will die out relatively quickly, while others may survive for long periods and perhaps give rise to succeeding generations which are capable of growing vigorously in the new environment. A choice of the most suitable organisms to use in testing a final formulation can be made by inoculating samples of the product without preservative with a wide range of bacteria and fungi, and selecting only those organisms which survive for more than 10 days for further tests on the formula with preservative. Bacterial counts and cultures for fungi made from uninoculated samples of the unpreserved product will show which organisms are intrinsic to the formula. Cultures of these should obviously be made for use in subsequent tests.

In all tests the inoculum should be in a form which interferes as little as possible with the properties of the emulsion. Minimum amounts of water should be used for making bacterial suspensions, to avoid adding appreciably to the aqueous phase, and the organisms ought to be washed free from residues of culture medium, so that on inoculation they are forced to metabolize the product to survive. Dry spores, rather than mycelium, suspended in small volumes of water are best for tests with fungi. The use of soil or other solid matter as a vehicle for the fungal inoculum is not to be recommended since the presence of particles could well lead to emulsion instability and thus prejudice a valid result.

Batches of the product with and without preservative are needed for final tests. An early comparison between the fate of the inoculum in the preserved and in the unpreserved product will give an indication of whether the preservative chosen is likely to fulfil its purpose, but a final conclusion about its efficacy cannot be made for several months. This is because of the extreme difficulty of estimating the effects of preservatives on fungi and spore-bearing bacteria. Samples of the product containing spores will invariably show growth when transferred to culture media because preservatives seldom have any effect on spores themselves. For this reason culturing from samples inoculated with spore-bearing organisms is much less informative than culturing from samples containing vegetative organisms. In the latter a gradual diminution in numbers can be traced over a period of time if the preservative is effective, but with fungi and spore-bearing organisms one can only wait for the appearance of visible spoilage, which sometimes takes several months to occur.

In one test carried out in the author's laboratory an oil-in-water emulsion containing a mixed preservative was inoculated with two varieties of Gram positive bacteria, two Gram negatives and six varieties of fungi. The Gram positive bacteria were never re-isolated after inoculation, the Gram negatives disappeared after about 2 weeks and none of the fungi showed visible growth in the product for 6 months. After 8 months, six of the uninoculated samples containing preservative showed copious growth of a fungus which had not been chosen for test purposes, and a month later 85 per cent of the fifty inoculated samples supported the same fungus. This organism was a laboratory contaminant which must have entered the product during the monthly inspection of samples since it did not appear in unopened jars. Its development showed, however, that although the product would probably have reached the consumer in good condition, it was not effectively enough preserved for a product which might be opened frequently over a long period in use.

No completely infallible test has yet been devised, and because of the length of time such tests as have been described take to complete, none but the most promising formulae can usually be subjected to them. This emphasizes the necessity for close attention to the prediction of preservative efficiency on a theoretical basis, and more realistic methods of component testing to aid preservative selection.

VIII. The Safe Use of Preservatives

Preservatives are more expensive than most other emulsion ingredients, and it is always advisable to use the lowest effective concentration. The cost, however, is secondary to the more important question of safety to the consumer.

If component testing to measure the efficacy of a certain preservative in the presence of chosen emulsion ingredients shows that several times the usual concentration is required to achieve the desired antimicrobial action because of physico-chemical binding, increased partitioning or factors influencing dissociation, it is wise to consider the toxicity of the preservative at the higher levels before proceeding. Although the preservative might be partially bound in the emulsion and the remaining fraction in the aqueous phase may represent no more than is safely used in other formulae, the ratio of bound to free preservative is very unlikely to remain unchanged when the product is used. Orally administered products will be changed on ingestion in such a way as to enable much of the total concentration of preservative to be absorbed by the gastro-intestinal tract. Thus from the point of view of toxicity, the *total* amount is important, in contrast to the considerations of preservation, where only that which is in an active form in the aqueous phase matters.

Similarly, emulsions which are applied to the skin will change in form during use; the water will evaporate and some of the preservative will become bound to the skin. This will disturb the original preservative equilibrium between the emulsion phases and may result in the liberation of preservative previously bound to the lipid phase or the emulsifier. In this way, preservative which was not available in the emulsion may become available on the skin and these high concentrations could well be toxic in use.

The concentrations at which preservatives cease to be safe in use have not been, and cannot be, defined, because there is no sharp dividing line between a toxic and a non-toxic concentration. There is, instead, a reasonably continuous spectrum of toxicity ranging from the very low concentrations to which very few people show any adverse reaction, to the high levels where both primary irritant and allergic responses will be much more numerous.

Primary irritation is a cutaneous inflammation brought about without the intervention of an antibody reaction. Although the mechanisms by which primary skin irritation occurs are not fully understood, it is believed that cutaneous inflammation is caused by interference with enzyme systems which are essential to the normal functioning of the skin. Strong primary irritants like mustard gas have been shown to interfere with enzyme systems such as hexokinase and pyruvate oxidase, but the mechanism of action of the many lesser irritants is not known. Many antimicrobial agents inhibit the metabolism of micro-organisms by interfering with their enzymatic activity, and many of the enzymes involved in microbial metabolism are the same as those present in the skin. It is thus likely that skin irritation brought about by contact with antiseptics and preservatives is caused at least in part by this mechanism, although others such as defatting of the skin probably operate as well.

Skin reactions which develop because of allergic sensitization only occur in certain hypersensitive individuals. These reactions are associated with certain genetic characteristics unlike the primary irritation response, which is non-specific. For example, almost everyone will react to the irritant effect of sulphuric acid on the skin, whereas only certain individuals react to traces of nickel or cobalt, which cause sensitization or allergic responses in some people. Rostenberg (1960) described a general scheme for the pathogenesis of allergic reactions. This indicated that the development of an eczematous sensitization requires, in addition to the allergen, a genetically appropriate individual. Table XV indicates that the two major factors in the genesis of any sensitization are (1) the intrinsic allergenicity of the compound, and (2) the genetic make-up of the host. The other factors influencing the reaction are the circumstances under which the subject comes into contact with the substance, and the concentration of the allergen.

Few of the preservatives used in emulsions are sensitizers at the very low concentrations normally necessary to prevent microbial spoilage, although, of course, isolated cases of reactions to well known compounds have inevitably occurred. Primary irritation is likewise extremely rare at the low levels used in the past.

With the advent of new emulsion ingredients which necessitate the use of either more powerful preservatives or higher concentrations of established compounds, new problems of toxicity may arise.

The toxicology of the *p*-hydroxybenzoate esters has been thoroughly studied and no primary irritation following their use at the usual preservative concentrations of up to about 0·3 per cent has been reported. For some years these esters have been used at between 5 and 10 per cent in powders, ointments and solutions to treat athlete's foot, and Bonnevie (1939) reported isolated cases of sensitization to the ethyl ester at high concentrations. Hjorth and Trolle-Lassen (1962) tested nineteen patients who had been sensitized to an ointment containing 14 per cent of mixed esters of *p*-hydroxybenzoate for their reactions to lower concentrations of each of the esters singly. Results with 0·5 and 0·1 per cent of the methyl, ethyl, propyl and benzyl esters showed very few reactions amongst the patients previously sensitized to very high concentrations. Hjorth concluded that sensitization is unlikely to be provoked by low concentrations, but the *p*-hydroxybenzoates used as preservatives may cause reactions in those previously sensitized by high levels.

Fryklof (1958) has reported skin reactions to sorbic acid used at the concentrations normally employed to preservative emulsions. The reaction appeared to be a primary irritation rather than a sensitization and was characterized by erythema and itching soon after application. It subsided and disappeared completely within 2 hours. Hjorth and Trolle-Lassen (1962) believe the current incidence of sensitivity to sorbic acid to be insignificant, but their studies of primary irritant reactions to this preservative tend to support those of Fryklof.

TABLE XV

Factors in the Genesis of Sensitization (from Rostenberg, 1960)

$$G^f . A^q \geqslant K = S$$

G = genetic make-up of host
A = intrinsic allergenicity of compound
f = adventitious factors influencing the ability of the host to be sensitized at the time
q = quantitative factors
k = some theoretical level which the product of $G^f . A^q$ must reach for a sensitization to be detectable clinically
S = detectable sensitivity

Sensitivity to mercury is widespread but Svendsen (1961) has shown that the organic mercury compounds do not always cause reactions in patients sensitized to mercury. Solutions of 0·1 per cent organic mercury compounds provoke primary irritant reactions in most people but 0·01 per cent appears bland in this respect. Sensitization to organic mercury compounds at the concentrations normally used as preservatives is rare, but there will be a greater risk of a higher incidence of both irritation and sensitization if higher concentrations are used in formulae which cannot be preserved with lower levels.

The quaternary ammonium compounds have been extensively tested for skin irritation and sensitizing properties. At concentrations below 0·1 per cent most of those commonly used as preservatives appear to cause little or no irritation, but Barail (1946, 1954) has demonstrated that higher concentrations cause erythema and drying of the skin. Resuggan (1952) examined the use of quaternaries as cosmetic preservatives and concluded that below 0·1 per cent they were safe, but might cause irritation at higher levels. Cruickshank and Squire (1949) have reported a number of cases of sensitization to cetrimide used at concentrations above 1 per cent.

Skin reactions to formaldehyde are very common, and it has not been extensively used as an emulsion preservative for many years. Nowadays it is tempting to revert to the use of formaldehyde because it is only slightly inactivated by non-ionic surface-active agents, but to do this might be a retrograde step.

There is comparatively little in the literature about the toxic thresholds of preservatives, partly because little research has been carried out, but mainly because the thresholds depend so much on the vehicle in which the preservative is incorporated. A certain concentration of a particular preservative may be quite harmless in one system, while the same level might evoke adverse skin responses in another because of the presence of substances which increase its penetration through the skin.

These problems introduce yet another dimension into the problems of preserving emulsions, and demand that the skill of the dermatologist or toxicologist be added to those of the physical chemist, and the microbiologist during the formulation of new emulsions which are difficult to preserve.

References

Aalto, T. R., Firman, M. C., and Rigler, N. E. (1953). *J. Amer. pharm. Ass., Sci. Ed.* **42**, 449.

Agar, A., and Alexander, A. E. (1949). *Trans. Faraday Soc.* **45**, 528.

Albert, A. (1942). *Lancet* **2**, 633.

Albert, A. (1945). *Brit. J. exp. Path.* **26**, 60.

Albert, A. (1951). "Selective Toxicity", Methuen Monograph. Methuen & Co., London.

Albert, A., Gibson, M. I., and Rubbo, S. D. (1953). *Brit. J. exp. Path.* **34**, 119.

Alexander, A. E., and Trim, A. R. (1946). *Proc. roy. Soc.* **B133**, 220.

Allawala, N. A., and Riegelman, S. (1953). *J. Amer. pharm. Ass., Sci. Ed.* **42**, 267.

Allawala, N. A., and Riegelman, S. (1954). *J. Amer. pharm. Ass., Sci. Ed.* **43**, 93.

Atkins, F. (1950). *Mfg Chem.* **21**, 51.

Autian, J., and Shaikh, Z. I. (1960). *Drug Stand.* **28**, 103.

Babicka, J. (1957). *Les Nouvelles Esthetiques* June–July 10.

Baker, J. H. (1959). *J. Soc. cosmet. Chem.* **10**, 133.

Baker, Z., Harrison, R. W., and Miller, B. F. (1941). *J. exp. Med.* **74**, 621.

Bandelin, F. J. (1958). *J. Amer. pharm. Ass., Sci. Ed.* **47**, 691.

Barail, L. G. (1946). *Amer. Dyest. Rep.* **35**, 521.

Barail, L. G. (1954). *Soap.* **30**, No. 8 149.

Barr, M., and Tice, L. F. (1957a). *J. Amer. pharm. Ass., Sci. Ed.* **46**, 217.

Barr, M., and Tice, L. F. (1957b). *J. Amer. pharm. Ass., Sci. Ed.* **46**, 219.

Barr, M., and Tice, L. F. (1957c). *J. Amer. pharm. Ass., Sci. Ed.* **46**, 221.

Barr, M., and Tice, L. F. (1957d). *J. Amer. pharm. Ass., Sci. Ed.* **46**, 442.

Barr, M., and Tice, L. F. (1957e). *J. Amer. pharm. Ass., Sci. Ed.* **46**, 445.
Bean, H. S., and Berry, H. (1951). *J. Pharm., Lond.* **3**, 639.
Bean, H. S., and Berry, H. (1953). *J. Pharm., Lond.* **5**, 632.
Bean, H. S., Richards, J. P., and Thomas, J. (1962). *Boll. chim-farm.* **101**, 339.
Beckett, A. H., and Robinson, A. E. (1958). *Soap Perfum. Cosm.* **31**, 454.
Beckett, A. H., Vahora, A. A., and Robinson, A. E. (1958a). *J. Pharm., Lond. Suppl.* **10**, 160T.
Beckett, A. H., Patki, S. J., and Robinson, A. E. (1958b). *Nature, Lond.* **181**, 712.
Beckett, A. H., Patki, S. J., and Robinson, A. E. (1959). *J. Pharm., Lond.* **11**, 421.
Bell, T. A., Etchells, J. L., and Borg, A. F. (1959). *J. Bact.* **77**, 573.
Bennett, E. C. (1962). "Developments in Industrial Microbiology", Vol. 3, p. 273. Plenum Press, New York.
Blaug, S. M., and Ahsan, S. S. (1961a). *J. pharm. Sci.* **50**, 138.
Blaug, S. M., and Ahsan, S. S. (1961b). *J. pharm. Sci.* **50**, 441.
Block, S. S. (1956). *Appl. Microbiol.* **4**, 183.
Boehm, E. (1933a). *Parfum. mod.* **27**, 373, 478.
Boehm, E. (1933b). *Drug Cosmet. Ind.* **32**, 510, 591.
Boehm, E., and Jones, E. (1957). *J. Soc. cosmet. Chem.* **8**, 1.
Bolle, A., and Mirimanoff, A. (1950). *J. Pharm., Lond.* **2**, 685.
Bonnevie, P. (1939). "Aetiologie und Pathogenese der Eksemkrankheiten". Busck, Copenhagen.
Bouchardy, M., and Mirimanoff, A. (1951). *Pharm. acta. Helv.* **26**, 69.
Briggs, A., and Cook, A. M. (1962). Paper presented to the Second Congress of the International Federation of Societies of Cosmetic Chemists. Pergamon Press, Oxford.
Bullock, K., and Keepe, W. G. (1951). *Pharm. J.* **167**, 188.
Chakovskoy, M., and Van Nechel (1956). *Bull. soc. chim. belge* **65**, 453.
Charles, R. D., and Carter, P. J. (1959). *J. soc. cosmet. Chem.* **10**, 383.
Cruickshank, C. N. D., and Squire, J. R. (1949). *Brit. J. industr. Med.* **6**, 164.
Cruickshank, G. A. (1956). *T.A.P.P.I.* **39**, 857.
Davies, G. E. (1949). *J. Hyg.* **47**, 271.
Davis, J. G. (1960). *J. Pharm., Lond. Suppl.* **12**, 29T.
Deeb, E. N., and Boenigh, J. W. (1958). *J. Amer. pharm. Ass., Sci. Ed.* **47**, 807.
Deeley, S. (1962). "Developments in Industrial Microbiology", Vol. 3, p. 267. Plenum Press, New York.
DeGray, R. J., and Killian, L. N. (1962). "Developments in Industrial Microbiology", Vol. 3, p. 296. Plenum Press, New York.
Deluca, P. P., and Kostenbauder, H. B. (1960). *J. Amer. pharm. Ass., Sci. Ed.* **49**, 430.
de Navarre, M. G. (1957). *J. Soc. cosmet. Chem.* **8**, 371.
de Navarre, M. G. (1959). *Amer. Perfum. Arom.* **73**, 40.
de Navarre, M. G. (1962). "The Chemistry and Manufacture of Cosmetics", 2nd edn. Vol. 2. 257 pp. D. Van Nostrand Co. Inc., Princeton, New Jersey.
de Navarre, M. G., and Bailey, H. E. (1956). *J. Soc. cosmet. Chem.* **7**, 427.
Einola, S. (1955). *Ann. Med. exp. Biol. Fenniae Suppl.* **33** suppl. 8, 54. pp.
Eisman, P. C. (1954). *Bull. Parent. Drug. Ass.* **8**, 1.
Eisman, P. C., Cooper, J., and Jaconia, D. (1957). *J. Amer. pharm. Ass., Sci. Ed.* **46**, 144.
Engler, V., and Mirimanoff, A. (1951). *Pharm. acta Helv.* **26**, 59.
Entrekin, D. N. (1961). *J. pharm. Sci.* **50**, 743.
Erlandson, A. L., and Lawrence, C. A. (1953). *Science* **118**, 274.

Ferguson, J. (1939). *Proc. roy. Soc. (Biol. Sci.)* *B***127,** 387.
Foter, M. J., and Nisonger, L. L. (1950). *Ann. N.Y. Acad. Sci.* **53,** 112.
Fryklof, L. E. (1958). *J. Pharm., Lond.* **10,** 719.
Gale, E. F., and Taylor, E. S. (1947). *J. gen. Microbiol.* **1,** 77.
Gershenfeld, L., and Pearlstein, D. (1939). *Amer. J. Pharm.* **111,** 277.
Gershenfeld, L., and Stedman, R. L. (1949). *Amer. J. Pharm.* **121,** 249.
Gingras, B. (1957). *Canad. J. Chem.* **35,** 599.
Glassman, H. N. (1950). *Ann. N.Y. Acad. Sci.* **53** (1) 91.
Goldstein, S. W. (1952). *J. Amer. pharm. Ass., Prac. Pharm. Ed.* **13,** 250.
Goodhart, F. W., and Martin, A. N. (1962). *J. pharm. Sci.* **51,** 50.
Gregg, R. M., and Zopf, L. C. (1951). *J. Amer. pharm. Ass., Sci. Ed.* **40,** 390.
Griffin, W. C. (1954). *J. Soc. cosmet. Chem.* **5,** 249.
Gundersen, K., and Jensen, H. L. (1956). *Acta Agric. scand.* **6,** 100.
Guttman, D., and Higuchi, T. (1955). *J. Amer. pharm. Ass., Sci. Ed.* **44,** 668.
Guttman, D., and Higuchi, T. (1956). *J. Amer. pharm. Ass., Sci. Ed.* **45,** 659.
Hadgraft, J. W. (1954). *J. Pharm., Lond.* **6,** 816.
Hall, C. S., and de Navarre, M. G. (1957). *Proc. sci. Sect. T.G.A.* No. 27. 29.
Hall, L. (1938). *Food Ind.* **10,** 424.
Hampil, B. (1928). *J. Bact.* **16,** 287.
Harris, W. A. (1961). *Aust. J. Pharm.* **42,** 583.
Hauser, E. A. (1950). *Ann. N.Y. Acad. Sci.* **53** (1) 18.
Herbold, M. (1943). *Amer. Perfum.* **45,** 36.
Hibbot, H. W., and Monks, J. (1961). *J. Soc. cosmet. Chem.* **12,** 2.
Higuchi, T., and Lach, J. L. (1954). *J. Amer. pharm. Ass., Sci. Ed.* **43,** 465.
Higuchi, T., Patel, K. P., Bonow, E. R., and Landsman, J. (1952). *J. Amer. pharm. Ass., Sci. Ed.* **41,** 293.
Hjorth, N., and Trolle-Lassen, C. (1962). *Amer. Perfum.* **77,** 43.
Hotchkiss, R. D. (1946a). *Ann. N.Y. Acad. Sci.* **46,** 479.
Hotchkiss, R. D. (1946b). *Ann. N.Y. Acad. Sci.* **46,** 377.
Hsiao, L., Dunning, H. N., and Lorenz, P. B. (1956). *J. phys. Chem.* **60,** 657.
Huppert, M. (1957). *Antibiotics Chemother.* **7,** 29.
Ingram, M., Ottaway, F. J. H., and Coppock, J. B. M. (1956). *Chem. & Ind.* **42,** 1154.
Jones, P. S., Thigpen, D., Morrison, J. L., and Richardson, A. P. (1956). *J. Amer. pharm. Ass., Sci. Ed.* **45,** 268.
Judis, J. (1962). *J. pharm. Sci.* **51,** 261.
Kamakaka, T. R. (1956). "Studies on the Bacterial Population of Two Phase Systems." Ph.D. Thesis, London.
Karabinos, J. V., Kapella, G. E., Ferlin, H. J., and Sawhill, D. L. (1955). *Euclides* **15,** 253.
Kim, H. K., and Autian, J. (1960). *J. Amer. pharm. Ass., Sci. Ed.* **49,** 227.
Kostenbauder, H. B. (1960). *Am. Perfumer* **75,** 28.
Kostenbauder, H. B. (1962). "Developments in Industrial Microbiology", Vol. 3. p. 286. Plenum Press, New York.
Kostenbauder, H. B., and Higuchi, T. (1956). *J. Amer. pharm. Ass., Sci. Ed.* **45,** 518.
Lachman, L., Weinstein, S., Hopkins, G., Slack, S., Eisman, P., and Cooper, J. (1962). *J. pharm. Sci.* **51,** 224.
Lawrence, C. A. (1950). *Ann. N.Y. Acad. Sci.* **53,** 66.
Lawrence, C. A., and Erlandson, A. L. (1953). *J. Amer. pharm. Ass., Sci. Ed.* **42,** 352.
Littlejohn, O. M., and Husa, W. J. (1955). *J. Amer. pharm. Ass., Sci. Ed.* **44,** 305.

Lord, C. F., and Husa, W. (1954). *J. Amer. pharm. Ass., Sci. Ed.* **43**, 438.
Maccacaro, G. A. (1961)."Progress in Industrial Microbiology", Vol. **3**, Heywood & Co., London.
Manowitz, M. (1961). "Developments in Industrial Microbiology", Vol. 2, p. 65. Plenum Press, New York.
Marcus, A. D., Wetstein, E., and Ruderman, M. (1956). *J. Amer. pharm. Ass. Pract. Pharm. Ed.* **17**, 453.
Marcus, E., Kim, H. K., and Autian, J. (1959). *J. Amer. pharm. Ass., Sci. Ed.* **48**, 457.
Matthews, C., Davidson, J., Bauer, E., Morrison, J. L., and Richardson, A. P. (1956). *J. Amer. pharm. Ass., Sci. Ed.* **45**, 260.
Maurice, P. (1952). *Proc. Soc. appl. Bact.* **15**, 144.
Meyers, D. B., Nadkarni, M. V., and Zopf, L. C. (1950). *J. Amer. pharm. Ass. Prac. Pharm. Ed.* **11**, 32.
Miller, B. F., Baker, Z., and Harrison, R. W. (1939). *Proc. Soc. exp. Biol.* **42**, 705.
Miyawaki, G. M., Patel, N. K., and Kostenbauder, H. B. (1959). *J. Amer. pharm. Ass., Sci. Ed.* **48**, 315.
Moore, C. D., and Hardwick, R. B. (1956). *Mfg. Chem.* **27**, 305.
Mulley, B. A., and Metcalf, A. D. (1956). *J. Pharm., Lond.* **8**, 774.
Neidig, C. P., and Burrell, H. (1944). *Drug Cosmet. Ind.* **54**, 408, 481.
Newton, B. A. (1960). *J. appl. Bact.* **23**, 345.
Okabayashi, T. (1953). *J. Ferment. Technol.* **31**, 292.
Okazaki, O., and Oshima, O. (1953). *J. pharm. Soc. Japan* **73**, 344.
Osman, H. G., and El-Mariah, A. (1960). *J. Amer. pharm. Ass., Sci. Ed.* **49**, 231.
Patel, N. K., and Kostenbauder, H. B. (1958). *J. Amer. pharm. Ass., Sci. Ed.* **47**, 289.
Pisano, F. D., and Kostenbauder, H. B. (1959). *J. Amer. pharm. Ass., Sci. Ed.* **48**, 310.
Poprzan, J., and de Navarre, M. G. (1959). *J. Soc. cosmet. Chem.* **10**, 81.
Price, P. B. (1950). *Ann. N.Y. Acad. Sci.* **53**, 76.
Prickett, P. S., Murray, H. C., and Mercer, N. H. (1961). *J. pharm. Sci.* **50**, 316.
Quisno, R. A., Irvin, W. G., and Foter, M. J. (1946). *J. Amer. pharm. Ass., Sci. Ed.* **45**, 317.
Rdzok, E. J., Grundy, W. E., Kirchmeyer, F. J., and Sylvester, J. C. (1955). *J. Amer. pharm. Ass., Sci. Ed.* **44**, 613.
Resuggan, W. L. (1952). *Soap Perfum. Cosm.* **25**, 610.
Ritter, H. W. (1956). *Appl. Microbiol.* **4**, 114.
Rostenberg, A. (1960). *J. Soc. cosmet. Chem.* **11**, 170.
Royce, A., and Sykes, G. (1957). *J. Pharm., Lond.* **9**, 814.
Sabalitschka, Th., and Boehm, E. (1929). *Arch. Pharm., Berl.* **267**, 272.
Sagarin, H. (1957). "Cosmetics: Science and Technology." Interscience Publishers Inc., New York.
Sawyer, C. N., and Ryckman, D. W. (1957). *J. Amer. Wat. Wks Ass.* **49**, 480.
Schick, M. J., Atlas, S. M., and Eirich, F. R. (1962). *J. phys. Chem.* **66**, 1326.
Schimmel, J., and Husa, W. J. (1956). *J. Amer. pharm. Ass., Sci. Ed.* **45**, 204.
Shafiroff, I. (1961). *Soap and Chem. Spec.* **37**, 75.
Simon, J. (1952). *New Phytol.* **51–52**, 163.
Sokolski, W. T., Chidester, C. G., and Honeywell, G. E. (1962). "Developments in Industrial Microbiology", Vol. 3, p. 179 Plenum Press, New York.
Svendsen, I. B. (1961). *Acta derm-venerol., Stockh.* **41**, 150.
Tamamushi, B., and Tamaki, K. (1959). *Trans. Faraday Soc.* **55**, 1007.
Tice, L. F., and Barr, M. (1958). *J. Soc. cosmet. Chem.* **9**, 171.

Tillman, W. J., and Kuramoto, R. (1957). *J. Amer. pharm. Ass., Sci. Ed.* **46**, 211.
Von Schelhorn, M. (1952). *Dtsch. LebensmittRdsch.* **48**, 15.
Von Schelhorn, M. (1953). *Food Technol., Champaign* **7**, 97.
Wagner, R. (1914). *Z. Gärphysiol.* **4**, 289.
Wailes, J. L. (1962). *J. pharm. Sci.* **51**, 165.
Walker, N. (1954). *Plant & Soil* **5**, 194.
Wedderburn, D. L. (1958). *J. Soc. cosmet. Chem.* **9**, 210.
Wolf, P. A., and Westveer, W. M. (1950). *Arch. Biochem.* **28**, 201.
Wyss, O. (1948). "Advances in Food Research", Vol. I, 373 pp. Academic Press Inc., New York.

CONTEMPORARY TRENDS IN HEAT STERILIZATION

G. R. Wilkinson and L. C. Baker
Allen & Hanburys Ltd., London, England

I. Historical

Although Pasteur in 1878 (Vallery-Radot, 1911) first outlined the requirements for achieving sterility, Schroeder and Von Dusch (1854) had made use of an early type of pressure cooker to bring about the sterilization of foods. Considerable activity took place about this period and Koch in 1880 (Perkins, 1956) modified an autoclave originally built by Charles Chamberland to produce the first practical equipment. This was used largely for biological and bacteriological media and it was in 1885 that Schimmelbusch (Perkins, 1956) made use of similar equipment for the sterilization of surgical dressings.

Although a number of workers examined the ways in which sterilization could be brought about, no positive work on the pharmaceutical use was carried out until 1944, when Savage (1944) investigated means by which surgical dressings could be rendered sterile with more certainty than previously achieved.

II. Time and Temperature Relationships

It fell to Rahn (1945) to examine the physical phenomena associated with sterilization and to propound the opinion that the curve relating the time at a temperature to kill bacteria was logarithmic and consistent with a first order reaction. An extremely important feature of his work has been overlooked until more recent times that statistically all bacteria cannot be killed, although the number of survivors may become very small. Examining a large number of organisms he determined the heat resistances of different species at the same temperature or the one species at the one temperature. He found that these figures were closely related and although not scientifically precise, it was possible to forecast the behaviour of specific organisms under specified circumstances. He eventually evolved a formula:

$$K_1 t_1 = \log \frac{\text{initial number}}{\text{survivors}} = K_2 t_2$$

the organisms which will develop very slowly after heat treatment and transfer to a suitable medium. If an enzyme or a single cell had been destroyed they would not exhibit this behaviour. Martin (1950) and Collier and Townsend (1956) have examined the effect of superheated steam and dry gases but have not elucidated the mechanisms of the method of kill.

The greater difficulty in killing spores has been considered to be due to a tough skin surrounding the protoplasm acting as an insulator and so preventing a necessary amount of energy to bring about denaturing of the protein reaching the centre of the spore.

IV. Determination of the Efficiency of Sterilization

Since the thermal death curve of bacteria is logarithmic, the efficiency of sterilization can be assessed by exhibiting a population of organisms with a known thermal death point to the sterilizing procedure and determining the number of survivors after selected periods. This is a much more satisfactory method than applying sterility tests to the product. This can be carried out in a number of ways, dependent upon the process being employed and the type of product undergoing control.

Spores of an organism such as *B. stearothermophilus*, after treatment at 85° C in water for 10 min, are shaken with glass beads and then poured through a plug of glass wool to remove aggregates. This suspension can be concentrated and washed by centrifuging, then redispersed in alcohol kept at 4° C. It may then be diluted with half-strength Ringer's solution and 5 per cent serum added. By using suitable dilutions volumes can be spread on aluminium foil so that a population of about 10^8 organisms is available for each sample. When dried at 56° C for 4 h they may be stored in paper envelopes or in screw-cap jars.

To recover the organisms after a test the foil can be shaken with glass beads and half-strength Ringer's and afterwards spread onto agar plates. This will give a suitable count if the organisms do not exceed 100 per plate for accurate work. If only approximations of the efficiency of an established method are required the foil can be dropped into a tube of broth, which is then cultured for a positive or negative growth (Kelsey, 1962).

If the survival curves are plotted it is possible to determine the time required to bring about the necessary degree of killing and for practical purposes the reduction brought about by 4 to 5 log phases is considered necessary (see Fig. 1). The British Pharmacopoeia requirement is about 3 for some organisms. Work is being carried out using P.V.A. cast film in which organisms can be suspended as a means for the ready recovery of viable organisms, as there is some little doubt as to whether all surviving organisms can be washed from the surface of aluminium foil.

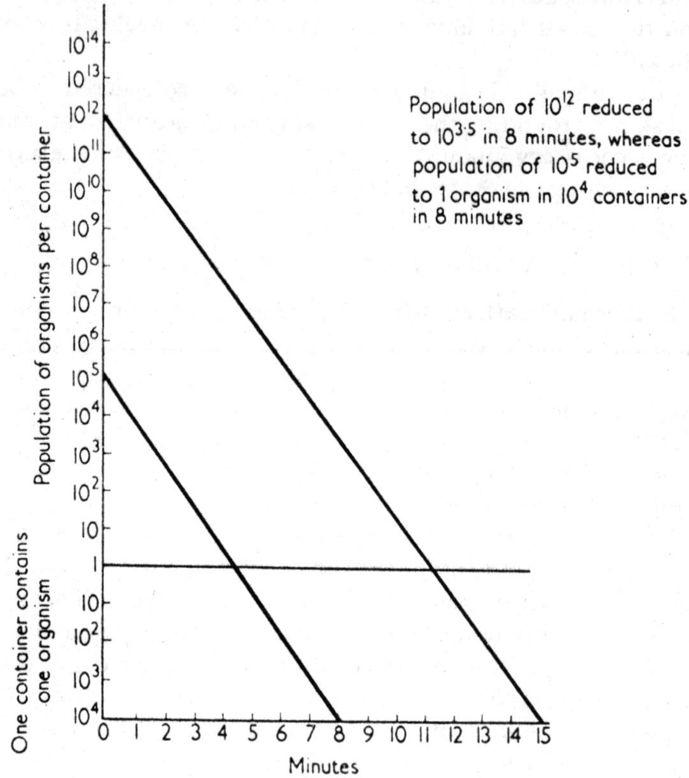

FIG. 1. Survival curve of bacteria at a constant sterilizing temperature.

V. Criticism of Sterility Tests

From consideration of curves produced from sterilizing times and numbers of survivors it can be seen (Powell, 1962) how a small number of organisms can remain dispersed in a large number of containers. Sterility tests can fail to pick up a chance contamination in a batch of solutions which have been sterilized, or suggest a level of contamination which does not reflect the facts. If the degree of contamination is such that 1 per cent of the containers, each of 1 l, contains one organism, the chances of proving this container non-sterile is one in 100,000, compared with the 0·2 or 0·3 per cent chance contamination which can occur during the practical manipulations required for such a sterility test (Fig. 1).

VI. Thermodynamic Considerations

Following from Rahn's work showing that sterilization by moist heat appears to follow a logarithmic function, it should be possible to calculate the rate of kill or the death rate constant k:

$$k = \frac{2 \cdot 303}{t} \log \frac{\text{initial bacteria}}{\text{bacteria at time } t}$$

This has been tested experimentally and closely follows the theoretical consideration. Higuchi and Busse (1950) were responsible and in 1952 Pfeifer and Vojnovich extended the basic observations into the realms of thermodynamics, evolving the formula:

$$\log {}^{t}d = \frac{0 \cdot 219E}{T} + K$$

E is the heat of activation and is in the range of 50 to 100 kcal for the most resistant micro-organisms and spores.

When organisms and spores are present in liquid or semi-solid aqueous media, other factors have an influence on the time required for sterilization. The pH of maximum heat tolerance is between 5 and 8 and up to 8 per cent of salts can also cause an increase in resistance.

VII. Inactivation of Viruses

The heat inactivation of viruses will not be discussed except to say that the causative organism of infective hepatitis which will withstand 10 h heating at 60° C is destroyed by the usual steam-sterilizing procedures (Neefe, 1946).

VIII. Sterilization at Sub-atmospheric Pressures

Work published by Alder and Gillespie (1961), who have been investigating the effect of steam at sub-atmospheric pressures with and without formalin, have produced results which at present do not fit into the present theories of sterilization by moist heat. By evacuating the chamber and introducing steam to absolute pressures just under 1 atm and keeping the temperature constant at about 100° C by means of heat from the jacket, they have been able to kill a number of strains of organisms, particularly staphylococci. It has also been shown that the same organisms will resist boiling water for very much longer periods. No theory has been advanced in explanation but this method provides a means of disinfecting easily damaged articles such as blankets.

IX. Materials of Pharmaceutical Interest Requiring Sterilization

The design of sterilizers is dependent upon the type of material which it is required to sterilize. If a sterilizer is used for a number of purposes for widely differing types of material, the design must be a compromise. Alternatively, small modifications which apparently increase its usability can render it almost useless. As far as pharmaceutical products are concerned they fall largely into the following types of preparations, some of which require special treatment during sterilization:

(*a*) Perfusion fluids or electrolytes.
(*b*) Topical fluids for use in operating theatres, wards and by patients in their own homes.
(*c*) Topically applied medicaments.
(*d*) Solutions for irrigation.
(*e*) Eye-drops and eye lotions.
(*f*) Parenteral injections
 (i) ampoules
 (ii) single-dose containers
 (iii) multi-dose containers.
(*g*) Sterilized powders.
(*h*) Sterilized creams, ointments and oils.
(*j*) Instruments.
(*k*) Glassware.
(*m*) Fabrics and dressings.
(*n*) Mixed loads and rubber tubing.

X. Basis of Autoclave Design

The simplest type of autoclave consists of a vessel which can be closed and in which steam can either be generated by introducing water and heating it with gas or electricity. Air is eliminated by a vent and pressure controlled by a safety valve or thermostat. For larger equipment a separate boiler is required and Fig. 2 gives the general arrangement of such an autoclave, which was in common use for all sterilization purposes and was only superseded for fabrics and perfusion fluids about 1955.

Once loaded and the steam turned on air is eliminated through a vent or the steam trap, which, once the load has reached about 100°, is closed and allows pressure to build up within the chamber.

The steam boiler required falls outside the scope of the present discussion, except to say that it must be capable of producing dry saturated steam at a pressure greater than that demanded in the autoclave.

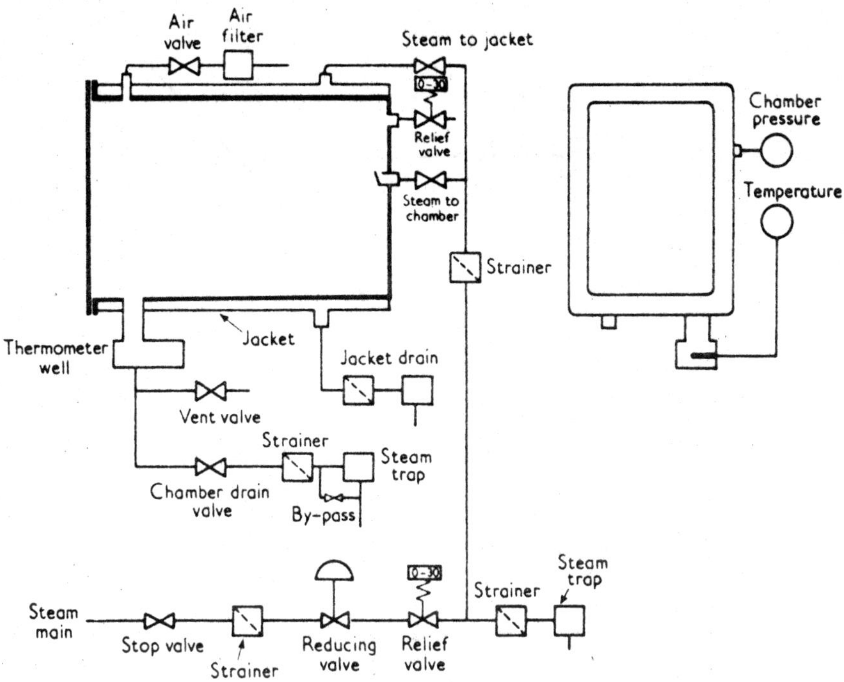

FIG. 2. Basic connections of a typical low pressure steam autoclave. The various features indicated are mentioned in the text.

XI. Steam

Steam is valuable for this pharmaceutical procedure, as it:

(*a*) has a high heat content,
(*b*) gives up this heat readily and at constant temperature,
(*c*) is clean and odourless,
(*d*) heats rapidly,
(*e*) penetrates fabrics,
(*f*) is cheap.

Steam is water vapour devoid of air under pressure, and its temperature is closely related to the pressure at which it exists. If steam is kept at the same pressure and heated to a higher temperature it is then said to be superheated. On the other hand, if there are suspended water droplets throughout the steam it is said to be wet or supersaturated.

The dryness of the steam is expressed in terms of a fraction and 1·0 is taken as dry saturated steam. A figure greater than 1·0 indicates superheat and a figure lower than 1·0 wetness. For practical sterilization purposes it is necessary to have steam in the region of 0·9 to 1·0 dryness

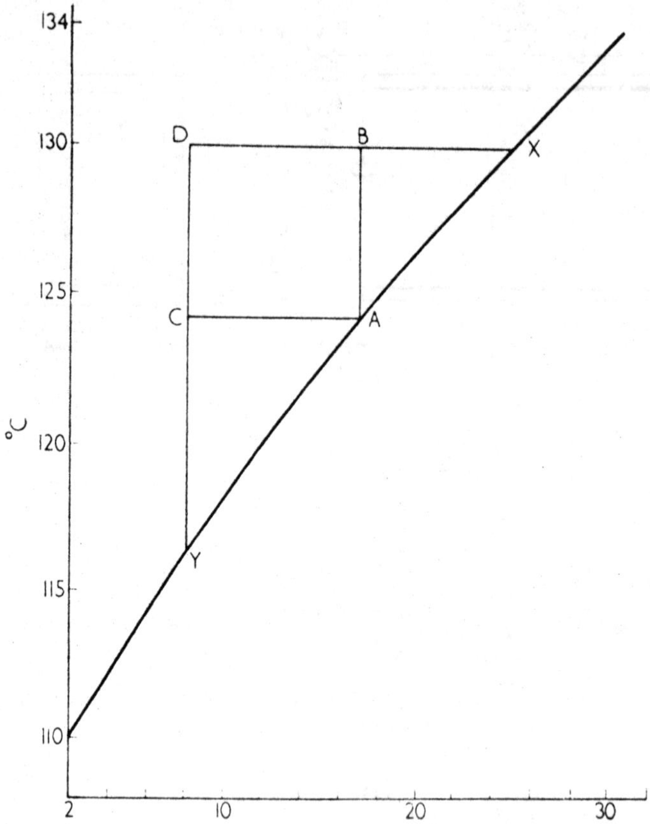

FIG. 3. Diagram showing the relation between pressure and temperature in steam. Steam at any point on the curve, such as point A, is saturated. If its temperature is raised to B, keeping pressure constant, it becomes superheated. If its pressure is lowered to C, keeping temperature constant, it is again superheated. If both events occur, it may reach a point such as D. This point can also be reached (*a*) by lowering the pressure of saturated steam from point X, or (*b*) by raising the temperature of saturated steam from point Y, the final state being exactly the same. The lowering of partial pressure may just as well be effected by mixing air with the steam, at the same total pressure, as by lowering the total pressure in pure steam (from Savage, 1959).

fraction (see Fig. 3). Superheated steam behaves more like a true gas and before it can be used to heat objects within a sterilizer must cool to saturated steam temperature. It is therefore inefficient as a source of heat. At saturated steam temperature, steam meeting a cold object gives up its latent heat and is converted to water at the same temperature. The dryness fraction can be determined by simple calorimetry. A large vessel full of water (20 to 50 gal) is counter-balanced on a platform scale and its temperature taken. Steam is then introduced by means of a pipe reaching the bottom and the rise in temperature recorded when a certain weight has been introduced. Reference to steam tables will give the amount of heat the steam should have produced and this can be compared with that actually produced. For further details of the method consult Lyle (1947). The heat is absorbed by the articles and causes them to be heated. It is because of this latent heat being readily available that steam is such a good heating agent for sterilization.

XII. Effect of Air during Sterilization and its Removal

Air need not be eliminated during sterilization procedures. Except when fabrics are being sterilized the pressure of air has no bad effects so long as thermometers are used to measure the temperature (Hoyt *et al.*, 1939; Savage, 1944). If the temperature is deduced from the pressure within the chamber, since both the air and steam will exert their own partial pressures, an erroneous reading will result (Gosset *et al.*, 1935). At 30 lb/in^2 10 per cent of air will produce 268° instead of 274°.

When fluids such as in categories (*a*) to (*f*) in Section IX are being sterilized, it is advantageous to introduce the steam in a turbulent manner so that it mixes with the air and brings about uniform heating through the load (Wilkinson and Peacock, 1961b) and care must be taken that steam does not impinge directly onto the containers, otherwise breakages due to a thermal shock can occur. Until the temperature of the load reaches 100° C it is possible to keep vents open to the atmosphere through which air can be eliminated, as all the steam is condensed within the chamber and none emerges until the load approaches 100° C.

If air is entrained in the incoming steam during the remainder of the sterilizing period it is liberated as the steam condenses and finds its way to the bottom of the chamber and can be eliminated by a suitable steam trap. Such a steam trap is known as a balanced-pressure thermostatic type, and has the advantage that it can be used over the range of sterilizing temperatures without adjustment. It consists of a bellows filled with a mixture of alcohol and water, which in contact with steam expands and holds the outlet valve closed (see Fig. 4). Since condensate is normally at the same temperature as the steam in the chamber it can be arranged to be a little cooler by mounting the trap at the end of about 2 ft of tubing, radiation from its outer walls bringing about the cooling effect. At the slightly lower temperature the bellows will contract, open the valve and allow the condensate to run out until replaced by steam. Steam will then cause the bellows again to expand and close the vent. This type of trap will eliminate large amounts of air until the bellows become heated, then they will not open when presented with small amounts of air. To eliminate small quantities of air it is usual to fit a by-pass to this type of trap. This may waste a little steam but ensures that the chamber is kept air-free. If the distance between the chamber and trap is reduced erratic behaviour can occur.

The temperature of the load lags considerably behind that of the chamber and this must be borne in mind when determining a suitable

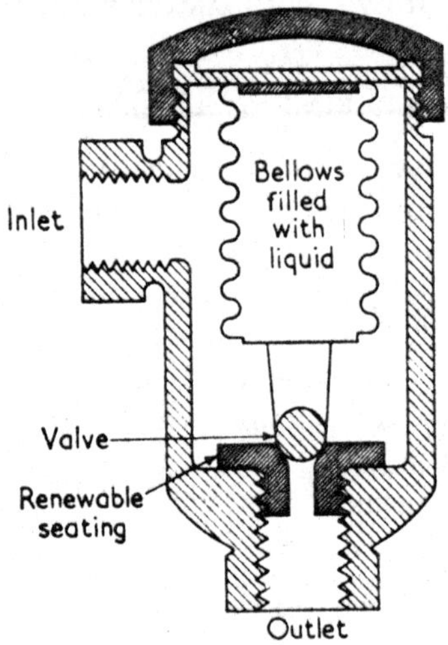

FIG. 4. Diagrammatic representation of a balance pressure thermostatic steam trap.

heating up and sterilizing period at a particular temperature. The rate of heating is dependent upon the pressure at which steam is supplied to the chamber from the main and this must also be controlled, otherwise varying rates of heating, and thus sterilization times, can be brought about, as it is the flow rate of the steam at this part of the cycle that is important. Buchi (1941) drew attention to the rate of heating in different sized containers and in highly viscous fluids, but this information was apparently overlooked until recently. This has been reflected in recommendations for the revision of the method for sterilizing fluids according to the British Pharmacopoeia. The previous wording could have lead to inadequate sterilization should certain fluids have heavy contamination and consideration not given to the question of viscosity.

Many present-day sterilizers are fitted with the bucket type of steam trap, where a float on the surface of the condensate controls the exit valve (see Fig. 5). Once sufficient condensate collects the float rises and opens the valve, and thereby allows it to escape. The level is lowered, the float then sinks and the valve shuts, so preventing any escape of steam. This procedure is repeated as long as condensate is being formed. This type of trap is extremely inefficient as regards the elimination of air.

Other steam traps make use of a bimetallic strip. These depend upon the temperature difference between the condensate and steam, bending and flexing a collection of bimetal elements which in turn open and close

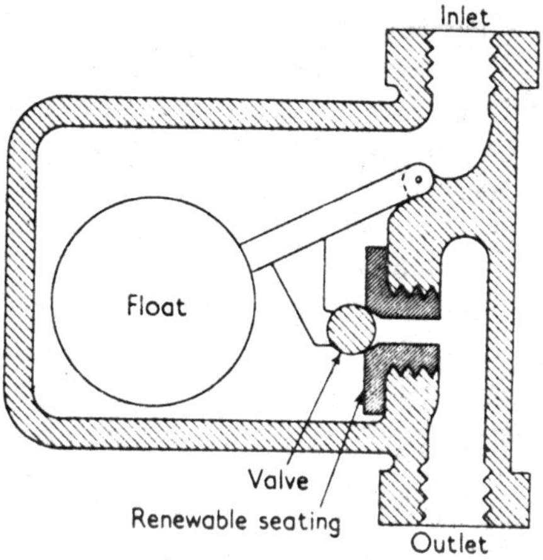

FIG. 5. Diagrammatic representation of a float operated steam trap.

a valve. This usually requires to be adjusted for each working pressure and is therefore inconvenient to use.

XIII. Protection against Undue Pressure

A pressure-relief valve set to 110 per cent of working pressure should be connected directly with the chamber to provide protection against undue pressure developing within the chamber and causing an explosion.

XIV. Cooling the Load within an Autoclave

When using small containers such as ampoules, because of their high specific surface, the rate of heating and cooling is fairly rapid and there is not much delay in being able to open the sterilizer safely. When containers of fluids are not hermetically sealed during the heating-up process, steam condenses inside them, heating the liquid and increasing its volume. If the pressure is slightly released this extra volume of water boils off and extracts the latent heat required from the rest of the liquid in the containers, the volume returning to its original value. This boiling off considerably reduces the temperature of the fluid and in most instances no further boiling takes place once atmospheric pressure has been achieved. This is not practicable, obviously, when dealing with sealed containers.

In the case of perfusion fluids, category (*a*) above, where an autoclave may hold 200 or 300 full 1-litre bottles, although the heating conditions are very similar, cooling can be protracted and may take as much as 16 or 24 h before the temperature falls to a point at which no pressure exists inside the bottles. The cooling can occur only by radiation from the containers and conduction through the walls of the autoclave. Under these circumstances it has been found advantageous to cool the bottles artificially. Various means have been employed, such as pumping compressed air through the chamber. This causes a certain amount of cooling, but because of its low specific heat, heat can be conveyed away from the bottles slowly. The alternative of using cold water suffered from the disadvantage that thermal shock to glass bottles caused breakages if a large temperature difference were used; if the temperature differential was reduced by heating the water the rate of cooling fell also (Wilkinson *et al.*, 1960). Means have been found of supplying water in the form of a very fine mist and by adjusting the flow of water to the rate at which heat is transferred through the glass from the contents, thermal shock can be avoided and bottles can be cooled rapidly. This principle has been made use of in equipment designed specifically for large volumes of fluids (Wilkinson *et al.*, 1960).

The autoclave is orthodox in construction except for an extra entry for cooling water and an oversize bucket-type steam trap. The arrangement is shown in Fig. 6*a*. When the steam is turned on a vent opens, through which the air is displaced by the incoming steam as the load temperature approaches 100°. This vent shuts when the temperature reaches 100°. Pressure builds up and heating by means of steam condensing continues for the sterilizing period and at this point in time the steam is turned off. Provision is then made for the introduction of compressed air at the same pressure as the steam within the chamber to prevent a vacuum forming when the steam is condensed by the incoming water, which is then applied to the spray heads within the sterilizer and the mist produced cools the load. The cooling period can be predetermined as long as the load is kept constant. Fuller details of this control equipment will be given later.

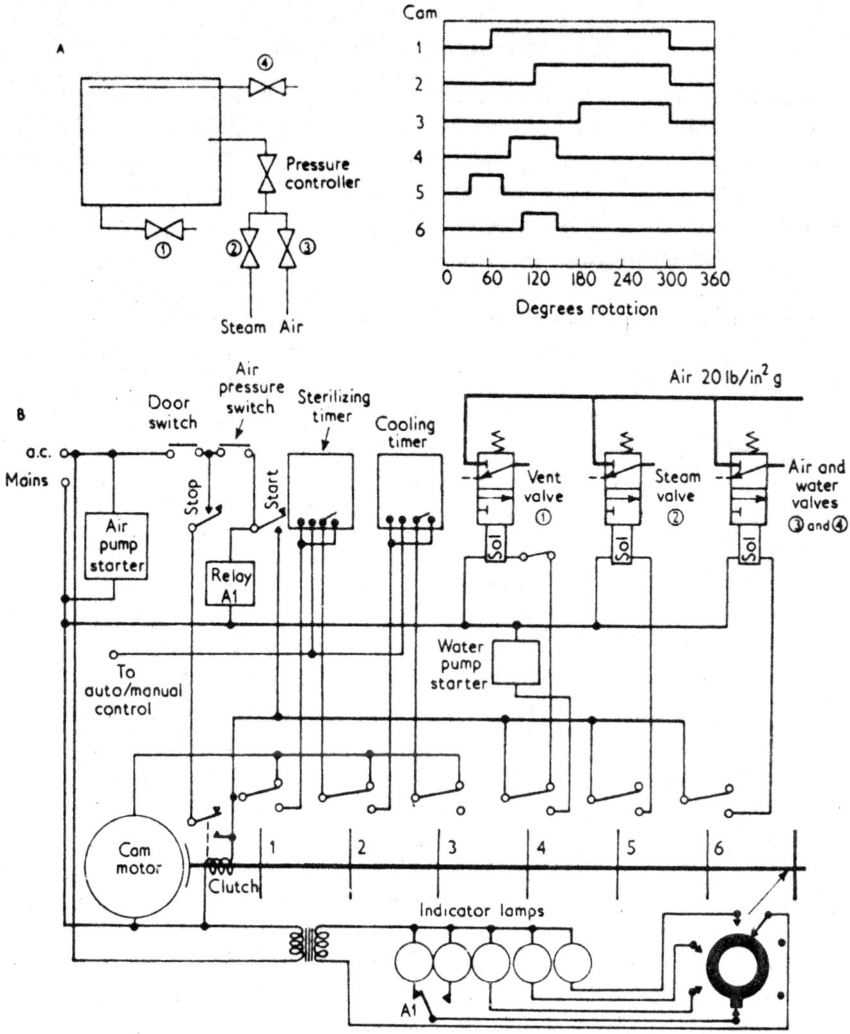

FIG. 6. (*a*) Arrangement of connections and valves required for automatic control of mist cooled fluids autoclave and a diagram of the sequence of operation of the valves. (*b*) Circuit of controller.

The advantages of this rapid cooling process are:

(*a*) The bottles are removed in a safe condition and are not liable to explode.

(*b*) There is much less damage to thermolabile materials such as glucose saline.

(*c*) The bottles can be handled readily immediately upon removal.

(*d*) The process is simplified and can be made completely automatic.

XV. Sterilization of Fabrics

Fabrics and dressing present many more difficulties, particularly that of steam penetration. To ensure certainty of penetration and bring about sterilization, steam must penetrate to every portion of the load and although this can be achieved by displacing the air by steam under the effect of gravity, the sterilizing period becomes uneconomically protracted. Furthermore, since the steam is condensing and heating the fabrics, these become moist and it is necessary for them to be dried out later. The Medical Research Council now considers downward displacement methods outmoded and unsafe for fabrics. Sterilization can only be considered efficient if the cycle is made to be consistent and if unskilled operators can achieve satisfactory results.

The first mention of high vacuum to assist steam penetration occurred in 1956 when work in Germany was reported and formed the basis of present thinking. Kanz (1955) reported that it was advisable to attain a vacuum of at least 93 per cent within 1 min and, if this could be attained, sterilization was practical within 15 min at 134°. A vacuum after the sterilizing procedure was said to assist in the drying of fabrics to their original moisture content. This work was investigated by Knox and Penikett (1958), who reported their findings to the Medical Research Council (1959) and recommended the introduction of the use of a vacuum greater than 29½ in Hg absolute as a standard requirement for dressings sterilizers. It was also stated that existing equipment exposed patients in hospitals to possible infection because of improperly sterilized articles.

Henry (1959), in the same year, examined the physical phenomenon related to high-vacuum procedure and work is at present being carried on to examine the effect of heat on the fibres and fabrics undergoing sterilization. The diminution of strength or heat tendering is a possible drawback to this method. There appears to be little damage but a series of experiments are in hand to check this point (M.R.C. Working Party).

XVI. Vacuum-Assisted Autoclaves for Fabrics

A British Standard Specification for a suitable sterilizer was issued in 1960 and a number of autoclaves have been built which comply with this specification. This class of autoclave comprises a chamber which can be evacuated to a pressure of under 20 mm Hg absolute by means of a vacuum pump and a system through which air can be filtered to equilibrate the chamber with atmospheric pressure at the end of the cycle. This Standard has now been shown to be inadequate and the procedure does not guarantee sterility. One way of overcoming the difficulties which has been put forward, (Wilkinson and Peacock, 1961a), is the introduction of steam to entrain remaining air which is then pumped out as an air/water vapour mixture.

XVII. Methods of Obtaining Vacuum within Autoclaves

To obtain the necessary vacuum various types of pump have been tried. Reciprocating pumps cannot produce an adequate degree of

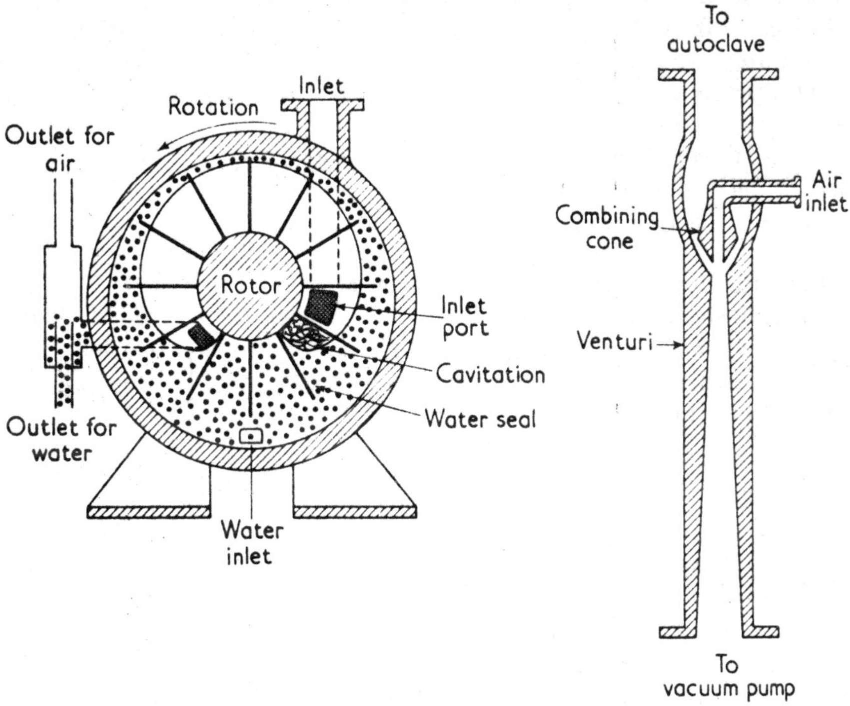

Fig. 7. Diagrammatic representation of water ring pump and air ejector suitable for use with vacuum assisted autoclaves (Ryaland Pumps Ltd.).

vacuum unless two-stage types are employed, and they suffer from difficulties of size and noise. Positive displacement vane types with oil as sealing agent have proved satisfactory except that extreme measures have to be taken to prevent condensate contaminating the oil, which must be maintained at a temperature of about 120° and as much moisture vapour as possible kept away from the pump (Alley Compressors Ltd.[1]).

Water ejectors have also been employed but they are only suitable for

[1] Alley Compressors Ltd., Cathcart, Glasgow, S.4.

vacuums down to about 30 mm Hg absolute. They are used on a small scale for drying loads after sterilization.

The most useful pump has been found to be the water-ring or water-seal pump backing an induced air ejector (see Fig. 7) (Ryaland Pumps Ltd.[1]).

The motor-driven rotor clears the periphery by a very small amount and the water is kept at a constant level. Some of the water is thrown outwards by centrifugal force and this annulus of water forms the seal. The chambers formed in the rotor are not symmetrical, therefore the air within them is compressed as the rotor rotates. The pockets then displace air from the inlet port to the outlet from which it emerges mixed with water to a simple constant level device which separates them.

This procedure operates until about 80 mm Hg absolute is achieved within the chamber. When this point is reached air is drawn in through the jet of the ejector and this produces a pressure drop across the venturi. By means of this the vacuum within the chamber can be reduced to as little as 5 mm Hg absolute.

With this type of equipment, apart from setting up and testing, automatic control is considered essential and in a revised British Standard Specification at present under consideration there will be no provision for manual control should the automatic controls fail. The Standard will set out a performance requirement rather than specify the method of attaining it.

XVIII. Control Systems for Autoclaves

The simplest form of controller is human, making use of manually operated valves with a thermometer to measure the temperature and a stopclock for timing a pre-arranged cycle. Valves controlling steam, air entry and blowdown or free steaming are the minimum required.

Even when an operator is adequately trained it is possible for errors to occur, resulting in accidents or damaged articles. To reduce the number of operations which the operator has to memorize, the valves can be operated by a camshaft which is turned through various stations for the various eras of the cycle. This system was instituted many years ago and is still in use. It has been further developed to include an electrically operated timer and electric motor for rotating the camshaft, but this is only applicable to very simple autoclaves and for a single pre-set cycle.

Autoclaves, particularly those for dressings and fluids, have become much more complex and safeguards and tests of its own efficiency must be built into the controller. This has led to the introduction of electrically

[1] Ryaland Pumps Ltd., Condor Works, Rusholme, Manchester 14.

and electronically operated systems which must be capable of working in hot humid conditions and be completely reliable, with the minimum of attention. Such controllers can have a number of pre-set cycles or have units which can be added on to extend their versatility. The behaviour of one such controller can be exemplified by the dressing cycle of a modern controller. Reference to the block diagram (Fig. 8) will give the various features which are considered essential for this type of controller and should be consulted together with this text.

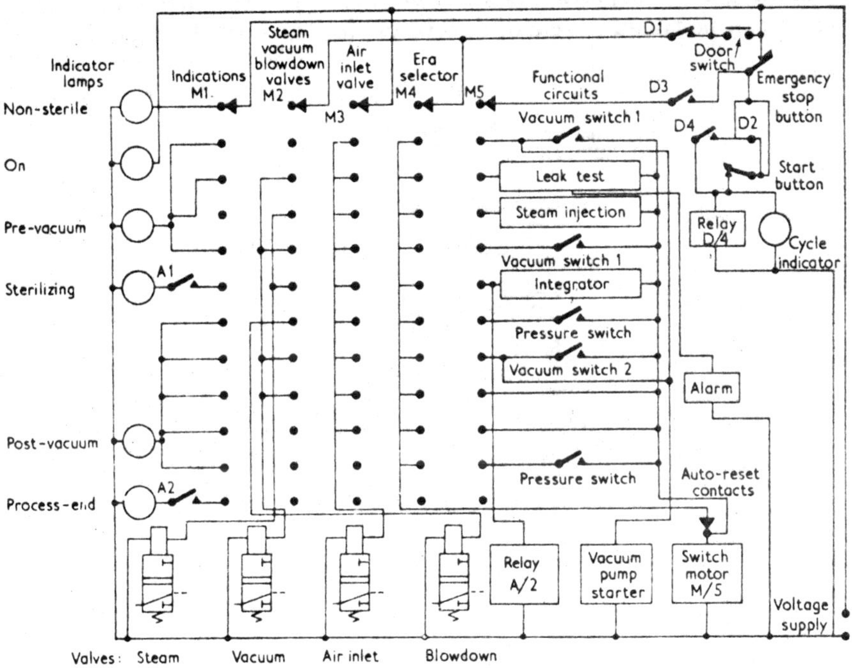

FIG. 8. Schematic diagram of an electrical controller for a jacketed steam heated dressings sterilizer.

Shutting and locking the sterilizer door energizes the controller and permits operation to take place. This is a safety device so that the controller cannot be started inadvertently. Pressing the "start" button causes the controller to switch on the vacuum pump and open the valve communicating with the chamber and at the same time holding all other valves closed. Pumping continues until a pressure of 20 mm absolute is obtained within the chamber. When this is achieved the pre-set vacuum switch closes and the vacuum pump is disconnected from the chamber by the vacuum valve closing. A timer is started and if the pressure within the chamber has not increased by more than 2 mm before the timer runs out, the controller continues to the next era. This is a test for any leak occurring due to the door not being correctly closed or one of the valves failing.

If the leak rate is satisfactory steam is introduced into the chamber to a pre-set pressure and is then pumped out by means of the vacuum pump; this steam entrains the remaining air and it is thus largely removed from the chamber. When the vacuum switch again reaches 20 mm Hg absolute, steam is introduced for the sterilizing period. This period can be timed in one or two ways: (*a*) for a fixed period above a

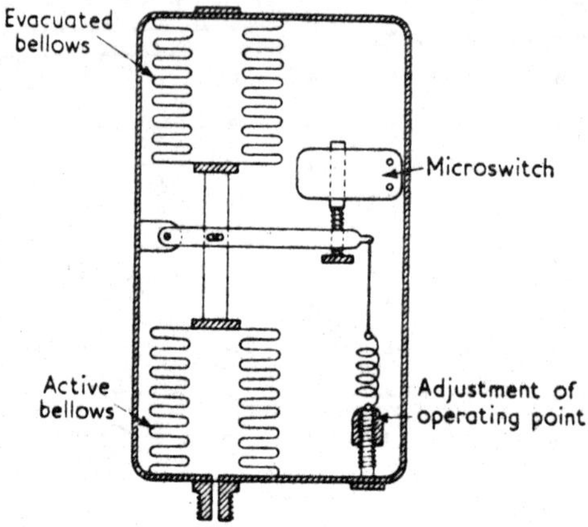

FIG. 9. Barometrically compensated vacuum switch.

given temperature, or (*b*) by means of an integrator which integrates the sterilizing dose between pre-set temperatures.

When one or other of these systems has been satisfied, steam is removed from the chamber, and when atmospheric pressure is reached the pump is again started and evacuation of the water vapour continues until a vacuum switch set at 30 mm Hg absolute stops the pump and allows air to enter the chamber through the filter. When pressure reaches atmospheric pressure an indication is given that the cycle has been completed. The vacuum switches used in the controller are compensated for changes in atmospheric pressure and one method of achieving this is to use two bellows in opposition, one evacuated and the other connected to the chamber (see Fig. 9). The switch is operated by movements of these bellows.

XIX. Controlling the Sterilizing Period and Integration of Time and Temperature

The simplest controller for the sterilizing timer consists of a contact thermometer usually obtaining its signal from a mercury-in-steel or vapour pressure bulb in the chamber drain in series with a time switch. The timer starts when a pre-set temperature is reached and stops if the temperature falls below the pre-set level. When the timer runs out the controller cycles to the next stage.

Since sterilization may be considered to commence at 121° and for fabrics this contact thermometer must be set at 134°, the time taken for the increase between these two temperatures is wasted. For this reason integrators making use of this heat have been employed.

Bacteria exposed to the temperatures of 121° for 15 min or 134° for 3 min will, for practical purposes, be killed. At intermediate temperatures between these limits the related time exists. Put another way, a certain amount of energy is required and this can be obtained rapidly by exposure for a short time at a high temperature or more slowly for a longer time at a lower temperature. The sterilizing curve relating time and temperature is shown in Fig. 10*b*. When plotted with a logarithmic scale for temperature a substantially straight line is produced over the range which we are considering. To explain the function of integrators the amount of energy required can be taken as 1 S unit which is the amount of energy available by exposure at any one fixed temperature for the appropriate time, or built up from a collection of times and temperatures. The manner in which 1 S unit can be built up is illustrated using a typical curve obtained from the temperature recorder of a sterilizer. In Fig. 10 the sterilizing time at temperature curve is adjacent to this trace obtained from the sterilizer recorder. The average temperature of every 15-sec duration of the period, which is the sampling time of the integrator, has been marked on the graph and has been entered in the second column of the table. The appropriate period for 1 S unit has been determined from the graph at these temperatures by drawing a horizontal line through the average sterilizing temperature until it meets the time at temperature curve, then dropping a vertical line and reading off the appropriate time along the base line. A table has been produced using these figures. Those obtained from the curve have been entered in column 3. The fraction of 1 S unit for each of these 15-sec periods has been worked out by dividing 0·25 by this time in minutes and is listed in column 5 of the table. In the final column is the cumulative total or integrated fraction of the sterilizing unit.

We are, in fact, integrating time and temperature. It will be seen that the sterilizing unit is achieved at about 5 min from the time a temperature of 121° C was reached. If the sterilizing curve is examined it will be seen that if timing had started when 134° C was reached, the time at sterilization temperatures would have been 7½ min.

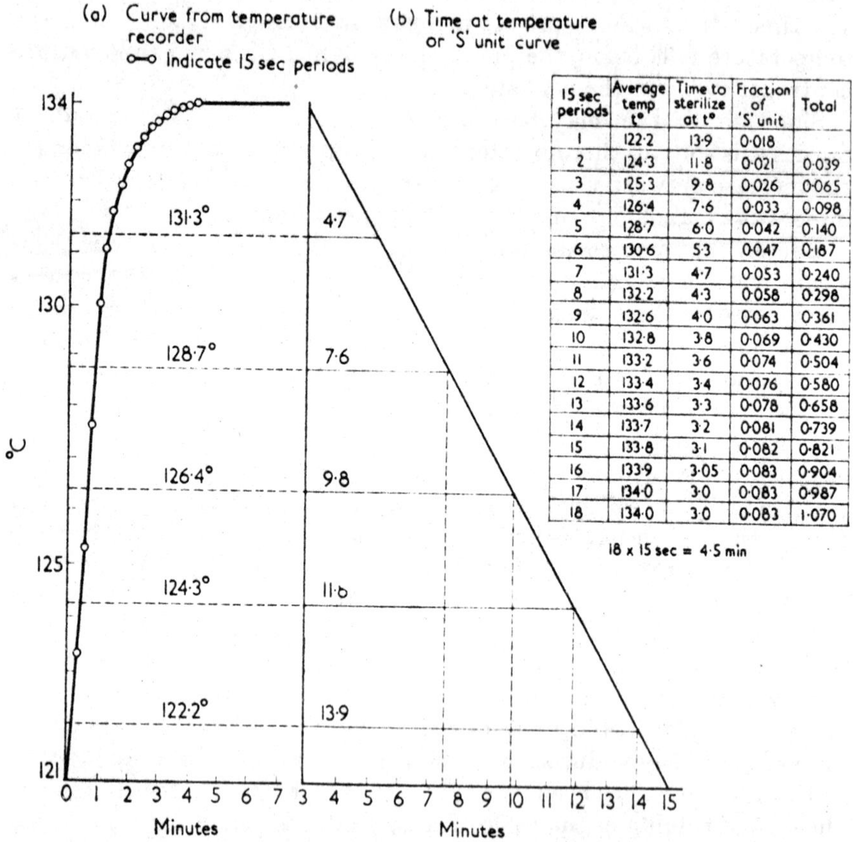

15 sec periods	Average temp t°	Time to sterilize at t°	Fraction of 'S' unit	Total
1	122·2	13·9	0·018	
2	124·3	11·8	0·021	0·039
3	125·3	9·8	0·026	0·065
4	126·4	7·6	0·033	0·098
5	128·7	6·0	0·042	0·140
6	130·6	5·3	0·047	0·187
7	131·3	4·7	0·053	0·240
8	132·2	4·3	0·058	0·298
9	132·6	4·0	0·063	0·361
10	132·8	3·8	0·069	0·430
11	133·2	3·6	0·074	0·504
12	133·4	3·4	0·076	0·580
13	133·6	3·3	0·078	0·658
14	133·7	3·2	0·081	0·739
15	133·8	3·1	0·082	0·821
16	133·9	3·05	0·083	0·904
17	134·0	3·0	0·083	0·987
18	134·0	3·0	0·083	1·070

FIG. 10. Graphical method of integrating time at temperature from a curve obtained from a temperature recorder fitted to an autoclave.

In the sterilizer controller the integrator is making these comparisons and calculations automatically and only when an S unit has been accumulated during the sterilizing part of the cycle does the controller turn off the steam and continue to the next era of the cycle. This means that should the temperature fall due to variations in steam pressure the sterilizing period is automatically extended.

XX. Types of Integrator

A number of integrators have been used, the crudest form being a make-and-break switch actuated by a bi-metallic strip which is alternately heated and cooled so that it makes and breaks a contact at a preset time interval (Drayton Regulator & Instrument Co. Ltd.[1]). This switch contact is in series with the feed to a time switch controlling the steam entry into the sterilizer. One contact of this make-and-break switch can be positioned at a variable distance from the other under the influence of a thermometer bulb within the sterilizer drain line. This alters the time, during which the time switch runs, according to the proportion of the make-and-break times and it is so adjusted that when the temperature is 134° C the timer is running constantly, but when at 121° C it runs for only one-fifth of its time. This extends the time required for the time switch to operate and so extends the sterilizing period. So between the ranges of 15 min at 121° C and 3 min at 134° C it should automatically compensate for any changes in temperature by running for an appropriate time. Instead of the bi-metallic strip another integrator uses a rotating cam, and in yet another, photo-electric cells mounted on a moving-coil galvanometer are used to produce a curve which follows approximately the time/temperature curve required and thereby influences the sterilizing time (West Instruments Ltd.[2]). The resistance bulb thermometer is used to supply the information to the galvanometer.

To date these integrators involving sensitive galvanometers and photo-electric cells (West Instruments Ltd.[2]) or thermally heated bi-metallic elements (Drayton Regulator & Instrument Co. Ltd.[1]) have been of delicate construction. These have not the sturdiness of the other components in the controller and have been subject to variation due to changes in ambient temperature. Additionally and most important, they have worked on a more or less linear relationship which does not match the time at temperature sterilizing curve required. Because of this, integration has fallen into disrepute.

An electronic unit has now been evolved which overcomes these difficulties. Figure 11*a* is a block diagram of its various circuits. As its sensing element it uses a stable platinum resistance thermometer bulb and the circuitry is completely transistorized on a printed circuit panel. The design ensures stability over widely varying ambient temperatures. By means of the circuitry it has been made to follow very closely the time at temperature curve required. Every 15 sec a waveform of the shape required to match the time at temperature curve

[1] Drayton Regulator & Instrument Co. Ltd., West Drayton, Middlesex.
[2] West Instruments Ltd., (Gulton Industries (Britain) Ltd.), Lower Bevendean 7, Sussex.

is produced. The resistance thermometer, through the necessary circuitry and relays, applies the actual temperature to the appropriate point on the curve and allows the timer to run for the appropriate time for that particular temperature and then stops it. Every 15 sec this procedure is repeated in exactly the same manner as was demonstrated

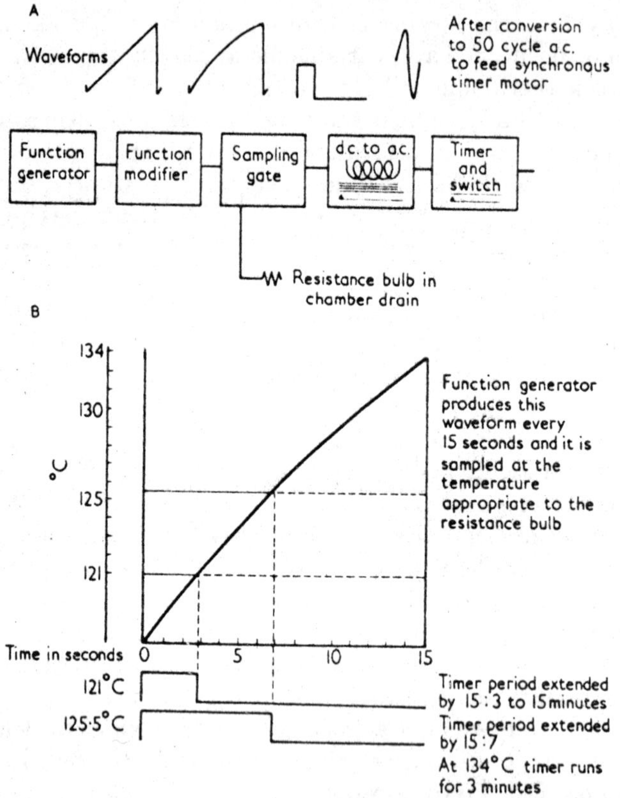

FIG. 11. (*a*) Block diagram of electronic integrator. (*b*) Variation of time with temperature determined by the integrator.

graphically. The timer is set so that if the temperature is constant at 134° C it will run out in 3 min and the stopping and starting is so arranged that at 121° C it requires 15 min to run out. The signals received by the relay to switch this timer on and off are shown in Fig. 11*b*. The curve covers one 15-sec period; the solid line indicates the period during which the timer runs and the dotted line the period during which it is stopped. It will be seen that as the temperature rises the solid line increases in length, that is, the timer runs for a longer period. Additional to this function the unit provides for switching on the recorder for the appropriate sterilizing time for any temperature between the pre-set limits.

XXI. Methods of Operating Autoclave Valves

In the case of some sterilizers the electrical impulses from the controller operate a motor to turn a camshaft, which in turn operates the necessary valves. In the case of others, solenoid or motor-operated valves are employed, but this type of operation can be unreliable and the valves are expensive.

The most convenient method is to use hydraulically or pneumatically operated valves of the diaphragm or piston type, operated by pneumatic or hydraulic relays from the electrical impulses originating in the control. The valves can be positioned where required rather than near the camshaft.

XXII. Further Type of Controller

A controller for operating a fluid sterilizer mentioned previously is somewhat simpler in construction, but more interlocks must be provided as it is necessary to establish that services are available and ready before they are actually connected to the sterilizer (see Fig. 6*b*).

Switching on the equipment starts the compressor and once the air reservoir reaches working pressure an indication is displayed that a cycle may be started. Shutting and locking the door energizes the controller and, when the "start" button is pressed, steam is admitted to the chamber and the pre-set sterilizing timer starts running. When the chamber and its contents are heated so that the outlet temperature reaches 100° C the temperature-sensitive switch in the drain closes the vent valve. Still under the control of the timer, steam continues to be admitted until the requisite period elapses. This period is pre-set to take care of the heating-up time and the sterilizing time for the particular load. At the end of the sterilizing period the controller turns off the steam and makes air available to the chamber through a common reducing valve so that it is at exactly the same pressure, and at the same time makes a contact to hold the vent valve closed. A little later the water pump is switched on and if pressure is developed within the feed line the valve will open and allow cooling water to be admitted to the spray heads. If pressure is not produced within 10 sec the controller will stay at the previous stage and ring an alarm bell until the fault is rectified. If water commences spraying the cooling-period timer starts and this continues until the timer runs out. At the end of the cooling period the compressed air is turned off and after a further short period the air inlet valve is opened and the water turned off. When the pressure within the chamber falls to atmospheric pressure the load may be removed from the chamber. Before the air inlet valve can open during the cooling period there must be air available to maintain pressure in the chamber when the cooling water condenses the steam, and there must be pressure on the up-stream side of the water valve so that the chamber pressure cannot be collapsed through this valve in the event of the failure of the water supply. Before commencing to time the cooling period water must be admitted to the chamber through the supply pipe, since the normal chamber pressure of approximately 20 lb/in^2 is not sufficient to operate the sensing switch which requires almost the full water pressure to make its contact. This interlocking ensures that the cooling period cannot be timed out unless cooling water has been admitted for the full cooling period. If there is an interruption in the flow of cooling water the alarm sounds and the timer stops. When the supply is reinstated the timer will recommence and the alarm is silenced, thus in the event of any failure of services the cooling cycle will be halted and if the services are not restarted within 10 sec a warning signal appears. In the event of an emergency, operating the stop button de-energizes all valves and drives the cam system to the non-sterile position. This system prevents the autoclave being inadvertently opened while the bottles within are sufficiently hot to render them dangerous. Should pressure remain within the chamber for any reason a safety lock makes it impossible to open the door.

XXIII. Problems Associated with Certain Loads

Considerable evidence has been built up within the past year that difficulties are experienced in drying fabrics when mixed with relatively large quantities of material with a high specific heat such as metal.

There is sufficient heat present in the metal objects to evaporate the condensate formed during the heating-up provided the fabric is in contact with the metal. Generally the condensate is absorbed into the fabric and evaporation does not occur although there is sufficient heat in part of the load. Rubber tubing in long lengths is also difficult material to dry within the lumen and falls into the same category.

Efforts have been made to alleviate this situation and the most satisfactory way is to introduce filtered warm air into the chamber and evacuate, so removing some of the moisture and repeating the effect over a number of cycles, greatly reducing the pressure of each pumping until some 30 mm is achieved. Under these circumstances drying can be considerably assisted. Suitable equipment is possible only with automatic controllers.

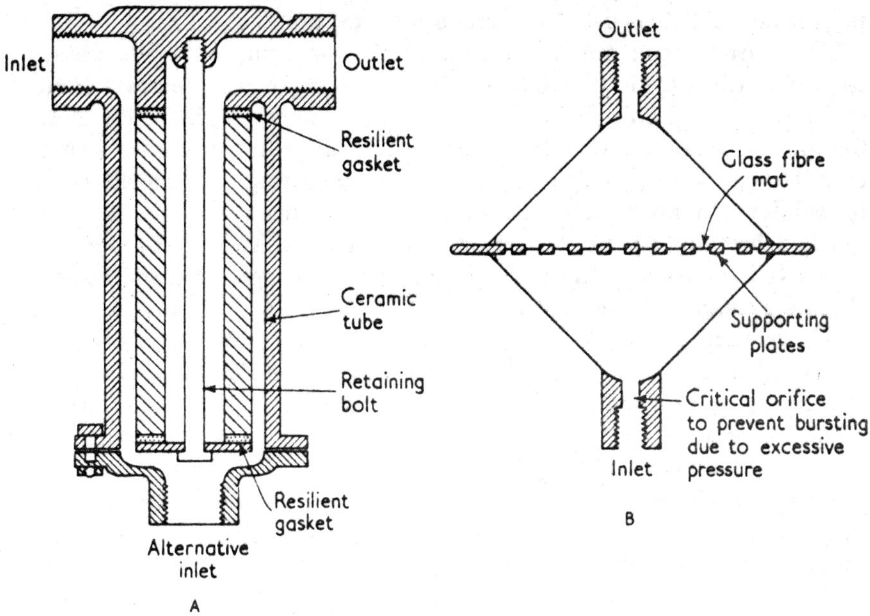

FIG. 12. Cross sections of ceramic and matted glass fibre filters.

XXIV. FILTERS

During the equilibration of the chamber with atmosphere whenever a vacuum is developed within the chamber, it is advisable to pass the incoming air through a filter to remove bacteria and dust particles. Originally, a cotton wool plug was used but this can be a breeding ground for bacteria when wet and has been shown by a number of workers to be ineffective. Ceramic filters made by sintering powders (see Fig. 12*a*) to produce a material of a standard porosity can be subjected to repeated sterilization without deterioration. These, together with filters constructed from glass fibre paper supported on perforated metal sheets have proved adequate in preventing the passage of bacteria (see Fig. 12*b*). Such filters will protect against a penetration of less than 0·0001 per cent of particles of 0·3 μ diameter when tested either by the methylene blue or sodium tests (Aerox Ltd.[1]).

XXV. CARE OF AUTOCLAVES

For an autoclave to operate satisfactorily all parts of it must be

[1] Aerox Limited, Cotswold Works, Chalford, Stroud, Glos.

maintained since small changes can bring about a severe reduction in performance. This is usually evidenced by failure to sterilize.

To ensure the continued working of valves and pumps it is necessary to protect them from the effects of particulate matter carried over in the steam or introduced by the breakage of containers. Strainers are therefore positioned on the upstream side of such valves and consist of a small chamber containing a piece of fine mesh gauge through which the steam or condensate must pass. In time these strainers become partially blocked bringing about a deterioration in the behaviour of the equipment. It is necessary, therefore, to inspect them regularly and remove them for cleaning when required.

Although it is now 7 years since Professor Howie drew attention to the danger of fitting autoclaves into drains without an air-break, many are still fitted in this manner. Under such circumstances polluted water could be drawn into the chamber if a vacuum is developed within it. Even if an air-break is fitted malfunction can be brought about by causing the condensate line to the steam trap to run uphill. This can cause waterlogging of the chamber before sufficient pressure is developed to drive out the condensate.

The door seal is a delicate system and the practice of trapping thermocouple leads between it and the door should not be tolerated. Permanent damage can occur to the door and at least the gasket will almost certainly require renewing. It is much easier and better to fit a proper entry for thermocouples. A suitable system has been described (Wilkinson and Peacock, 1962) and consists of a Kontite fitting in which is clamped a rubber bung drilled with holes for the thermocouples and retained by a washer.

Over a period of time wear and fatigue can cause pressure gauges and dial thermometers to alter in calibration, and failure to check them at regular intervals can lead to inexplicable failures or to unnecessary adjustments. It is usual to keep one instrument as a standard and to use it only when the others are undergoing calibration. Both pressure gauges and thermometers should be calibrated at their normal working indication.

If the chamber is jacketed and the autoclave is used daily it is inadvisable to turn off the steam supply to the jacket at night. If the jacket cools air can be drawn into it through the steam trap and under certain circumstances can be transferred to the chamber during subsequent sterilization cycles.

Failure to provide adequate removal of condensate at a point close to where the steam enters the chamber can cause condensate to be carried over during the periods of slow steam flow and cause wet loads.

XXVI. Steam Pressure Reducing Valves for Autoclaves

The behaviour of a sterilizer can be influenced by the fitting of different types of reducing valves. In one type a diaphragm is balanced against the pressure downstream of it and a spring adjusts the flow of incoming steam accordingly. Adjustment of the spring provides for pre-setting at a given pressure. With this type of reducing valve, well before the steam pressure downstream approaches the set value, the valve commences to close and the pressure build-up is slowed down as working pressure is reached. This means that time is lost in reaching sterilizing pressure if,

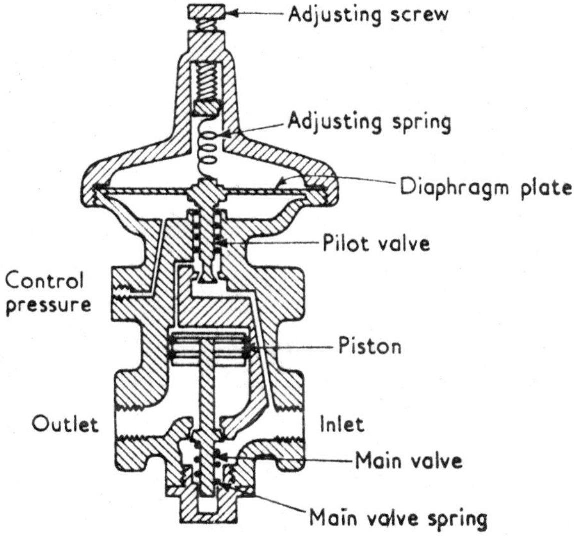

FIG. 13. Diagrammatic cross section of a pilot operated reducing valve.

in fact, the chamber ever does. This type of reducing valve is perfectly satisfactory for large steam flows where a critical setting is not necessary or for primary reducing valves where the load is constant.

A more suitable type of reducing valve is the pilot-operated type where a very small diaphragm and valve system working on the same principal admits steam to a cylinder and piston which work the main valve (see Fig. 13). The pilot valve is much more sensitive and more accurately follows changes in pressure. When working properly the main valve will stay fully open until the chamber reaches working pressure and then will maintain the chamber to well within 0·5 lb differential. This type of valve will function over the whole range of demand, which is usually at least a 10 : 1 change between first turning on and standby.

The most satisfactory type of reducing valve for steam is the pressure controller type (see Fig. 14). In this a Bourdon tube or capsule is used to sense the pressure within the chamber and a small tube is occluded by a vane attached to the pressure measuring system. Air at constant pressure is emitted from this tube and as it is occluded pressure builds up within the supply pipe and this is sensed by a valve which in turn relays an amplified pressure to a diaphragm operated valve which actually controls the steam entry. This valve has ports which are "V" shaped so that the control becomes greatest when the valve is almost

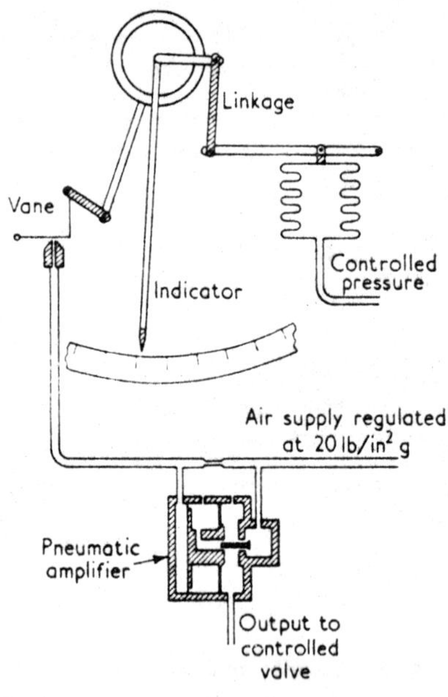

FIG. 14. Diagrammatic representation of pressure operated control valve.

closed. It is also capable of dealing with wide variations of demand. With this type of controller it is possible to maintain very accurately pressure and therefore temperature within sterilizer chamber, which can be set to any pressure by turning a knob. They suffer from the disadvantage that a compressed air supply is necessary but their efficiency far outweighs this extra requirement.

XXVII. Testing the Behaviour of Autoclaves

Modern advances in sterilization methods have drawn attention to the need for greater knowledge of the behaviour of the contents of an autoclave than has previously been considered necessary. In some instances the supplies themselves must be capable of being checked. These requirements fall under the following headings:

(1) Temperature;
(2) Pressure;
(3) Steam Flow;
(4) Water Flow;
(5) Safety Testing.

A. TEMPERATURE MEASUREMENT

Although this can be done by several methods, including maximum and minimum thermometers, the most satisfactory method has been found to be a strip-chart recorder of the self-balancing potentiometric type, using thermocouples, or in a few instances resistance bulbs, to determine the temperature. The thermocouple junctions, having small mass, respond rapidly and can be positioned accurately within bottles or fabrics, or other materials within the autoclave. It is usual to employ at least a 6-point recorder, using thermocouples in the following positions:

(*a*) Chamber drain.
(*b*) Free within the chamber, away from the walls.
(*c*) In the steam supply line to the autoclave.
(*d*), (*e*) and (*f*) At different parts within the load.

In this type of instrument the small voltage from the thermocouple, which is usually iron-constantan, is fed into an amplifier and applied to a potentiometer network, the slider of the ratio arm of the potentiometer being driven by a motor which receives its power from the amplifier. The circuit is so arranged that the motor will drive the slider on the ratio arm and at the same time the pointer or indicator, until it balances exactly the input voltage from the thermocouple (see Fig. 17). It therefore works as a null-point indicator and various possible sources of error such as varying potentiometer voltage can be cancelled out. Cold junction compensation of the thermocouples can be obtained by immersing a similar thermocouple in melting ice, but is more usually automatic. This automatic compensation is obtained by inserting in one of the standard ratio arms a copper coil which is in close physical proximity to the thermocouple terminations. This coil responds to any temperature changes in the thermocouple junctions and, because of its resistance characteristics, offsets any voltage developed. These instruments are reliable but must be regularly checked against a standard mercury-in-glass thermometer, preferably near the temperature at which measurement is most critical. This type of instrument can also be used for checking hot-air ovens and also for infra-red ovens, but in this case the thermocouple junction must be embedded in the article whose temperature one wishes to measure. Circular chart recorders are available but it has been found that the chart is much more difficult to interpret.

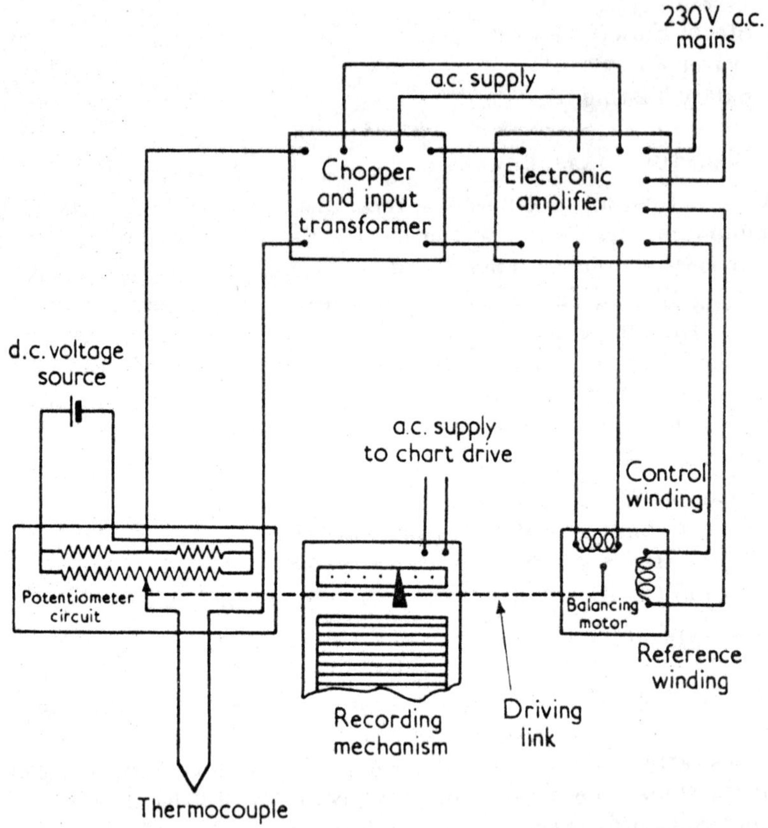

FIG. 15. Block diagram of potentiometric recorder with thermocouple input. A standard cell (not shown) is periodically connected into the potentiometer circuit and compares with a portion of the voltage source. The circuit is arranged to correct itself to maintain the voltage source constant.

B. PRESSURE

Absolute pressure measurement of the order of 0 to 500 mm Hg are now commonly required. The simplest gauge to use is a mercury manometer but these suffer from difficulty in transport and the effect of water condensing on the mercury. The most convenient gauge is the capsule gauge (see Fig. 16). This consists of a metallic bellows containing a spring which has been evacuated to an extremely low absolute pressure and sealed, positioned within a case which is capable of withstanding 0 to 1 atm absolute pressure. The bellows is attached to a magnifying mechanism and thence to a pointer which moves over a dial calibrated in millimetres of mercury absolute. A suitable range is 0 to 50 or 0 to 100 mm Hg absolute. When vacuum is applied within the case the capsule expands under the influence of the spring and the pointer moves around the dial to the appropriate reading. Using these gauges on autoclaves, they frequently become contaminated with moisture which can be seen

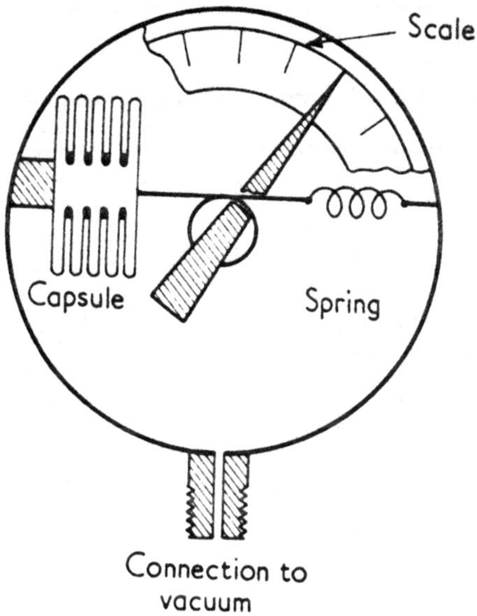

Fig. 16. Dial gauge for measuring absolute pressure.

as globules or even pools inside. If this should happen the gauge is temporarily useless, but may be made usable again by placing within a desiccator containing anhydrous calcium chloride and evacuating to a millimetre or two of mercury absolute. After a few hours under these conditions the water will have been removed and the gauge is once more usable.

C. STEAM FLOW

Instruments for measuring steam flow are generally made for large equipment and to deal with flow rates in excess of 1000 lb of steam/h. Since much of the equipment normally encountered uses between 5 and 500 lb of steam/h, this available equipment can prove either unsuitable or too expensive. A steam meter has been described (Lyle, 1947) which can be modified to accommodate the types of flow encountered and consists of an orifice plate and a mercury manometer, one limb of which is connected upstream and the other downstream on the orifice plate. The instrument can be calibrated in terms of steam flow by weighing the amount of condensate produced in measured times at constant indications and the figures later used to measure unknown steam flows. An

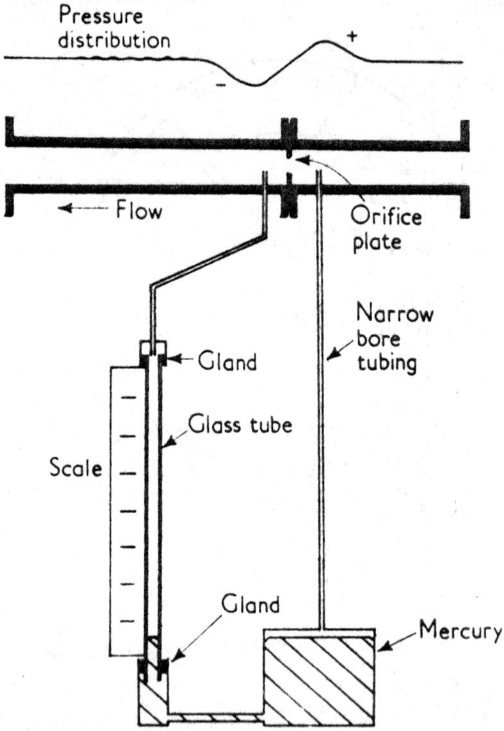

FIG. 17. Principle of steam flow meter.

instrument constructed on these principles, with an orifice plate with a hole $\frac{1}{2}$ in in diameter in a steam pipe 1 in in diameter, covers the range of about 50 to 350 lb of steam/h (see Fig. 17).

D. WATER FLOW

With some water-sealed pumps and with water-cooled equipment it is at times valuable to know the rate at which water is flowing through the equipment. This can be obtained conveniently by measuring the amount of water produced in a given time. This, however, only produces an average flow rate. If the flow rate is changing the instantaneous flow can only be measured by some type of dynamic flowmeter. Most of these types of meter depend upon a plummet suspended in the water which flows in an upward direction through a tapered tube (see Fig. 18). The tubing is either graduated directly in water flow at a particular temperature or in arbitrary units which when applied to a table or nomogram

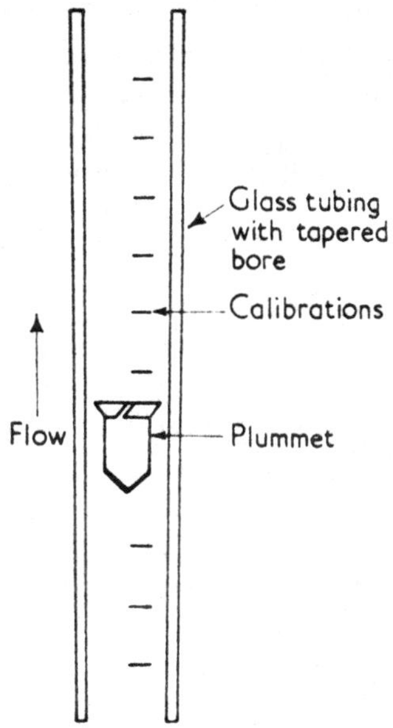

FIG. 18. Flow meter suitable for water.

give the actual fluid flow at a measured temperature. It is important when measuring condensate, or other water which has been heated, to interpose between the source and the measuring point a water surface condenser, otherwise some may be lost due to flash evaporation.

E. SAFETY TESTING

Whenever any work is carried out on an autoclave it is advisable to test it for safety before it is brought into use. This entails a pressure test using water, the pressure being applied by a small piston hand pump. The pressure is read from a suitable gauge on the equipment or a special test gauge attached for the purpose. Before this testing takes place it is necessary to blank off any equipment on the autoclave which would be damaged by excessive pressures. Reference to B.S. 3220: 1960 will give the test pressure and this is usually about twice the working pressure. At this pressure there should be no permanent distortion or leaks developed.

Much discussion is at present taking place in an attempt to standardize a test which was put forward by Bowie (M.R.C. Working Party, 1963) for routine testing of dressing sterilizers. In this test self-adhesive tape printed with a design in ink, which is sensitive to moisture and temperature is applied in the form of a cross to the tenth towel of a stack of thirty towels packed in a dressing casket to B.S. 2798: 1956. After being exposed to sterilizing conditions within an autoclave the tape is examined, and if there is uniform colouration at all points the equipment is considered to be working satisfactorily. If air has not been adequately eliminated, an area about the centre of the cross is lighter in colour.

XXVIII. Design

The foregoing has discussed the theoretical background of present-day sterilizing equipment. It is now proposed to consider the problems confronting designers, translating these requirements into concrete form.

It should be noted at this point that boiling water as a means for sterilizing instruments and utensils has been shown to be inadequate (Nuffield, 1958). Boiling water sterilizers are not capable of killing spores and unless supplied with distilled water cause deposits to form on instruments. Pressure type bulk-water sterilizers (Howie and Kelsey, 1962) have been proved to be a source of contamination and are falling into disrepute. Neither type is likely to be included in future projects. It is suggested that in future all sterile tap water such as is used during surgery and for external purposes will be supplied in 1-litre capacity glass, plastic or aluminium containers, sterilized either in industrial pharmaceutical factories, in pharmaceutical departments or in media kitchens of laboratories where such water is employed.

The primary concept is therefore of sterilizers capable of withstanding internal pressures and conditions varying between steam at 64 lb/in^2 absolute and 5 mm Hg absolute. In this it is further required to ensure that dry saturated steam is conveyed to all surfaces of the load placed therein.

This sterilizing equipment can be considered in three main groups:

(*a*) Autoclaves for processing bottled fluids and solutions.
(*b*) Autoclaves for fabrics, dressings, clothing and wrapped instruments and utensils.
(*c*) Autoclaves for unwrapped instruments and utensils.

XXIX. Steam Supply

It has been shown that a fundamental requirement is a satisfactory steam supply and this can only be obtained if the supply mains are correctly designed and maintained.

It is generally accepted that steam and condensate mains of the type generally to be found in modern industrial plants and institutions are suitable for supplying steam for sterilizing purposes. The primary requirement is for them to be correctly sized and laid. The necessary data for pipe sizing are available in published form (Institution of Heating and

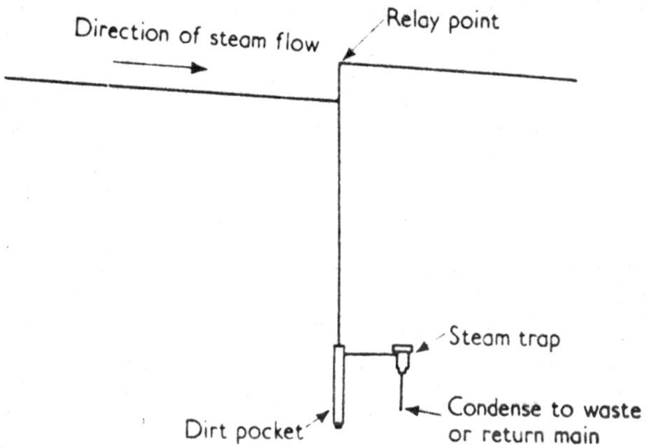

Fig. 19. Steam main relay point.

Ventilation Engineers Guide, 1959). The following points are, however, not obvious to anyone with only limited contact with the problem but they can have an important bearing on efficiency.

Particular care must be taken in installing steam mains to ensure that condensate formed by radiation losses is removed. Horizontal runs should be avoided and all pipes should be laid to a slight fall so that condensate will run by gravity to steam traps, and all vertical rising pipes should have a drain connection with a steam trap and a scale pocket at the lowest point (see Fig. 19). Steam connections from a horizontal steam main should be made from the top of the pipework so that condensate will remain in the main and not be carried in the branch line, as would be the case if the connections were made in the bottom of the main line.

The formation of condensate can be reduced if the pipework is properly insulated. In permanent installations thermal insulation is usually an asbestos compound applied as a wet paste and covered after drying by a hard setting compound, which will produce a smooth surface to protect the softer inner layer and provide a clean easily painted outer skin. A very good alternative is rigid preformed sections in various sizes made from a variety of insulating substances such as asbestos or resin-bonded glass fibres, with an outer coating of tough cloth or hard plastic material. This sectional insulation is also useful where alterations are frequent. The sections are usually fastened by metal clips, and since it can readily be assembled in confined spaces it is very suitable for use in ducts or ceiling voids, although it is not considered to be as efficient as the wet compounds, but has the advantage of being removable for maintenance purposes and is easily restored.

Recent investigations have shown that some air can be present in steam mains feeding sterilizers, causing fluctuating temperatures while indicated pressure remains constant. Air can be released in a boiler from feed water, but this problem can usually be overcome by properly designed feed-water treatment equipment.

Attention has been drawn earlier to the requirement for dry steam. The water particles in wet steam arise from two causes: improperly drained steam lines and from water carried over from the boiler into the pipework; this latter condition, known as "priming", usually arises if unsuitable feed-water treatment is used or if the concentration solids in solution in the boiler water is allowed to become excessive. Some types of feed water treatment require the "blowdown" valve on the boiler to be opened to allow a proportion of the water to be blown away to waste once a day; others require a small continuous blowdown. Unless this simple operation is carried out, these solids or "boiler mud" can be carried into the pipelines and valves in sufficient quantity to cause failures.

These matters are properly the province of steam design engineers but much useful information can be obtained from "The Efficient Use of Steam" (Lyle, 1947).

XXX. Control Systems

It is essential that sterilizing equipment should, as far as possible, be suitable for use by unskilled labour. Controls must be reduced to the minimum and so arranged that minimum responsibility and decision is required from operating staff.

Until recently most autoclaves were constructed with individual handwheel-operated valves directly on supply pipes or at points scattered around the plant. On others they were grouped at the front, but in either case it was necessary to open or shut a number of valves to change over from one phase of an operating cycle to another. Contemporary manually operated sterilizers are made so that pipework is led to a group of valves operated by a camshaft so arranged that by turning it step by step through one revolution a predetermined cycle can be completed. Only the reading of simple gauge indication and timing by means of a stop-clock is required from the operator.

The control valves used should have easily accessible renewable valve seatings.

This type of controller is mostly used for downward displacement autoclaves intended for a variety of situations, by operators of widely varying physical capabilities. The operating handwheel and camshaft assembly must therefore be sturdy to withstand strong operators and yet be sufficiently free moving to allow young girls to operate the equipment. To achieve this careful attention must be paid to bearings, cam profile design and considerable care taken during both assembly and final fitting on to the autoclave.

The simplest form of automatic control is the substitution of an electric driving motor for the operating handwheel in the camshaft controller described above. Operation of the motor is usually determined during the sterilizing cycle by a contact-head thermometer. This is a mercury-in-steel or vapour-pressure system linked to a circular indicating dial, the pointer acting as a switch in conjunction with an assembly of fixed and movable contacts which may be set to any temperature shown on the scale. The operating motor is held stationary until the pointer makes contact, completing the circuit and allowing current to flow, thus causing the operating motor to turn the camshaft on to the next stage. Similarly, during the vacuum phase of the cycle it can be controlled by a contact-head pressure gauge. This type of controller has the advantage of minimizing the risks of valves used and permitting the use of a simple handwheel attachment for manual operation in the event of electrical failure.

A more advanced system which has been in use for some years for dressing sterilizers makes use of a small camshaft unit operating small pilot valves which feed water or compressed air to diaphragm-operated valves placed at the appropriate places in the service pipelines. This type of controller overcomes the problem of complicated pipework by decentralizing the main control valves, allowing shorter pipework runs and permitting easy access for maintenance and servicing. This is now being superseded by an electrical controller where electrically operated pilot valves control the supply of operating fluid to the control valves.

The positioning of controls and indicators is of great importance, particularly for manually operated sterilizers. A study of ergonomic considerations and "applied common sense" suggests that a control panel may be considered as a page of reading matter. Indicators which require to be read before or at the commencement of a cycle should be placed at the top left and those to be used later placed in reading order to the left. The operating handles should be placed in positions where their relationship to their associated indicator is unequivocal.

Considerable study has been made of the readability of gauge dials over the whole indicated range but it is an additional advantage if required valves are shown by coloured marks or coloured sectors. Handwheels or valve handles should be positioned so that they can be comfortably reached without bending or stretching.

Where recorders are fitted it should be possible to read and change charts from a standing position.

Automatic control mechanisms are usually push-button operated. For ease of operation the operating buttons should be clearly marked, particularly where alternative programmes are built into the controller. Each programme requires a button for selection and an emergency stop button is included for obvious reasons. The addition of a diagram or symbol to the legend on the button or marking plate assists in eliminating errors of selection. Illuminated buttons or an annunciator panel can be used as a means of showing which programme has been selected while the cycle is in progress.

XXXI. Autoclave Room

Hitherto, door seals against pressure and vacuum have been made from solid woven asbestos material or from a square section of rubber core with a woven asbestos outer covering. These have a comparatively short life and are prone to adhere to the door surface and lose their sealing properties unless great care is taken in use. Circular-section one-piece rubber rings are now regularly available; these are sometimes referred to as "O" ring seals. They have the advantage of a comparatively long life and do not require so much pressure between the surfaces to be sealed as asbestos packings. This has the effect of reducing the effort required to operate the door-closing mechanism (see Fig. 20).

Power-operated door-closing mechanisms are now available either as an electro-mechanical mechanism, using shafts and bevel gears mounted on the head ring, operating on, but not connected to, the door; or as an electro-hydraulic device utilizing hydraulic rams acting directly upon radial arms or wedges.

Taking a broad view of planning projects in hand, both for the pharmaceutical industry and hospitals, it is probable that power-operated doors

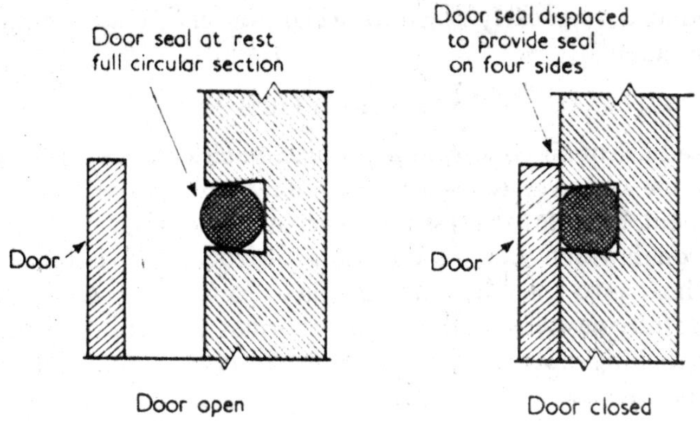

FIG. 20. Diagrammatic arrangement of autoclave door seal.

may be required in conjunction with fully mechanized loading and handling equipment in large-scale sterilizing plants.

XXXII. NOISE OUTPUT

Considerable attention has recently been focused upon the problems raised by excessive noise in hospitals and industrial plants, and autoclaves have not escaped this examination.

It is known that exposure to loud noise can cause permanent loss of hearing and, at comparatively lower levels of sound output, working efficiency is impaired, and the ability to understand speech is diminished, particularly in conditions of changing sound level. It is, however, difficult to assess the nuisance value of noise as personal tolerance varies widely.

The noisiest component of a dressing sterilizer is usually the vacuum pump. In this respect water-ring pumps having only rotating moving parts are less liable to a higher sound level output than oil-seal pumps with reciprocating components. The provision of anti-vibration and sound-absorbing mounting for the pump assembly and flexible pipe connections can do much to reduce the transmission of noise to the structure of a building. Provision of acoustic treatment to the walls and ceilings of rooms or recesses containing autoclaves can also materially restrict the passage of airborne sound to other departments. It is important to recognize that measurement of noise taken from any piece of apparatus will vary with its environment. For instance, sound level measurements taken from a sterilizer in a manufacturer's works may not be realized in its ultimate site. Since noise can be transmitted both through the air and through the fabric of the building, it must be considered at a very early stage in design, otherwise appropriate steps cannot be taken.

XXXIII. Heat Output

Increased use of air conditioning in pharmacies and hospital buildings both at home and overseas is an additional factor in sterilizer design.

Equipment built into recesses or permanent casings with large front panels through which controls and doors protrude, will, in some measure, transmit heat into the surrounding space, particularly from autoclave doors. Carefully designed and installed thermal insulation, together with suitable panelling material, can reduce the heat emission. "Formica", or similarly faced material is superior to mild or stainless steel sheet for the purpose, and glass fibre reinforced polyester laminate or "Fibreglass" has proved an ideal material for individual sterilizer front panels and door covers.

Although it is necessary to prevent heat from radiating into the space in front of an autoclave enclosure, it is equally necessary to prevent a high temperature build-up in the recess itself. The electrical components of most control systems suffer deterioration in ambient temperatures exceeding 50°. Temperatures of this order have frequently been observed where no provision for ventilation of a recess has been made.

It must also be remembered that maintenance and service engineers may be required to spend time working in the recess on one of a group of autoclaves while the others continue working. It is impossible to generalize about the ventilation requirements of sterilizer enclosures except to say that air average ambient temperature in the region of 20° to 30° should be the aim.

Necessity to keep the overall dimensions of autoclaves as compact as possible has been briefly noted above. In a well-designed sterilizer all components such as valves, steam traps, strainers and the like will be so positioned that the minimum of effort is required to dismantle them, and test connections, thermocouple entries, gauge and similar connections must be readily accessible when the sterilizer and pipework is hot. However, it is possible to nullify the effect of such design features if insufficient space is available when equipment is installed. Sufficient space for a maintenance fitter to work comfortably must be allowed around each side of an enclosed autoclave. Restricted working space can extend the working time required to service valves and pipework, etc., and to carry out adjustments to control equipment. There is also a tendency on the part of maintenance staff to postpone necessary servicing if working conditions are difficult. Both these factors will tend to increase the cost of servicing and maintenance.

The points raised above are particularly apposite when the design of double-ended autoclaves are considered. The purpose of such autoclaves is to provide a means of feeding sterile goods from one section of a department to another. In a central sterile supply department goods can be loaded directly from preparation areas into one end and from the opposite end directly into a sterile store. Theatre suites have been recently planned so that utensils and autoclaves can be passed through double-ended autoclaves into an ante-room opening directly into the theatre, which is included in the aseptic area. In pharmaceutical departments, solutions can be prepared and loaded into double-ended autoclaves and passed through into a clean storage area for checking, labelling and despatch.

XXXIV. Hot-air Sterilization

Hot air ovens have been used for sterilizing glassware for many years. The simplest form was a copper box with a door on its front standing over a gas ring. Temperature control was by means of a gas thermostat inserted into the chamber. Many of these are still in use.

Electrically heated ovens have also been developed with the heaters in the base or at either side of the chamber. These suffer from the fault of poor temperature distribution. Other similar ovens have had an electrically driven fan positioned either at the bottom or back of the chamber to circulate the air (see Fig. 21). In most instances the fan is inadequate and temperature distribution is still poor. A further disadvantage is that this type of oven cannot be used for sterilizing powders except in sealed containers, as these are blown about in the air stream.

To obtain more satisfactory temperature distribution it is advantageous to position the heaters in a separate chamber and circulate air over them and the thermostat and then through the chamber (see Fig. 22). This system has been in use for many years but is the subject of a recent British Patent (Chirana, Czechoslovakia [1]).

Any oven which is used for sterilizing purposes should comply with B.S. 3421. This specification gives details of a test by means of which the ovens can be assessed. The test consists of loading the oven with jars containing a non-volatile liquid and measuring the temperature at selected points, and then comparing these temperatures with that indicated by the fixed thermometer. The purpose of the liquid is to damp out any rapid fluctuation in local temperatures.

The greatest advance has been in the use of infra-red heat as the source of heat. Ovens have been produced where the oven contents are heated

[1] Chirana, n.p., 48–50 Gottwaldova, Brno, Czechoslovakia.

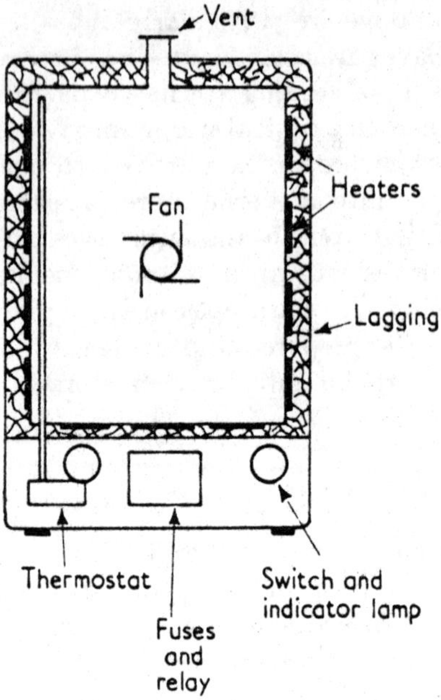

FIG. 21. Cross section of electrically heated oven with circulating fan.

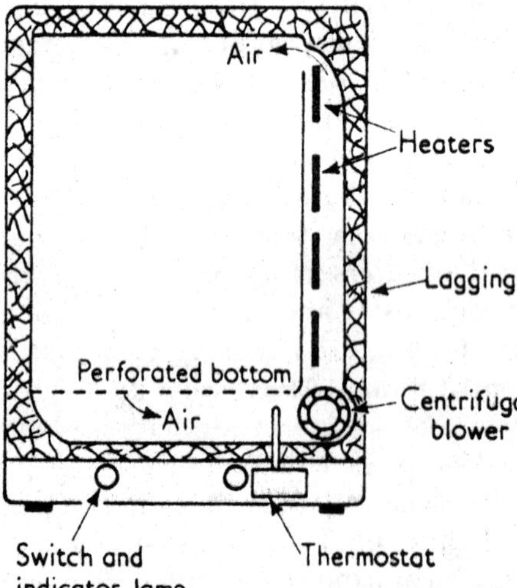

FIG. 22. Cross section of electrically heated oven with forced air circulation.

by infra-red radiators above the shelves but these suffer from the problem of difficulties of temperature control.

For the sterilization of hypodermic syringes two types of equipment relying upon infra-red heating have been devised. The syringes are sealed into aluminium tubes, each of which forms its own sterilizing chamber. For small quantities these tubes are placed into holes drilled into a thermostatically controlled hot-plate. Large quantities are processed on conveyor belts which can be moved at a constant rate under infra-red heaters. The rate of travel can be adjusted empirically to produce a suitable degree of heating to raise the interior of the tubes to sterilizing temperature. Various sizes of syringes can be processed at the same speed by packing them in tubes with different finishes to modify their rate of heating. These infra-red heaters are very sensitive to small changes in voltage and it is necessary to feed them through voltage regulators or constant-voltage transformers.

References

Alder, V. G., and Gillespie, W. A. (1961). *J. clin. Path.* **14**, 515.

Ball, C. O. (1923). *Bull. nat. Res. Coun., Wash.* 37.

Buchi, Von J. (1941). *Pharm. acta Helv.* **16**, 1.

Collier, C. P., and Townsend, C. T. (1956). *Food Techn., Champaign* **10**, 477–481.

Gosset, A., Hauduroy, P., and Rouche, P. (1935). *C. R. Soc. Biol., Paris* **119**, 682.

Henry, P. S. H. (1959). *J. appl. Bact.* **22**, 159–173.

Higuchi, T., and Busse, L. W. (1950). *J. Amer. pharm. Ass.* **39**, 411–412.

Howie, J. W., and Kelsey, J. C. (1962). *Lancet* 991.

Hoyt, A., Chaney, A. L., and Cavell, K. (1939). *Quart. J. Pharm.* **12**, 315.

Institution of Heating and Ventilation Engineers (1959). "Guide to Current Practice", London.

Kanz, E. (1955). *Chirurg* **26**, 110–119.

Kelsey, J. C. (1959). "Report of a Symposium on The Operation of Sterilising Autoclaves", 25 pp. The Pharmaceutical Press, London.

Kelsey, J. C. (1962). Personal Communication.

Knox, R., and Penikett, E. J. K. (1958). *Brit. med. J.* i, 680.

Lyle, O. (1947). "The Efficient Use of Steam", Her Majesty's Stationery Office, London.

Martin, W. M. (1950). *Canner* **111**, 12–16.

Medical Research Council (1959). *Lancet* i, 425.

Medical Research Council Working Party (1963).

Neefe, J. R. (1946). *Med. Clin. N. Amer.* **30**, 1407–1443.

Nuffield Provincial Hospitals Trust (1958). "Present Sterilising Practice in Six Hospitals." London.

Perkins, J. J. (1956). "Principles and Methods of Sterilisation", 340 pp. Chas. C. Thomas, Springfield, Illinois.

Powell, D. B. (1962). Personal communication.

Rahn, O. (1945). *Bact. Rev.* **9**, 1–47.

Savage, R. M. (1944). *Quart. J. Pharm.* **17**, 165 and *Pharm. J.* **153**, 63.

Savage, R. M. (1959). Report of a Symposium "The Operation of Sterilising Autoclaves", 25 pp. The Pharmaceutical Press, London.

Schroeder, H., and Von Dusch, T. (1854). *Liebigs Ann.* **89**, 232–241.

Vallery-Radot, R. (1911). "The Life of Pasteur", 274 pp. Constable, London.
Wilkinson, G. R., and Peacock, F. G. (1961a). *J. Pharm., Lond. Suppl.* **13**, 67T.
Wilkinson, G. R., and Peacock, F. G. (1961b). *J. Pharm., Lond. Suppl.* **13**, 72T.
Wilkinson, G. R., and Peacock, F. G. (1962). *Lancet*, **488**.
Wilkinson, G. R., Peacock, F. G., and Robins, E. L. (1960). *J. Pharm., Lond.* **12**, 197.

AUTHOR INDEX

Numbers in italics refer to the page on which references are listed at the end of each article.

SUBJECT INDEX

I